Problem Solving Questions in Toxicology

P K Gupta

Problem Solving Questions in Toxicology

A Study Guide for the Board and other Examinations

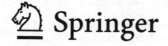

P K Gupta
Former Chief of the Division of Pharmacology and Toxicology, Indian Veterinary
Research Institute, Izatnagar
Director of the Toxicology Consulting Group; President of the Academy of Sciences
for Animal Welfare
Bareilly, India

ISBN 978-3-030-50411-3   ISBN 978-3-030-50409-0   (eBook)
https://doi.org/10.1007/978-3-030-50409-0

This Springer imprint is published by the registered company Springer Nature Switzerland AG
The registered company address is: Gewerbestrasse 11, 6330 Cham, Switzerland

Dedicated to my wife Rakesh, sons Vikas and Pankaj and grandson Dhruvik

PK Gupta

Preface

This book, "Toxicology: Problem Solving Question," is aimed to make the study of toxicology simple and understandable. It is a general experience that theoretical description does not attract as much attention and interest; at the same time, the information learnt through questions and their satisfactory replies make the topics easier to grasp them.

The book is subdivided into 8 units consisting of 24 chapters dealing with various aspects of toxicology such as historical glimpse and stalwarts, general toxicology, principles of toxicology, mechanism of toxicity, disposition of toxicants, toxicokinetics of xenobiotics, target organ toxicity, chemical carcinogenesis, genetic toxicology, developmental toxicology, pesticides, metals and micronutrients, solvents, gasses, and vapors, toxicology of nanomaterials, toxic effects of calories, plant toxicity, biotoxins and venomous organisms, poisonous foods and food poisonings, radiation and radioactive materials, food toxicology, ecotoxicology, environmental toxicology, analytical and clinical toxicology, and occupational toxicology. Each chapter is supported by suitable explanations, figures, and tables wherever necessary along with a brief overview, key points, and relevant problem solving text in the question format followed by multiple-choice questions (MCQs) along with their answers.

Thus this book provides understandable specialized topic in toxicology through questions and answers compiled at one place. The answers are in the form of text along with few diagrams and their explanations which will be extremely useful for self-study to the reader for the examination point of view. As toxicology remains one of the major thrust areas to be studied in any health science department, the book holds a global audience for undergraduates as well as graduates in pharma, veterinary, medical, environmental sciences, and allied subjects in academia and industry having the international market.

Who will be benefitted?

- The book targets both entrance exams and course exams. The information used in content is updated and very relevant in the current scenario.
- As question and answer book, it would be extremely useful for teachers, students, and scientists in academia and industry for their course exams.
- Question and detailed answer type content enables the book to be used both for subjective as well as objective exams.

Thus, the main strength of the book is that it reflects the breadth and multidisciplinary nature of toxicology with self-study approach to the subject that is needed to improve engagement with and understanding of the subject having a very wide audience.

Toxicology is a rapidly evolving field. Suggestions and comments are welcome to help the author improve the contents of the book. Please also suggest the deficiencies that need to be covered at drpkg_brly@yahoo.co.in or drpkg1943@gmail.com if you have any topics you feel should be better covered in any future editions.

Bareilly, India   P. K. Gupta

Contents

Part I

General and Principles of Toxicology

A Historical Glimpse and Stalwarts

Abstract

In the distant past, our observational skills did not extend beyond our senses. Now toxicology being a science-based discipline, its scope and current status has established deep routes that include the study of the adverse effects of chemical, physical, or biological agents on living organisms and the ecosystem, including the prevention and amelioration of such adverse effects. Today, the branch of toxicology is a highly interdisciplinary science that borrows from and intersects with other branches of science such as chemistry, biology, pharmacology, medicine, physiology, biochemistry, molecular biology, pathology, and environmental science. This chapter briefly describes the overview, key points, and relevant text that are in the format of problem-solving study questions followed by multiple-choice questions (MCQs) along with their answers related to the contribution of historical stalwarts and various regulations for control, manufacture, and use of a vast number of chemicals for health and protection of animals and human beings.

Keywords

Toxicology · Historical stalwarts · Poison · Questions and answers · Toxins · Regulations · Legislations · MCQs

1 Introduction

Today, the branch of toxicology is a highly interdisciplinary science that borrows from and intersects with other sciences such as chemistry, biology, pharmacology, medicine, physiology, biochemistry, molecular biology, pathology, and environmental science. The chapter briefly describes an overview, key points, and relevant text that is in the format of problem-solving study questions followed by multiple-choice questions (MCQ's) along with their answers related to the contribution of historical stalwarts, their important discoveries, and various regulations for control, manufacture, and use of a vast number of chemicals for health and protection of animals and human beings.

2 Overview

Knowledge of venoms and plant extracts for hunting, warfare, and assassination presumably predates recorded history. Thus the history of the evolution of the science of toxicology from the original concepts of Paracelsus through the early development of analytical chemistry and its contributions to the detection of toxic substances in foods and drugs, have led to modern regulatory rules for public protection. The legal actions taken to protect against adulteration of food prior to the

P K Gupta, *Problem Solving Questions in Toxicology*, https://doi.org/10.1007/978-3-030-50409-0_1

early steps by the US Department of Agriculture that concluded with the passage of the 1906 Pure Food and Drugs Act are systematically documented. The legal and often litigious controversies over the claimed carcinogenicity of chemical substances are documented with comments on the Delaney dilemma and the role of in vitro tests in toxicology. One of the oldest known writings, the Ebers Papyrus (circa 1500 B.C.), contains information pertaining to many recognized poisons, including hemlock, aconite, opium, and metals such as lead, copper, and antimony. During middle ages, Paracelsus described all substances are poisons; there is none that is not poison. The right dose differentiates poison from remedy. Subsequently experimental toxicology accompanied the growth of organic chemistry and science developed rapidly during the nineteenth century. Toxicology has drawn its strength and diversity to borrowing from almost all the knowledge and techniques from most branches of biochemistry, biology, chemistry, mathematics, medicine, pharmacology, physiology, and physics and applies safety evaluation and risk assessment to the discipline of toxicology. Currently, several dozens of professional, governmental, and other scientific organizations with thousands of members and over hundred books and journals are dedicated to toxicology and related disciplines.

Key Points

- Hippocrates is regarded as the "father of rational medicine." He believed that disease came naturally and not from superstitions and God.
- Toxicology applies safety evaluation and risk assessment to the discipline.
- The right dose differentiates a poison and a remedy.
- A rare congenital deformity, after the thalidomide taken during early pregnancy, formed the basis of strict regulatory requirement for reproductive and development toxicology and creation of Environmental Protection Agency (EPA) in 1970.

---

3   Problem-Solving Study Questions

3.1   Historical Stalwarts

Q. Who is regarded as father of rational medicine?

Hippocrates (460–375 BC) is regarded as the "father of rational medicine." He created the Hippocratic Oath. He believed that disease came naturally and not from superstitions and GOD. He advocated hot oil as an antidote in poisoning and induced vomiting to prevent absorption of the poisons.

Q. Who was Paracelsus?

Theophrastus Paracelsus Bombastus Von Hohenheim (1493–1541), a first-century Roman physician, promoted a focus on the toxicon, the toxic agent, as a chemical entity. He recognized the dose–response concept and in one of his writings stated, "All substances are poisons, there is none which is not a poison. The right dose differentiates a poison and a remedy."

Q. What is the contribution of Friedrich Serturner?

Friedrich Serturner (1783–1841) was a German pharmacist who isolated the specific narcotic substance from opium and named as morphine after Morpheus, the Roman God of sleep.

Q. Who is the father of toxicology?

M.J.B. (Mathieu Joseph Bonaventure) Orfila (1787–1853), a Spanish physician, is considered as a "father of toxicology."

Q. Describe in brief the contributions of M.J.B. Orfila (1787–1853)?

He established toxicology as a discipline distinct from others and defined toxicology as the study of poisons. He advocated the practice of autopsy followed by chemical analysis of viscera to prove that poisoning has taken place. His "treatise" Traite des Poisons published in 1814 laid the foundations of forensic toxicology.

Q. Who is the father of experimental pharmacology?

Describe in brief his contributions.

Francois Magendie (1783–1855) is known as the "father of experimental pharmacology," a pioneer French physiologist and toxicologist studied the mechanism of action of emetine, morphine, quinine, strychnine, and other alkaloids.

Q. Who was Claude Bernard?
Claude Bernard (1813–78) was a French physiologist who is considered the "father of modern experimental physiology." Claude Bernard's first important works were carried out on the physiology of digestion, particularly the role of the pancreas exocrine gland, of the gastric juices, and of the intestines. In addition to this, Bernard also made other important contributions to the neurosciences.

Q. Who was Louis Lewin (1854–1929)?
Louis Lewin (1854–1929) was a German scientist who took up the task of classifying drugs and plants in accordance with their psychological effects. He also published many articles and books dealing with toxicology of methyl alcohol, ethyl alcohol, chloroform, opium, and some other chemicals. His important publications are Toxicologist's View of World History and A Textbook of Toxicology.

Q. Who discovered the insecticidal properties of dichlorodiphenyltrichloroethane (DDT)?
Paul Hermann Muller in 1939 discovered the insecticidal properties of DDT. He was awarded Nobel Prize in 1948 "for his discovery of the high efficiency of DDT as a contact poison against several arthropods".

Q. Who is the "father of nerve agents"?
Gerhard Schrader (1903–90) was a German chemist who accidentally developed the toxic nerve agents sarin, tabun, soman, and cyclosarin while attempting to develop new insecticides. Schrader and his team, thus, introduced a new class of synthetic insecticides and defined the structural requirements for insecticidal activity of anticholinesterase compounds. He is known as the "father of nerve agents."

Q. What is phocomelia in children?
A rare congenital deformity in which the hands or feet are attached close to the trunk. The limbs are grossly underdeveloped or absent. This condition was a side effect of the drug thalidomide taken during early pregnancy.

Q. Who is Wilhelm Röntgen?
Nonetheless, precautions are necessary because radiation hazards can be devastating. Wilhelm Röntgen discovered X-rays, electromagnetic energy waves with wavelengths some 1000 times shorter than those of light. He also learned that X-rays could penetrate human flesh.

Q. Who is Henri Becquerel?
In 1896, Henri Becquerel discovered that uranium salts naturally emitted similar rays.

Q. Who is Marie Curie
Marie Curie was a physicist, a chemist, and a pioneer in the study of radiation. She and her husband, Pierre, discovered the elements polonium, thorium, and radium. They and Henri Becquerel were awarded the Nobel Prize in Physics in 1903, and Marie received the Nobel Prize in Chemistry in 1911 named the phenomenon "radioactivity." Tragically, her death was attributed to aplastic anemia, likely contracted from her extensive work with radioactive materials because X-rays could penetrate human flesh.

3.2 Food and Drug Acts

Q. Which year Department of Agriculture was established in the United States?
The Department of Agriculture, which eventually gave rise to the Food and Drug Administration (FDA), was established under Abraham Lincoln in 1862.

Q. Which year Pure Food and Drugs Act was enacted in the United States?
The Pure Food and Drugs Act of 1906 was the first of a series of significant consumer protection laws which was enacted by Congress in the twentieth century and led to the creation of the Food and Drug Administration. In 1938, Federal Food, Drug, and Cosmetic Act (FFDCA) was enacted. The functions include approve investigational new drug (IND)

applications to initiate clinical trials; approve pharmaceuticals for marketing under a new drug application (NDA); and regulate chemical exposures in skin creams, lotions, powders, and makeup products.

Q. Which year Pure Food and Drugs Act and the Meat Inspection Act was passed in the United States?

Pure Food and Drugs Act and the Meat Inspection Act were passed in 1906 by the then president Theodore Roosevelt.

Q. Which law (s) in the United States regulates the use of additives (flavors, texturing agents, preservatives, processing aids, etc.) that can be used in food?

The laws that regulate approval of new direct additives (flavors, texturing agents, preservatives, processing aids, etc.) that can be used in food and to determine additives that are generally recognized as safe (GRAS) and do not require FDA approval for use include:

1938, Federal Food, Drug, and Cosmetic Act (FFDCA)

1958, Delaney Clause

1996, Food Quality Protection Act (FQPA)

3.3 Pesticides and Chemical Warfare Agents

Q. Which was the first nerve agent synthesized?

Tabun was the first nerve agent synthesized in 1937 by the IG Farben scientist.

Q. Who synthesized the first nerve agent, tabun?

The first nerve agent, tabun, was synthesized by Gerhard Schrader during his research to discover new organophosphate insecticides.

Q. Who was Paul Hermann Müller?

Paul Hermann Müller in 1939 recognized DDT as an insecticide. His discovery won him the Nobel Prize in Physiology in 1972. DDT was extremely effective in preventing the spread of malaria in developing countries. It was the chemical of choice for controlling insect populations in the United States as well.

Q. Who is Rachel Carson (1907–64)?

The work and research of Rachel Carson brought to the attention of environmental scientists and to the public about the long term effects of DDT, when she published her findings in the book *Silent Spring* in 1962.

3.4 Environmental Exposures and Legislation

Q. When and why Environmental Protection Agency (EPA) was created?

Environmental Protection Agency (EPA) was created in 1970, in response to the welter of confusing, often ineffective *environmental protection* laws enacted by states and communities. President Richard Nixon *created* the *EPA* to fix national guidelines and to monitor and enforce them.

Q. Name some of environmental legislations in the United States?

In the United States, significant environmental legislation administered by the EPA includes the Federal Insecticide, Fungicide, and Rodenticide Act (FIFRA) (1947), which regulates pesticides, the Clean Air Act (1970), the Clean Water Act (1972), the Safe Drinking Water Act (1974), and the Resource Conservation and Recovery Act (RCRA) (1976), giving the agency the authority to control hazardous waste from "cradle to grave," all strengthened in various ways with amendments since their initial implementation.

Q. What is the Toxic Substances Control Act (TSCA) and when it was passed?

The Toxic Substances Control Act (TSCA) is a US law passed by the US Congress in 1976 and administered by the US Environmental Protection Agency. The law regulates the introduction of new or already existing chemicals.

Q. What are the major laws in the United States responsible to establish exposure standards for pesticides, water, and air pollutants and hazardous wastes"?

The major laws are:

1947, Federal Insecticide, Fungicide, and Rodenticide Act (FIFRA)

1970, Clean Air Act

1972, Clean Water Act

1976, Resource Conservation and Recovery Act (RCRA)

1976, Toxic Substances Control Act

1980, Comprehensive Environmental Response, Compensation and Liability Act (CERCLA)—Creation of Superfund

1984, Federal Hazardous and Solid Waste Amendments

2016, The Lautenberg Chemical Safety Act amends the Toxic Substances Control Act (TSCA), the nation's primary chemicals management law for Chemical Safety for the 21st Century Act

3.5 REACH Regulation

Q. What is REACH regulation?

The Registration, Evaluation, Authorization and Restriction of Chemicals (REACH) is a European Union regulation dated December 18, 2006. REACH requires all companies manufacturing or importing chemical substances into the European Union in quantities of one ton or more per year to register these substances with the European Chemicals Agency (ECHA) in Helsinki, Finland.

Since REACH applies to some substances that are contained in products ("articles" in REACH terminology), any company importing goods into Europe could also be affected.

3.6 Occupational Safety and Health Regulation in the United States

Q. Who is responsible for Occupational Safety and Health in the United States?

For Occupational Safety and Health, the Bureau of Mines, for example, was created in 1910, within the Department of the Interior and health and safety were within its purview. The National Safety Council was established in 1911. An Office of Industrial Hygiene and Sanitation was established within the Public Health Service in 1914.

Q. What is Occupational Safety and Health Administration (OSHA)?

The Occupational Safety and Health Administration (OSHA) was created by President Nixon also in 1970 with the first guidelines for standards of safety following in 1972. Thus OSHA is the regulatory agency that establishes limits to chemical exposures in the workplace and investigates workplace hazards {e.g., permissible exposure limits (PELs) and short-term exposure limits (STELs)}.

Q. What is National Institute for Occupational Safety and Health (NIOSH)?

The National Institute for Occupational Safety and Health (NIOSH). NIOSH conducts research to help to reduce workplace illnesses and accidents.

5.0 Sample MCQ's (choose the correct statement, it may be one, two or none)

Q.1. Which one of the following statements regarding toxicology is true?

    A. Modern toxicology is concerned with the study of the adverse effects of chemicals on ancient forms of life.

    B. Modern toxicology studies embrace principles from such disciplines as biochemistry, botany, chemistry, physiology, and physics.

    C. Modern toxicology has its roots in the knowledge of plant and animal poisons, which predates recorded history and has been used to promote peace.

    D. Modern toxicology studies the mechanisms by which inorganic chemicals produce advantageous as well as deleterious effects.

    E. Modern toxicology is concerned with the study of chemicals in mammalian species.

Q.2. Knowledge of the toxicology of poisonous agents was published earliest in the ---

    A. Ebers Papyrus

    B. De Historia Plantarum

    C. De Materia Medica

    D. Lex Cornelia

    E. Treatise on Poisons and Their Antidotes

Q.3. Paracelsus, physician–alchemist, formulated many revolutionary reviews that remain integral to the structure of toxicology, pharmacology, and therapeutics today. He focused on the primary toxic agent as chemical entity and articulated the dose–response relation. Which one of the following statements is not attributable to Paracelsus?

A. Natural poisons are quick in their onset of actions.
B. Experimentation is essential in the examination of responses to chemicals.
C. One should make distinction between the therapeutic and toxic properties of chemicals.
D. These properties are sometimes but not always indistinguishable except by dose.
E. One can ascertain a degree of specificity of chemicals and their therapeutic or toxic effects.

Q.4. The art of toxicology requires years of experience to acquire, even though the knowledge base facts may be learned more quickly. Which modern toxicologist is credited with saying that "you can be toxicologist in two easy lesions, each of 10 years?"

A. Claude Bernard
B. Rachel Carson
C. Upton Sinclair
D. Arnold Lehman
E. Oswald Schmiedeberg

Q.5. Which of the following statements is correct?

A. Claude Bernard was a prolific scientist who trained over 120 students and published numerous contributions to the scientific literature.

B. Louis Lewin trained under Oswald Schmiedeberg and published much of the early work on the toxicity of narcotics, methanol, and chloroform.
C. An *Introduction to the Study of Experimental Medicine* was written by the Spanish physician Orfila.
D. Magendie used autopsy material and chemical analysis systematically as legal proof of poisoning.
E. Percival Potts was instrumental in demonstrating the chemical complexity of snake venoms.

Q.6. Regulatory toxicology aims at guarding the public from dangerous chemical exposures and depends primarily on which form of study?

A. Observational human studies
B. *Controlled laboratory animal studies*
C. Controlled human studies
D. Environmental studies

Q.7. The scientist referred to as "father of toxicology" is --------

A. Bombastus Von Hohenheim
B. Friedrich Serturner
C. Claude Bernard
D. M.J.B. Orfila

Q.8. DDT which is used to control malaria and typhus was discovered by -----

A. Bombastus Von Hohenheim
B. Friedrich Serturner
C. Paul Hermann Muller
D. M.J.B. Orfila

Q.9. The person who is known as "father of nerve agents" is ------------

A. Friedrich Serturner
B. M.J.B. Orfila
C. Rachel Carson
D. Gerhard Schrader

Q.10. The author of the book Silent Spring in which the detrimental effect of DDT and other pesticides on environment were highlighted was ------

    A. Bombastus Von Hohenheim
    B. Friedrich Serturner
    C. Paul Hermann Muller
    D. M.J.B. Orfila
    E. None of above

Answers
1. B.   2. A.   3. A.   4. D.   5. B.   6. B.
7. D.   8. C.   9. D.   10. E

Further Reading

Gallo MA (2015) History and scope of toxicology. In: Klaassen CD, Watkins JB III (eds) Casarett & Doull's essentials of toxicology, 3rd edn. McGraw-Hill, New York, pp 1–4

Gupta PK (2014) Essential concepts in toxicology. PharmaMed Press (A unit of BSP Books Pvt. Ltd), Hyderabad

Gupta PK (2016) Fundamentals of toxicology: essential concepts and applications, 1st edn. BSP/Elsevier, San Diego

Gupta PK (2018) Illustrative toxicology, 1st edn. Elsevier, San Diego

Gupta PK (2019) Concepts and applications in veterinary toxicology: an interactive guide. Springer-Nature, Cham

Gupta PK (2020) Principles of toxicology in: brain storming questions in toxicology. Francis and Taylor CRC Press, Boca Raton

Gupta RC (ed) (2018) Veterinary toxicology: basic and clinical principles, 3rd edn. Academic Press/Elsevier, San Diego

Fruncillo RJ (2011) 2,000 Toxicology board review questions. Xlibris Publishers, Bloomington

General Toxicology

2

Abstract

Modern toxicology is a science-based toxicology; the scope and future of toxicologists are very bright because this branch of science will further expand as people and animals will continue to be poisoned by more and different chemicals. Toxic agents are classified in a number of ways depending on the interests and needs of the classifier. There is no single classification applicable for the entire spectrum of toxic agents and hence combinations of classification systems based on several factors may provide the best rating system. Classification of poisons may take into account both the chemical and biological properties of the agent; however, exposure characteristics are also useful in toxicology.

Keywords

Sub-disciplines of toxicology · Toxicity rating · Delayed toxicity · Toxic effects · Classification of toxic agents · Irreversible toxic effects · Hazards · Risk assessment · MCQs · Questions and answers

1 Introduction

The modern toxicology is a science-based toxicology; the scope and future of toxicologists are very bright because this science will further expand as people and animals will continue to be poisoned by more and different chemicals. Toxic agents are classified in number of ways depending on the interests and needs of the classifier. There is no single classification applicable for the entire spectrum of toxic agents, and hence combinations of classification systems based on several factors may provide the best rating system. Classification of poisons may take into account both the chemical and biological properties of the agent; however, exposure characteristics are also useful in toxicology. Given the space limitations, the chapter covers the overview, key points, and relevant text that is in the format of problem-solving study questions followed by multiple-choice questions (MCQ's) along with their answers.

2 Overview

Toxicology is traditionally associated with chemical exposures. There is no single classification that is applicable to the entire spectrum of toxic

P K Gupta, *Problem Solving Questions in Toxicology*, https://doi.org/10.1007/978-3-030-50409-0_2

chemicals. Instead, a combination of classification systems is generally needed to best characterize toxic substances. Exposure to various chemicals involves the assessment of risks to human health and scientific examination and evaluation of information in four areas: the hazardous nature of agents in the environment; the degree of human exposure to such agents; the response of people's health to exposure, and the risk management. The product of a risk assessment is information about the likelihood of health degradation following an exposure to hazardous agents.

Key Points

- *Poison*, as a noun is the Latinized form of the Greek word, meaning "arrow poison," dates back to the Old French *poison* or *puison*.
- Toxicology studies the agents responsible for adverse effects, the mechanisms involved, the damage that may ensue, testing methodologies to determine the extent of damage, and ways to avoid or repair it.
- Poison is a broader term which includes any/every substance causing harmful effects to living beings. Toxicant is any toxic substance introduced into the environment, e.g., a pesticide, metals, solvents, gases, etc. Toxins a poison of plant or animal origin, especially one produced by or derived from microorganisms. This could be of plant (plant toxin), fungal (mycotoxin), animal (zootoxin), or bacteria (—endo and exo toxins) origin.
- Toxic agents are classified in number of ways depending on the interests and needs of the classifier. There is no single classification applicable for the entire spectrum of toxic agents
- Risk is defined as the probability of an adverse outcome based upon the exposure and potency of the hazardous agent(s).

---

3 Problem-Solving Study Questions

3.1 About Toxicology

Q. Can you elaborate toxicology?

(a) Toxicology studies the agents responsible for adverse effects, the mechanisms involved, the damage that may ensue, testing methodologies to determine the extent of damage, and ways to avoid or repair it. Thus toxicology is traditionally associated with chemical exposures, such as the effects of drugs, industrial chemicals, pesticides, food additives, household products, and personal care items. Other agents such as radiation and substances derived from biological organisms are equally relevant to the field.

(b) Toxinology, a sub-discipline of toxicology, studies biological exposures, such as insect stings, poisonous mushrooms and plants, venomous snakes, and aquatic life.

(c) The third category of toxicology is concerned with physical hazards, such as radiation and noise.

Q. What is Toxicon?

It is the Latinized form of the Greek word, meaning "arrow poison." *Poison*, as a noun, dates back to the Old French *poison* or *puison*, meaning, originally, a drink, especially a medical drink, but later signifying more of a magical potion or poisonous drink.

Q. What is toxin?

Toxic substances produced biologically are known as toxins. Thus, technically, chemicals such as formaldehyde or asbestos, say, would *not* be considered toxins.

Explanation: There are any number of other terms which could be used to delineate the broader category of substances which are toxic, regardless of origin. Examples are *toxicant*, *toxic agent*, and *toxic substance*.

Q. Define xenobiotic.

Xenobiotic: Xenobiotics (xeno is a Greek word which means "strange or alien") are the substances which are foreign to the body and are biologically active. These cannot be broken down to generate energy or be assimilated into a biosynthetic pathway. It is a very wide class and structurally adverse agents, both natural and synthetic chemicals such as drugs, industrial chemicals, pesticides, alkaloids, secondary plant metabolites and toxins of molds, plants and animals, and environmental pollutants.

3.2 Types of Toxicants

Q. Define poison.
Poison is derived from Latin "potus," a drink that could harm or kill. It is any substance which when taken inwardly in a very small dose or applied in any kind of manner to a living body depraves the health or entirely destroys life. Although the word toxicant has essentially the same medical meaning, there are psychological and legal implications involved in the use of the word poison that makes manufacturer reluctant to apply it to chemicals, particularly those intended for widespread use in large quantities, unless they are required to do so by law. The term toxicant is more acceptable to both manufacturer and legislators.

Q. Define toxicant.
Toxicant is synonym of poison, produced by living organism in small quantities, and is generally classified as biotoxin. These may be phytotoxins (produced by plants), mycotoxins (produced by fungi), zootoxins (produced by lower animals), and bacteriotoxins (produced by bacteria).

Q. Define different types of toxins.
(a) Endotoxins are found within bacterial cells.
(b) Exotoxins: elaborated from bacterial cells.

Q. Define venom.
Venom is a toxicant synthesized in a specialized gland and ejected by the process of biting or stinging. Venom is also a zootoxin but is transmitted by the process of biting or stinging.

Q. What is the difference between "poison," "toxicant," and "toxin"?
Poison is a broader term which includes any/every substance causing harmful effects to living beings.
Toxicant is any toxic substance introduced into the environment, e.g., a pesticide, metals, solvents, gases, etc.
Toxins a poison of plant or animal origin, especially one produced by or derived from microorganisms. This could be of plant (plant toxin), fungal (mycotoxin), animal (zootoxin) or bacteria (bacteriotoxins—endo and exo toxins) origin.

Q. How "toxicosis" differs from "toxicity"?
Toxicosis is the disease or condition (effect) which results due to exposure to a poison, whereas, "toxicity" is the degree of the disease or condition. However, the term toxicity is also used to mean the adverse effects of a poison.

Q. Define pollutant.
It is any undesirable substance to solid, liquid, or gaseous matter resulting from the discharge or admixture of noxious materials that contaminate the environment and contributes to pollution.

3.3 Sub-disciplines of Toxicology

Q. What are the sub-disciplines of toxicology?
(a) Biochemical toxicology
(b) Reproductive toxicology
(c) Development toxicology
(d) Teratology
(e) Genetic toxicology
(f) Clinical toxicology
(g) Forensic toxicology
(h) Analytical toxicology
(i) Nutritional toxicology
(j) Veterinary toxicology
(k) Environmental toxicology
(l) Occupational (industrial) toxicology
(m) Regulatory toxicology
(n) Mechanistic toxicology
(o) Aquatic toxicology

(p) Ecotoxicology
(q) Food toxicology
(r) Formal toxicology
(s) Descriptive toxicology
(t) Nanotoxicology

Q. Define occupational (industrial) toxicology.
Occupational (industrial) toxicology is concerned with health effects from exposure to chemicals in the workplace. It deals with the clinical study of workers of industries and environment around them.

Q. Define regulatory toxicology.
It deals with administrative functions concerned with the development and interpretation of mandatory toxicology testing programs and controlling the use, distribution, and availability of chemicals used commercially and therapeutically. For example, Food and Drug Administration (FDA) regulates drugs, cosmetics, and food additives. Regulatory toxicology gathers and evaluates existing toxicological information to establish concentration-based standards of "safe" exposure. The standard is the level of a chemical that a person can be exposed to without any harmful health effects.

Q. Define regulation.
Regulation is the control, by statute, of the manufacture, transportation, sale, or disposal of chemicals deemed to be toxic after testing procedures or according to criteria laid down in applicable laws.

Q. Define food toxicology.
It deals with natural contaminants, food and feed additives, and toxic and chemoprotective effects of compounds in food. Explanation: food toxicology is involved in delivering a safe and edible supply of food to the consumer. During processing, a number of substances may be added to food to make it look, taste, or smell better. Fats, oils, sugars, starches, and other substances may be added to change the texture and taste of food. All of these additives are studied to determine if and at what amount they may produce adverse effects. A second area of interest includes food allergies.

Almost 30% of the American people have some food allergy. For example, many people have trouble digesting milk and are lactose intolerant. In addition, toxic substances such as pesticides may be applied to a food crop in the field, while lead, arsenic, and cadmium are naturally present in soil and water and may be absorbed by plants. Toxicologists must determine the acceptable daily intake (ADI) level for those substances.

Q. Define formal toxicology.
It deals with the formal toxicological studies which are prerequisite for release of a new drugs/chemical, e.g., calculation of lethal dose 50 (LD50) and minimum toxic dose.

Q. Define descriptive toxicology.
Descriptive toxicology is concerned with gathering toxicological information from animal experimentation. These types of experiments are used to establish how much of a chemical would cause illness or death. The US Environmental Protection Agency (EPA), the Occupational Safety and Health Administration (OSHA), and the Food and Drug Administration (FDA) use information from these studies to set regulatory exposure limits.

Q. Define mechanistic toxicology.
Mechanistic toxicology makes observations on how toxic substances cause their effects. The effects of exposure can depend on a number of factors, including the size of the molecule, the specific tissue type, or cellular components affected, whether the substance is easily dissolved in water or fatty tissues, all of which are important when trying to determine the way a toxic substance causes harm and whether effects seen in animals can be expected in humans.

Q. Define nutritional toxicology.
Nutritional toxicology is the study of toxicological aspects of food/feed stuffs and nutritional products/habits.

Q. Define toxicodynamics.
It deals with the study of biochemical and physiological effects of toxicants and their mechanism of action.

Q. Define toxicokinetics.

It deals with the study of absorption, distribution, metabolism, and excretion of toxicants in the body.

Q. Define toxicovigilance.

It deals with the process of identification, investigation, and evaluation of various toxic effects in the community with a view of taking measures to reduce or control exposures involving the substances that produce these effects.

Q. Define toxinology.

It deals with assessing the toxicity of substances of plant and animal origin and those produced by pathogenic bacteria/organism.

Q. Define toxicoepidemiology.

It refers to the study of quantitative analysis of the toxicity incidences in organisms, factors affecting toxicity, species involved, and the use of such knowledge in planning of prevention and control strategies.

3.4 Toxicity, Frequency, and Duration of Exposure

Toxic and toxicity are relative terms commonly used in comparing one chemical with another.

Q. Define toxicity.

It is a state of being poisonous or capacity to cause injury to living organisms.

Q. Define toxicosis.

It is the condition or disease state that results from exposure to a toxicant. The term toxicosis is often used interchangeably with the term poisoning or intoxication.

Q. Define toxic effects.

These are undesirable effects produced by a toxicant/drug which are detrimental to either survival or normal functioning of the individual.

Q. Define side effects.

These are undesirable effects which result from the normal pharmacological actions of drugs. These results may not be detrimental or harmful to the individual.

Q. Define plant toxins.

Different portions of a plant may contain different concentrations of chemicals. Some chemicals made by plants can be lethal. For example, taxon, used in chemotherapy to kill cancer cells, is produced by a species of the yew plant.

Q. Define animal toxins.

Animal toxins can result from venomous or poisonous animal releases. Venomous animals are usually defined as those that are capable of producing a poison in a highly developed gland or group of cells and can deliver that toxin through biting or stinging. Poisonous animals are generally regarded as those whose tissues, either in part or in their whole, are toxic. For example, venomous animals, such as snakes and spiders, and poisonous animals, such as puffer fish or oysters, may be toxic to some individuals when contaminated with *Vibrio vulnificus*.

Q. What is toxicity?

The word "toxicity" describes the degree to which a substance is poisonous or can cause injury. The toxicity depends on a variety of factors: dose, duration, and route of exposure (see Module Two), shape and structure of the chemical itself, and individual human factors.

Q. What is toxic?

This term relates to poisonous or deadly effects on the body by inhalation (breathing), ingestion (eating), or absorption, or by direct contact with a chemical.

Q. What is a toxic symptom?

This term includes any feeling or sign indicating the presence of a poison or foreign substance in the system/body.

Q. What are toxic effects?

This term refers to the health effects that occur due to exposure to a toxic substance, also known as a poisonous effect on the body.

Q. How does toxicity develop?

Before toxicity can develop, a substance must come into contact with a body surface such as the skin, eye, or mucosa of the digestive or respiratory tract. The dose of the chemical, or the amount one comes into contact with, is important when discussing how "toxic" a substance can be.

Q. Define acute toxicity.

Acute toxicity is defined as an exposure to a chemical for less than 24 hours. The exposure usually refers to a single administration; repeated exposures may be given within a 24-hour period for some slightly toxic or practically nontoxic chemicals. Acute exposure by inhalation refers to continuous exposure for less than 24 hours, most frequently for 4 hours.

Q. Define repeated exposure.

Repeated exposure is divided into three categories:

(a) Subacute

(b) Subchronic

(c) Chronic

Subacute exposure to a chemical is for 1 month or less, subchronic for 1–3 months, and chronic for more than 3 months (usually this refers to studies with at least 1 year of repeated dosing).

Explanation: Acute or repeated exposure can be by any route, but most often they occur by the oral route, with the chemical added directly to the diet. In human exposure situations, the frequency and duration of exposure are usually not as clearly defined as in controlled animal studies. However, almost same terms are used to describe general exposure situations. Thus, workplace or environmental exposures may be described as acute (occurring from a single incident or episode), subchronic (occurring repeatedly over several weeks or months), or chronic (occurring repeatedly for many months or years).

Q. Repeated oral toxicity of a compound is tested in rats for a period of 28 days. What kind of toxicity is being studied here?

It is termed as subacute toxicity.

Q. Define cumulative toxicity.

It is a progressive toxicity or harmful effect produced by summation of incremental injury resulting from successive exposures, e.g., liver fibrosis produced by ethanol.

Q. What are harmful or adverse effects?

Harmful or adverse effects are those that are damaging to either the survival or normal function (s) of the individual.

3.5   Classification of Toxic Agents

Toxic agents are classified in a number of ways depending on the interests and needs of the classifier. There is no single classification applicable for the entire spectrum of toxic agents, and hence combinations of classification systems based on several factors may provide the best rating system. Classification of poisons may take into account both the chemical and biological properties of the agent; however, exposure characteristics are also useful in toxicology.

Q. Classify toxic agents.

In toxicology, compounds are classified in various ways, by one or more of the following classes:

(a) Use, e.g., pesticides (atrazine), solvents (benzene), food additives (NutraSweet), metals, and war gases.

(b) Effects, e.g., carcinogen (benzo[a] pyrene), mutagen (methylnitrosamine), and hepatotoxicant (CHCl3).

(c) Physical state such as oxidant (ozone), gas (CO_2), dust (Fe_2O_3), and liquid (H_2O).

(d) Chemistry such as aromatic amine (aniline) and halogenated hydrocarbon (methylene chloride).

(e) Sources of toxicants, e.g., plant or animal or natural.

(f) Mechanism of action: cholinesterase inhibitor (malathion), methemoglobin producer (nitrite), etc.

Q. Classification based on sources of toxicants

(a) Plant toxins

(b) Animal toxicants

(c) Mineral toxicants

(d) Synthetic toxicants

(e) Physical or mechanical agents

Q. Classification based on physical state of toxicants

(a) Gaseous toxicants

(b) Liquid toxicants

(c) Solid toxicants

(d) Dust toxicants

Q. Classification based on target organ or system
  (a) Neurotoxicants
  (b) Hepatotoxicants
  (c) Nephrotoxicants
  (d) Pulmotoxicants
  (e) Hematotoxicants
  (f) Dermatotoxicants
  (g) Development and reproductive toxicants
Q. Classification based on chemical nature/ structure of toxicants
  (a) Metals
  (b) Non-metals
  (c) Acids and alkalis
  (d) Organic toxicants (carbon compounds other than oxides of carbon, the carbonates, and metallic carbides and cyanides)
Q. Classification based on analytical behavior of toxicants
  (a) Volatile toxicants
  (b) Extractive toxicants
  (c) Metals and metalloids
Q. Classification based on type of toxicity
  (a) Acute
  (b) Subacute
  (c) Chronic
Q. Classification based on toxic effects
  (a) Carcinogens
  (b) Mutagens
  (c) Teratogens
  (d) Clastogens
Q. Classification based on their uses
  (a) Insecticides
  (b) Fungicides
  (c) Herbicides
  (d) Rodenticides
  (e) Food additives, etc.
Q. Classification based on symptoms produced
  (a) Corrosive poisons
  (b) Irritant poisons
  (c) Systemic poisons
  (d) Miscellaneous poisons
In addition, there are other types of classifications that are based on the environmental and public health considerations and so on.

3.6 Toxicity Rating and Spectrum of Effects

Q. Describe briefly the term "toxicity rating."
A system of "toxicity rating" has been evolved for common poisons. The higher the toxicity rating for a particular substance (over a range of 1–6), the greater is the potency. The toxicity rating based on toxic potential of substances (super toxic, extremely toxic, very toxic, moderately toxic, slightly toxic, and practically nontoxic).
Q. What will be the toxicity rating of a toxic compound having LD50 values more than 1000 mg/kg?
Practically nontoxic
Q. What will be the toxicity rating of a toxic compound having LD50 values less than 1000 mg/kg?
Mild/slightly toxic
Q. What will be the toxicity rating of a toxic compound having LD50 values less than 500 mg/kg?
Moderately toxic
Q. What will be the toxicity rating of a toxic compound having LD50 values less than 50 mg/kg?
Highly toxic
Q. What will be the toxicity rating of a toxic compound having LD50 values less than 1 mg/kg?
Severe/extremely toxic
Q. What are local toxic effects?
Local effects are those that occur where contact is first made by the toxicant and the biological system. Such effects are produced by the ingestion of toxic substances or the inhalation of irritant materials. For example, chlorine gas reacts with lung tissue at the site of contact, causing damage and swelling of the lungs, with possibly fatal consequences, even though very little of the chemical is absorbed into the bloodstream.
Q. What are systemic toxic effects?
Systemic effects require the absorption and distribution of a toxicant from its entry point to a

distant site where the deleterious effects are produced. Most chemicals that produce systemic toxicity do not cause a similar degree of toxicity in all organs; instead, they usually elicit their major toxicity in only one or two organs.

Q. What is target toxicity?

Some chemicals elicit their major toxicity in only one or two organs. The target organ of toxicity is not always the site of the highest concentration of the chemical. For example, lead accumulates in bones, but its toxic effects occur in soft tissues, particularly the brain. Instead, the bones act as a reservoir that can leach and release stored lead and cause neurological injury even years after exposure. The insecticide dichlorodiphenyltrichloroethane (DDT) concentrates in adipose tissue due to its lipophilic chemical property but produces no known toxic effects in that tissue. However, the primary target organs for toxicity of DDT are the brain and female reproductive system referred to as the *target organs* of toxicity for a particular chemical.

Q. What is nontarget toxicity?

Some chemicals also disrupt the population of some of the valuable soil invertebrates like earthworms, predatory mites, centipedes, and carabid beetles. Such chemicals are known as to produce nontarget toxicity. Accumulation of pesticides in resistant or tolerant species may provoke episodes of toxicity to organisms higher in the food chain.

Q. What are reversible toxic effects?

Some toxic effects of chemicals are reversible, and a toxic response to be reversed largely depends on the ability of an injured tissue to adapt, repair, and regenerate. Therefore, for tissues such as the liver and gastrointestinal tract that have a high ability to regenerate, many injuries are reversible. Within days of exposure to the hepatotoxicants acetaminophen, the liver mounts an adaptive response that includes the proliferation of remaining centrilobular hepatocytes and the differentiation of oval stem cells.

Q. What are irreversible toxic effects?

Some toxic effects of chemicals are irreversible. For example, the CNS has a much more limited ability to divide and replace damaged neurons making damage largely irreversible. This is exemplified by the persistent loss of neurons that utilize the neurotransmitter, dopamine, which results in Parkinson's-like symptoms observed in patients exposed to the neurotoxin 1-methyl-4-phenylpyridinium (MPP+). Likewise, cancers and birth defects caused by chemical exposures, once they occur, are often also considered irreversible toxic effects.

Q. What is immediate toxicity?

During immediate toxicity, the toxic effects of a chemical can develop rapidly after a single exposure such as exposure to hydrogen cyanide or nerve gas, sarin. Exposure to high doses of these chemicals can have rapid effects on the cardiovascular, respiratory, and neurological systems culminating in death within minutes. Because of their high toxicity and expeditious actions, hydrogen cyanide, sarin, and similar chemicals have been used as chemical warfare agents.

Q. What is delayed toxicity?

Delayed toxicities of chemicals may take months or years to be recognized. There are a number of examples of delayed toxicities due to xenobiotic exposure. Women were prescribed diethylstilbestrol (DES) during pregnancy in order to prevent preterm birth. The daughters of these women have a greatly increased risk of developing vaginal cancer. Also, delayed neurotoxicity is observed after exposure to some organophosphate insecticides that act by covalent modification of an enzyme referred to as *neuropathy target esterase* (NTE), a neuronal protein with serine esterase activity.

3.7   Other Terms Used in Toxicology

Q. What are haptens?

Haptens are allergenic only when bound to protein.

Q. Define cheminformatics.

Cheminformatics (also known as chemoinformatics, chemioinformatics, and chemical informatics) is the use of computer and informational techniques applied to a range of problems in the field of chemistry. These in silico techniques are used in, for example, pharmaceutical companies in the process of drug discovery.

Q. Define end point study record.

End point study record or IUCLID (International Uniform Chemical Information Database) format of the technical dossier is used to report study summaries and robust study summaries of the information derived for the specific end point according to the REACH regulation.

Q. Define end point of study design.

End point: an observable or measurable inherent property/data point of a chemical substance. For example, a physical chemical property like vapor pressure or degradability or a biological effect that a given substance has on human health or the environment, e.g., carcinogenicity, irritation, and aquatic toxicity.

Q. Define in vitro test.

In vitro test: literally stands for "in glass" or "in tube," refers to the test taking place outside of the body of an organism, usually involving isolated organs, tissues, cells, or biochemical systems.

Q. Define in vivo test.

In vivo test: a test conducted within a living organism.

Q. Define in silico test.

In silico: in silico (a phrase coined as an analogy to the familiar phrases in vivo and in vitro) is an expression used to denote "performed on computer or via computer simulation." It means scientific experiments or research conducted or produced by means of computer modeling or computer simulation.

Q. Define IUCLID flag.

IUCLID flag: an option used in the IUCLID software to indicate submitted data type (e.g., experimental data) or its use for regulatory purposes (e.g., confidentiality).

Q. Define prediction model.

Prediction model is a theoretical formula, algorithm, or program used to convert the experimental results obtained by using a test method into a prediction of the toxic property/effect of the chemical substance.

Q. Define quantitative structure–activity relationship (QSARs) and structure–activity relationship (SARs).

QSARs and SARs: theoretical models that can be used to predict in a quantitative or qualitative manner the physical, chemical, biological (e.g., (eco)toxicological), and environmental fate properties of compounds from knowledge of their chemical structure. A SAR is a qualitative relationship that relates a (sub)structure to the presence or absence of a property or activity of interest. A QSAR is a mathematical model relating one or more quantitative parameters, which are derived from the chemical structure, to a quantitative measure of a property or activity.

Q. Define test or assay, validation test, and validation.

Test (or assay): an experimental system setup to obtain information on the intrinsic properties or adverse effects of a chemical substance. Validation test: a test for which its performance characteristics, advantages, and limitations have been adequately determined for a specific purpose. Validation: the process by which the reliability and relevance of a test method are evaluated for the purpose of supporting a specific use.

Q. Define vertebrate animal.

Animals that belong to subphylum Vertebrata; chordate with backbones and spinal columns is known as a vertebrate animal.

Q. Define accidental poisoning.

Accidental poisoning may occur when human beings or animals take toxicant accidentally or is added unintentionally in food or through in its feed, fodder, or drinking water. Such toxicants come from either natural or man-made sources. The natural sources include ingestion of toxic plants, biting or stinging by poisonous reptiles, ingestion of food contaminated with toxins, and contaminated water with minerals. Man-made sources include therapeutic agents, household products, and agrochemicals.

Q. Define malicious poisoning.

It is the unlawful or criminal killing of human beings or animals by administering certain toxic/poisonous agents. Incidence of such poisonings is more prevalent in human beings and less in animals.

3.8   Hazard and Risk Assessment

Terms Used in Risk Assessment

Q. Define risk.

Risk is defined as the probability of an adverse outcome based upon the exposure and potency of the hazardous agent(s).

Q. Define safety.

Means practical certainty that injury will not result from the use of a substance under specified condition of quantity and manner of use.

Q. Define benefit-to-risk ratio.

This implies that even a toxic agent may warrant use if its benefits for a significant number of people are much greater than the dangers.

Q. Describe briefly risk assessment.

Risk assessment is a quantitative assessment of the probability of deleterious effects under given exposure conditions. It requires an integration of both qualitative and quantitative scientific information. For example, qualitative information about the overall evidence and nature of the end points and hazards are integrated with quantitative assessment of the exposures, host susceptibility factors, and the magnitude of the hazard. A description of the uncertainties and variability in the estimates is a significant part of risk characterization and an essential component of risk assessment.

Q. Define human health risk assessment.

The EPA defines human health risk assessment as "the process to estimate the nature and probability of adverse health effects in humans who may be exposed to chemicals in contaminated environmental media, now or in the future."

Q. Define hazard.

It is the qualitative description of the adverse effect arising from a particular chemical or physical agent with no regard to dose or exposure. The term hazard is related to the risk, but it mainly expresses likelihood or probability of danger, irrespective of dose or exposure.

Or

A property or set of properties of the chemical substance that may cause an adverse health or ecological effect provided if there is an exposure at a sufficient level.

Q. Define acceptable risk.

It is the probability of suffering a disease or injury during exposure to a substance, which is considered to be small but acceptable to the individual.

Q. Define acceptable exposure.

It is the unintentional contact with a chemical or physical agent that results in the harmful effect.

Q. Define margin of exposure.

Margin of exposure is defined as the ratio of the no-observed adverse effect level (NOAEL) for the critical effect to the theoretical, predicted, or estimated exposure dose or concentration.

Q. Define threshold limit values (TLVs).

The TLVs refer to the airborne concentration of a substance to which it is believed a worker can be exposed day after day for a working lifetime without adverse effects. These values are expressed as time weight concentration for 7- to 8-hour workday and for 40 weeks.

Q. Define no-observed effect level/concentration (NOEL/NOEC).

NOEL/NOEC is the highest dose level/concentration of a substance that under defined conditions of exposure causes no effect (alteration) on morphology, functional capacity, growth, development, or life span of the test animals.

Q. Define no-observed adverse effect level/concentration (NOAEL/NOAEC).

NOAEL/NOAEC is the highest dose level/concentration of a substance that under defined conditions of exposure causes no-observable/detectable adverse effect (alteration) on morphology, functional capacity, growth, development, or life span of the test

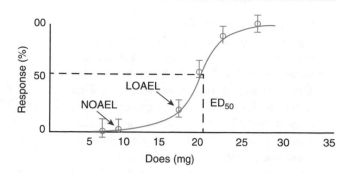

Fig. 2.1 NOAEL and LOAEL

animals. NOAEL/NOAEC is a variant of NOEL/NOEC that specifies only that the effect in question is adverse (Fig. 2.1).

Q. Define lowest observed adverse effect level/concentration (LOAEL/LOAEC).

LOAEL/LOAEC is the highest exposure level/dose level/concentration of a substance under defined conditions of exposure; an observable/detectable effect (alteration) on morphology, functional capacity, growth, development, or life span of the test animals is observed.

Q. Define reference dose/concentration (RfD/RfC).

For noncancerous effects, oral intake (RfD) or an inhalation RfC for airborne materials is calculated using the NOAEL or LOAEL as a starting point. These values are developed from experimentally determined NOAEL or LOAEL.

Risk Assessment Evaluation

Q. Describe briefly the requirement of data for preliminary evaluation of risk assessment in human health.

The type of data required for preliminary evaluation include the following:

(a) Physiochemical processes	(Observed effects on humans)
(b) Toxicity	(Derived from animal studies)
(c) Release/transport/uptake	(Applicable to expected dosage)
(d) Chemical physical interaction	(Most current to support specific conclusions)

Q. What are the basic elements involved in the process of risk assessment?

Four steps used in risk analysis include:

(a) Hazard identification

(b) Dose–response evaluation

(c) Exposure assessment

(d) Risk characterization

Explanation: The initial step is hazard identification, which identifies the chemical that presents a risk to human health. This is a qualitative step, which involves a thorough evaluation of current scientific evidence, including animal studies, human studies, epidemiological studies, and cellular studies. If a chemical is identified as a potential hazard to human health, the process continues.

The second step of risk analysis is the dose–response evaluation, which is a quantitative step. This step measures the magnitude of the response at different doses. If available, human studies showing the potency of the agent, or its ability to produce negative health effects in humans, are also assessed.

The next step is the exposure assessment. This step seeks to estimate people's level of exposure. Exposure refers to the amount of a substance in the environment, and such an estimation includes the length of exposure, duration of exposure, and route of exposure, among other considerations. The difference between the actual dose, or level of a substance taken in, and the amount of the substance measured (exposure) is included in this assessment. This assessment must also quantify various properties of a substance, e.g., volatility, as well as the group exposed and whether the exposure is continuous, intermittent, short term, long term, or chronic. The final step is risk characterization. This step uses all of the previously gathered information through the first three steps and creates a picture of risk that describes its likelihood, severity, and consequences. This characterization includes an estimate of the negative effects, e.g., deaths or cancer cases per 100,000 people. The final step also takes into account any limitations and/or uncertainties that were involved in creating the estimate.

Q. Name four steps involved in hazard identification used for risk assessment process.
Hazard identification involves the following four steps:
(a) Epidemiology
(b) Animal studies
(c) Short-term assays
(d) Structure activity relationship

Q. Name three steps involved in dose–response assessment used for risk assessment process.
Dose–response assessment involves the following three steps:
(a) Quantitative toxicity information collected
(b) Dose–response relationship established
(c) Extrapolation of animal data to human

Q. Name three steps involved in exposure assessment used for risk assessment process.
Exposure assessment involves the following three steps:
(a) Identification of exposed populations
(b) Identification of routes of exposure
(c) Identification of degree of exposure

Q. Name three steps involved in risk characterization used for risk assessment process.
Risk characterization involves the following three steps:
(a) Estimation of the potential for adverse health effects to occur
(b) Evaluation of uncertainty
(c) Risk information summarized

Q. Discuss at least three limitations inherent in risk analysis.
Limitations to risk analysis include:
(a) Uncertainty of effect
(b) Variability of exposure
(c) Possibility of multiple exposures
Explanation: Often, too little is known about any substance to provide any real assurance. Despite laboratory testing and careful risk analysis, uncertainty will remain. Interpersonal variability may also strongly affect a specific individual's risk, as a general overview may not identify people who may be more sensitive to exposures than others, and thus may have a higher "safe" dose. Multiple exposures are difficult to study, although they certainly exist in the real world. In addition, any additive effects are ignored, which may heighten the risk and which are sure to occur outside of the laboratory. However, despite its limitations, risk analysis is still an important tool to explore and understand risks in the modern world.

Establishment of an ADI or Acceptable RfD

Q. How ADI (human dose) is calculated?
Once the critical study demonstrating the toxic effect of concern has been identified, the selection of the NOAEL results from an objective examination of the data available on the chemical in question. The ADI is then derived by dividing the appropriate NOAEL by a safety factor (SF) as follows:

$$\text{ADI}(\text{human dose}) = \text{NOAEL}(\text{experimental dose})/\text{SF}$$
$$\text{or UF} \times \text{MF}.$$

where SF (safety factor) or the uncertainty factor (UF) and modifying factor (MF) is typically equal to 100.
Explanation: Generally, the SF (UF × MF) consists of multiples of 10, each factor representing a specific area of uncertainty inherent in the available data. For example, a factor of

10 may be introduced to account for the possible differences in responsiveness between humans and animals in prolonged exposure studies. A second factor of 10 may be used to account for variation in susceptibility among individuals in the human population. The resultant SF of 100 has been judged to be appropriate for many chemicals. For other chemicals, with data bases that are less complete (e.g., those for which only the results of subchronic studies are available), an additional factor of 10 (leading to a SF of 1000) might be judged to be more appropriate. For certain other chemicals, based on well-characterized responses in sensitive humans (as in the effect of fluoride on human teeth), an SF as small as 1 might be selected.

Q. How an acceptable RfD is established for risk assessment?

Acceptable RfD is established by the following relationship.

$$RfD = NOAEL / (UF \times MF)$$

where the uncertainty factor (UF) and modifying factor (MF) are typically equal to 100. For cancer end points, the only strictly safe exposure level is at zero dose, although for very small doses the risk is extremely low and is not considered significant.

Explanation: Approaches for characterizing dose–response relationships include identification of effect levels such as LD50 (dose producing 50% lethality), LC50 (concentration producing 50% lethality), ED10 (dose producing 10% response), as well as NOAELs. NOAELs have traditionally served as the basis for risk assessment calculations, such as RfDs or ADI values. RfDs or RfCs are estimates of a daily exposure to an agent that is assumed to be without adverse health impact in humans. The ADIs are used by WHO for pesticides and food additives to define "the daily intake of chemical, which during an entire lifetime appears to be without appreciable risk on the basis of all known facts at that time." RfDs and ADI values typically are calculated from NOAEL values by dividing uncertainty (UF) and/or modifying factors (MF). Tolerable daily intakes can be used to describe intakes for chemicals that are not "acceptable" but are "tolerable" as they are below the levels thought to cause adverse health effects. These are calculated in a manner similar to ADI. In principle, dividing by the uncertainty factors allows for interspecies (animal-to-human) and intraspecies (human-to-human) variability with default values of 10 each. An additional uncertainty factor is used to account for experimental inadequacies—e.g., to extrapolate from short exposure—duration studies to a situation more relevant for chronic study or to account for inadequate numbers of animals or other experimental limitations. If only a LOAEL value is available, then an additional tenfold factor commonly is used to arrive at a value more comparable to a NOAEL. Traditionally, a safety factor of 100 is used for RfD calculations to extrapolate from a well-conducted animal bioassay (tenfold factor animal-to-human variability) and to account for human variability in response (tenfold factor human-to-human variability). Assumption is made that exposure below a certain level, the NOAEL, will have no adverse health consequences. An acceptable RfD is then established.

5.0 Sample MCQ's (choose the correct statement; it may be one, two, or none)

Q.1. Regulatory toxicology aims at guarding the public from dangerous chemical exposures and depends primarily on which form of study?

  A. Observational human studies
  B. Controlled laboratory animal studies
  C. Controlled human studies
  D. Environmental studies

Q.2. Risk from a public health perspective is best described as which of the following?

A. Undesirable end point is reached.
B. A possibility of a bad outcome.
C. Likelihood of an unwanted outcome combined with uncertainty of when it will occur.
D. A bad outcome is assured and its mechanism is well understood.

Q.3. Which of the following statements is true regarding risk analysis?

A. It is a field of study that has been around for the last century.
B. It was developed by the pharmaceutical companies in response to concerns over new medications.
C. It is a relatively new field of study, spurred by new technologically based risks.
D. It was largely a private sector venture.

Q.4. Which of the following are tools used in risk analysis?

A. Toxicology
B. Epidemiology
C. Clinical trials
D. All of the above

Q.5. Which of the following are common end points?

A. Death
B. No-observable effect level
C. No-observable adverse effect level
D. Lowest observable adverse effect level
E. All of the above

Q.6. The LD50 is best described as which of the following?

A. The dose at which 50% of all test animals die
B. The dose at which 50% of the animals demonstrate a response to the chemical

C. The dose at which all of the test animals die
D. The dose at which at least one of the test animals dies

Q.7. The effective dose is best described as which of the following?

A. The dose at which 50% of all test animals die
B. The dose at which some of the animals demonstrate a response to the chemical
C. The dose at which all of the animals demonstrate a response to the chemical
D. The dose at which 50% of all test animals demonstrate a response to the chemical

Q.8. Extrapolation is best described as which of the following?

A. Using known information to reach a conclusion
B. Using known information to infer something about the unknown
C. Using speculative information to infer something about the known
D. A "best guess" approach

Q.9. Which of the following assumptions is NOT correct regarding risk assessment for male reproductive effects in the absence of mechanistic data?

A. An agent that produces an adverse reproductive effect in experimental animals is assumed to pose a potential reproductive hazard to humans.
B. In general, a non-threshold is assumed for the dose–response curve for male reproductive toxicity.
C. Effects of xenobiotics on male reproduction are assumed to be similar across species unless demonstrated otherwise.
D. The most sensitive species should be used to estimate human risk.
E. Reproductive processes are similar across mammalian species.

Q.10. Which of the following statements is true?
   A. Chemical carcinogens in animals are always carcinogens in animals.
   B. A chemical that is carcinogenic in humans is usually carcinogenic in at least one animal species.
   C. From a regulating perspective, carcinogens are considered to have a threshold dose–response curve.
   D. Arsenic is an example of a chemical that is carcinogenic to humans and nearly all species treated.

Q.11. The RfD is generally determined by applying which of the following default procedures?

   A. An uncertainty factor of 100 is applied to the NOAEL in chronic animal studies.
   B. A risk factor of 1000 is applied to the NOAEL in chronic animal studies.
   C. A risk factor of 10,000 is applied to the NOAEL in subchronic animal studies.
   D. An uncertainty factor between 10,000 and 1 million is applied to the NOEL from chronic animal studies.
   E. Multiplying the NOAEL from chronic animal studies by 100.

Q.12. Which of the following concerning the use of the "benchmark dose" in risk assessment is NOT correct?

   A. Can use the full range of doses and responses studied
   B. Allows the use of data obtained from experiments where a clear "no-NOAEL has been attained"
   C. May be defined as the lower confidence limit on the 10% effective dose
   D. Is primarily used for the analyses of carcinogenicity data and has limited utility for analyses of developmental and reproduction studies that generate quantal data
   E. Is not limited to the values of the administered doses

Q.13. Administration by oral gavage of a test compound that is highly metabolized by the liver vs. subcutaneous injection will most likely result in -----

   A. Less parent compound present in the systemic circulation
   B. More local irritation at the site of administration caused by the compound
   C. Lower levels of metabolites in the systemic circulation
   D. More systemic toxicity
   E. Less systemic toxicity

Q.14. The phrase that best defines "toxicodynamics" is the

   A. Linkage between exposure and dose
   B. Linkage between dose and response
   C. Dynamic nature of toxic effects among various species
   D. Dose range between desired biological effects and adverse health effects
   E. Loss of dynamic hearing range due to a toxic exposure

Q.15. Which of the following toxicity can occur due to single exposure?

   A. Acute toxicity
   B. Subacute toxicity
   C. Subchronic toxicity
   D. Chronic toxicity

Q.16. Which of the following assumptions is NOT correct regarding risk assessment for male reproductive effects in the absence of mechanistic data?

   A. An agent that produces an adverse reproductive effect in experimental animals is assumed to pose a potential reproductive hazard to humans.
   B. In general, a non-threshold is assumed for the dose–response curve for male reproductive toxicity.
   C. Effects of xenobiotics on male reproduction are assumed to be similar

across species unless demonstrated otherwise.

D. The most sensitive species should be used to estimate human risk.

E. Reproductive processes are similar across mammalian species.

Answers

1. B.   2. C.   3. C.   4. D.   4. E.   6. A.
7. D.   8. B.   9. B.   10. C.   11. A.
12. D.   13. A.   14. B.   14. A.   16. B.

Further Reading

Eaton DL, Gilbert SG (2015) Principles of toxicology. In: Klaassen CD, Watkins JB III (eds) Casarett &Doull's essentials of toxicology, 3rd edn. McGraw-Hill, New York, pp 5–20

Gupta PK (2014) Essential concepts in toxicology. PharmaMed Press (A unit of BSP Books Pvt. Ltd), Hyderabad

Gupta PK (2016) Fundamentals of toxicology: essential concepts and applications, 1st edn. BSP/Elsevier, San Diego

Gupta PK (2018) Illustrative toxicology, 1st edn. Elsevier, San Diego

Gupta PK (2019) Concepts and applications in veterinary toxicology: an interactive guide. Springer-Nature, Cham

Gupta PK (2020) Principles of toxicology in: brain storming questions in toxicology. Francis and Taylor CRC Press, Boca Raton

Gupta RC (ed) (2018) Veterinary toxicology: basic and clinical principles, 3rd edn. Academic Press/Elsevier, San Diego

Fruncillo RJ (2011) 2,000 Toxicology board review questions. Xlibris Publishers, Bloomington

Principles of Toxicology

3

Abstract

Several factors such as age, strain, species variation, pregnancy, physical state and chemical properties of the toxicant, and environmental factors can greatly influence the toxicity of a specific compound. The dose–response relationship, or exposure-response relationship, describes the change in effect on an organism. The relationship between dose and response is usually established when the chemical/drug effect at a particular dose has reached a maximum or a steady level. The chemical effects do not develop instantaneously or continue indefinitely; they change with time. Many toxicants/xenobiotics exert their effects by interacting with specific receptors in the body. Interaction between chemicals may result in an inhibition (*antagonism*) or may produce a more pronounced effect than would be expected by addition or by potentiation.

Keywords

Dose–response relationship · Response curve · Graded doses · Quantal dose · Therapeutic index · Margins of safety · Potency · Efficacy · Principles of toxicology · Factors affecting toxicity · Interactions · Receptors · Question and answer bank · MCQ's.

1 Introduction

The dose is the total amount of chemical absorbed during an exposure. Dose depends on the concentration of the chemical and duration (contact time) of the exposure. Several factors such as age, strain, species variation, pregnancy, physical state and chemical properties of the toxicant, and environmental factors can greatly influence the toxicity of a specific compound. The dose–response relationship, or exposure–response relationship, describes the change in effect on an organism. The relationship between dose and response is usually established when the chemical/drug effect at a particular dose has reached a maximum or a steady level. This chapter deals with the overview, key points, and relevant text that is in the format of problem-solving study questions followed by multiple-choice questions (MCQs) along with their answers.

2 Overview

The Dose Makes the Poison Evaluating clinical effects based on the amount of exposure is a basic *toxicology principle* called dose–response. The dose is the total amount of chemical absorbed during an exposure. Dose depends on the concentration of the chemical and duration (contact time) of the exposure. Factors that influence

P K Gupta, *Problem Solving Questions in Toxicology*, https://doi.org/10.1007/978-3-030-50409-0_3

chemical toxicity include the dosage, duration of exposure (whether it is acute or chronic), route of exposure, species, age, sex, and environment. It is essential to toxicology to establish dose–effect and dose–response relationships. In medical (epidemiological) studies, a criterion often used for accepting a causal relationship between an agent and a disease is that effect or response is proportional to dose.

Several dose–response curves can be drawn for a chemical—one for each type of effect. The dose–response curve for most toxic effects (when studied in large populations) has a sigmoid shape. There is usually a low-dose range where there is no response detected; as dose increases, the response follows an ascending curve that will usually reach a plateau at a 100% response. The dose–response curve reflects the variations among individuals in a population. The slope of the curve varies from chemical to chemical and between different types of effects. There is no necessary correlation between acute and chronic toxicity. ED_{50} (effective dose) is the dose causing a specific effect other than lethality in 50% of the animals. For some chemicals with specific effects (carcinogens, initiators, mutagens), the dose–response curve might be linear from dose zero within a certain dose range. This means that no threshold exists and that even small doses represent a risk. Above that dose range, the risk may increase at greater than a linear rate. High peak exposures may be more harmful than a more even exposure level. Interaction between chemicals may result in an inhibition (*antagonism*) or may produce a more pronounced effect than would be expected by addition or by potentiation.

Key Points

- Several factors such as age, strain, species variation, pregnancy, physical state and chemical properties of the toxicant, and environmental factors can greatly influence the toxicity of a specific compound.
- The individual or "graded" dose–response relationship describes the response of an individual organism to varying doses of a chemical.
- A quantal dose–response relationship characterizes the distribution of responses to different doses in a population of individual organisms.
- For natural or endogenous chemicals that are required for normal physiological function and survival (e.g., vitamins and essential trace elements such as chromium, cobalt, zinc, manganese, and selenium), the "graded" dose–response relationship in an individual over the entire dose range can be U-shaped, known as non-monotonic dose–response curves.
- Hormesis, a "U-shaped" dose–response curve, results with some xenobiotics that impart beneficial or stimulatory effects at low doses but adverse effects at higher doses.
- A ligand of low affinity requires a higher concentration to produce the same effect than ligand of high affinity.
- Agonists, partial agonist, antagonist, and inverse agonist have same or similar affinity for the receptor.

3   Problem-Solving Study Questions

3.1   Terms Used in Relation to Dose and Dose–Response

Q. Define parts per million.
   Just as per cent means out of a hundred, so parts per million or ppm means out of a million. Usually describes the concentration of something in water or soil. One ppm is equivalent to 1 milligram of something per liter of water (mg/l) or 1 milligram of something per kilogram soil (mg/kg).
Q. How 1000 ppm is equivalent to 0.1%? Explain.

1000 ppm is 0.1% because $1000/1 \times 10^6 \times 100 = 0.1\%$

Q. Define lethal dose (LD).

LD is the lowest dose that causes death in any animal during the period of observation. Various percentages can be attached to the LD value to indicate doses required to kill 1% (LD1), 50% (LD50), or 99% (LD99) of the test animals in the population.

Q. Define lethal dose 50 (LD50).

LD50 is also known as median lethal dose (MLD). It is the dose of the toxicant that causes death of the 50% animals under defined conditions like species, route of exposure, and duration of exposure. It is a commonly used measure of toxicity.

Q. Define lethal concentration (LC).

LC is the lowest concentration of the compound in feed (or water in case of fish) that causes death during the period of observation. It is expressed as milligrams of compound per kilogram of feed (or water).

Q. 61. Define lethal concentration 50 (LC50).

LC50 is the concentration of the compound in feed (or water in case of fish) that is lethal to 50% of exposed population. It mainly expresses acute lethal toxicity.

Q. Define maximum allowable or admissible/acceptable concentration (MAC).

MAC is regulatory value defining the upper limit of concentration of certain atmospheric contaminants allowed in the ambient air of the work place.

Q. Define maximum residue limit/maximum residue level: (MRL).

MRL is the maximum amount of a pesticide or grog (mainly veterinary pharmaceutical) residue that is legally permitted or recognized as acceptable in or on food commodities and animal feeds. Although both the terms have the same meaning, in practice the term maximum residue limit is used for the pesticide residue, while the term maximum residue level is applicable for the drug residue.

Q. Define maximum tolerated dose (MTD).

MTD is the highest dose/amount of a substance that causes the toxic effects but no morality in the test organism. In chronic toxicity study, the MLD can cause limited toxic effects in the test organism, but it should not decrease the body weight more than 10% compared with control group or produce the overt toxicity (death of cells or organ dysfunction). The value is often denoted by LD0.

Q. Define maximum tolerated concentration (MTC).

MTC is the highest concentration of a substance in an environment medium that causes the toxic symptoms and no mortality in the test organism.

Q. Define absolute lethal dose (LD100).

LD100 is the lowest dose of substance that under defined conditions is lethal to 100% exposed animals. The value is dependent on the number of organisms used in its assessment.

Q. Define absolute lethal concentration (LC100).

LC100 is the lowest concentration of substance in an environment medium that under defined conditions is lethal to 100% exposed organisms or species.

Q. Define acceptable daily intake (ADI).

ADI is the estimated amount of substance in food or drinking water that can be ingested daily over a lifetime by humans without appreciable health risk. Acceptable daily intake is normally used for food additives (the term tolerable daily intake is used for contamination).

Q. What do you mean by alternative tests (other than use of animals)?

Alternative test is an alternative technique that can provide the same level of information as current animal tests but which use fewer animals, cause less suffering, or avoid the use of animals completely. Such methods, as they become available, must be considered wherever possible for hazard characterization and consequent classification and labeling for intrinsic hazards and chemical safety assessment.

Q. Name different routes of drug administration.
   (a) GI tract (ingestion, oral, or diet)
   (b) Lungs (inhalation)
   (c) Parenteral routes (IV, IP, IM, SC, intra dermal, i.e., other than intestinal canal)

Q. Describe briefly different routes of drug administration in descending order of effectiveness.
   IV > inhalation > IP > SC > IM > intradermal > oral (per OS) > dermal > diet.

Q. Discuss the route (s) having highest toxicity.
   Generally, toxicity is the highest by the route that carries the compound to the bloodstream most rapidly. However, a compound could be more toxic orally than parenterally if an active product is formed in the GI tract. The GI absorption of a compound varies widely. The difference between oral and parenteral LD50s gives some indication as to the extent of absorption of a compound. The IV toxic dose is greatly influenced by the rate of injection.

Q. Define benefit-to-risk ratio.
   This implies that even a toxic agent may warrant use if its benefits for a significant number of people are much greater than the dangers.

Q. What is the difference between lethal dose (LD) and lethal concentration (LC)?
   Both LD and LC cause death in exposed population. LD refers to the "lethal dose" of the toxicant administered to the animal in any route. LC refers to the "lethal concentration" of toxicant present in feed, water, or air.

Q. What is the meaning of the subscripts in the terms LD50 or 99 and LC50?
   The subscripts indicate the % of mortality (deaths) in exposed population.

Q. For a given compound, between MTD and NOAEL, which one will be higher?
   NOAEL is the highest dose which will not cause any adverse effect, but MTD refers to the highest dose which will cause adverse effects. Hence, MTD is higher than NOAEL (MTD is also referred to as LD).

Q. What is the relationship between various toxicity doses with respect to given compound?
   LD > MTD > NOAEL > NOEL > ADI > MRL

Q. What is a dose?
   The dose is the actual amount of a chemical that enters the body. The dose received may be due to either acute, subacute, or chronic (long-term) exposure.

Q. What is dose–response?
   Dose–response is a relationship between exposure/dose and response/effect that can be established by measuring the response relative to an increasing dose. This relationship is important in determining the toxicity of a particular substance. It relies on the concept that a dose, or a time of exposure (to a chemical, drug, or toxic substance), will cause an effect (response) on the exposed organism. Usually, the larger the dose, the greater is response, or the effect. This is the meaning behind the statement "the dose makes the poison."

Q. What is the threshold dose?
   Threshold dose is exposure level below which the harmful or adverse effects of a substance are not seen in a population. This dose is also referred to as the no observed adverse effect level (NOAEL) or the no effect level (NOEL). These terms are often used by toxicologists when discussing the relationship between exposure and dose. However, for substances causing cancer (carcinogens), no safe level of exposure exists, since any exposure could result in cancer.

Q. What do you mean by lethal dose 50 (LD50) and median lethal dose (MLD)?
   Lethal dose 50 (LD50), also called median lethal dose (MLD), is the dose that is lethal to 50% of animals exposed to a given toxicant under defined conditions.

Q. What do you mean by three Rs in toxicology or animal research?
   Three Rs stand for Replacement, Reduction, and Refinement. These ethical principles are widely adhered to throughout the world as a way to significantly limit the number of animals used in scientific experimentation. The term *alternatives*, as an approximate synonym for the three Rs, was coined by the distinguished physiologist David Smyth in 1978.

3.2   Dose–Response Relationship

Q. Describe time–effect relationship of a toxicant?

The relationship between dose and response is usually established when the chemical/drug effect at a particular dose has reached a maximum or a steady level (Fig. 3.1). The chemical effects do not develop instantaneously or continue indefinitely; they change with time. There are three distinct phases and a fourth phase that may be present or pronounced with some chemicals while absent with others. These include:

(a) Time of onset of action
(b) Time to peak effect
(c) Duration of action

Phase I: Time of onset of action (Ta)—following the administration of a chemical agent to a system, there is a delay in time before the first signs of chemical effects are manifested. The lag in onset is of finite time, but for some chemicals, the delay may be so short that it gives the appearance of an instantaneous action. There are various reasons responsible for the chemical effect to reach an observable level.

Phase II: Time to peak effect (Tb)—the maximum response will occur when the most resistant cell has been affected to its maximum or when the chemical has reached the most inaccessible cells of the responsive tissue.

Phase III: Duration of action (Tc)—the duration of action extends from the moment of onset of perceptible effects to the time when an action can no longer be measured. It will depend upon the rate at which it is metabolized, altered, or otherwise inactivated or removed from the body.

Phase IV: Residual effects (Td)—even after its primary actions are terminated, many chemicals are known to exert a residual action. It is not always possible to determine whether the residual effect is caused by a persistence of minute quantities of the chemical or by persistence of subliminal effects.

Q. What is dose–response relationship?

The dose–response relationship, or exposure–response relationship, describes the change in effect on an organism caused by differing levels of exposure (or doses) to a stressor (usually a chemical) after a certain exposure time (Fig. 3.2). This may apply to individuals (e.g., a small amount has no significant effect, a large amount is fatal) or to populations (e.g., how many people or organisms are affected at different levels of exposure).

Explanation: This type of relationship is useful in measuring the incremental responses of a compound and can be seen in an individual organism, e.g., contraction of small intestine produced by carbachol, convulsions produced by strychnine, and inhibition of cholinesterase produced by OP insecticides. This type of relationship is useful in studying the efficiency of therapeutic drugs or toxic symptoms produced by a toxicant(s). This is a typical dose–response curve in which the percentage of organisms or systems responding to a chemical is plotted against the dose.

Q. What are different types of dose–response relationships?

Dose–response relationship is of two types:
(a) Graded or gradual
(b) Quantal (all-or-none) such as death

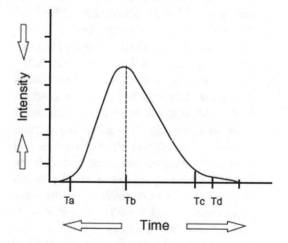

Fig. 3.1 Hypothetical curve showing time effect relationship of a toxicant. Ta, latency time; Tb, peak time; Tc, persistence time; Td, residual effect

Fig. 3.2 A typical
dose–response curve in
which the percentage of
organisms or systems
responding to a chemical
is plotted against the
dose

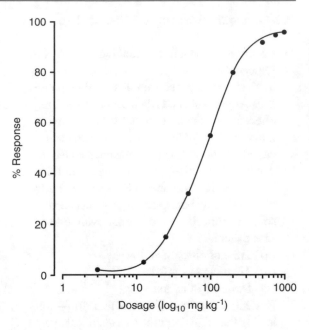

Q. What is a graded or gradual dose–response
   relationship?
   The individual dose–response relationship,
   which describes the response of an individual
   organism to varying doses of a chemical,
   often referred to as a "graded" response
   because the measured effect is continuous
   over a range of doses (Fig. 3.1).

Q. What are the assumptions of graded dose–
   response relationship?
   The graded dose–response relationship is
   based on following presumptions:
   (a) The pharmacological/toxicological effect
       is a result of the known drug/toxicant.
   (b) There is a molecular or receptor site(s)
       with which the drug/toxicant interacts to
       produce the response.
   (c) The production of a response and the
       degree of response are related to the con-
       centration of the drug/toxicant at the
       molecular or receptor site.
   (d) The concentration of the drug/toxicant at
       the molecular or receptor site in turn is
       related to the administered dose of the
       agent.
   (e) The effect of drug/toxicant is propor-
       tional to the fractions of molecular or
       receptor site occupied by the agent;

therefore, by increasing or decreasing
the dose, the response also increases or
decreases, respectively. The maximal
effect occurs when the drug/toxicant
occupy all molecular or receptor sites.

Q. What is a quantal or all-or-none dose–
   response relationship?
   Quantal dose–response relationship is one
   involving an all-or-none response, i.e., on
   increasing the dose of a compound, the
   response is either produced or not. This relationship is seen with certain responses that
   follows all-or-none phenomenon and can't be
   graded, e.g., effective dose, death (Fig. 3.2).
   Explanation: In toxicology, quantal dose–
   response relationship is extensively used for
   the calculation of lethal dose (LD) because in
   it we observe only mortality. The quantal
   dose–response relationship is always seen in
   a population because the assumption is made
   that individual responds to maximal possible
   or not at all. Both are graphs from the same
   set of experimental data. The log dose scale
   results in a more linear representation of the
   data and is more desirable since we will use
   the linear portion of the curve (from approximately 16–84%) to calculate toxic potency
   (Fig. 3.2). This graph does not show the

intensity of effect but rather the frequency with which any dose produces the all-or-none phenomenon. A widely used statistical approach for estimating the response of a population to a toxic exposure is the "effective dose" (ED) or "toxic dose" (TD) or "lethal dose" (LD). Generally, the midpoint, or 50%, response level is used, giving rise to the "ED50" or "TD50" or "LD50" value is chosen. However, any response level, such as an ED01, ED10, or ED30 or TD01, TD10, or TD30 or LD01, LD10, or LD30, could be chosen (Fig. 3.3). The figure also shows comparison of effective dose (ED), toxic dose (TD), and lethal dose (LD).

Q. How you can compare effective dose (ED), toxic dose (TD), and lethal dose (LD)? Show with the help of a plot, log dose versus percentage of population responding in probit units.

Explanation: From Fig. 3.3 one can approximate a TI by using median doses. The larger the ratio, the greater relative safety is assumed. The ED50 is approximately 20, and the TD50 is about 60; thus, the TI is 3, a number indicating that reasonable care in exposure to the drug is necessary to avoid toxicity. However, the use of the median effective and median toxic doses is not without disadvantages, because median doses do not reflect the slopes of the dose–response curves for therapeutic and toxic effects.

Q. Explain LD50 with the help of a plot.

LD50 is the dose of a compound which is lethal for 50% of the population exposed to that compound. The value is determined from the dose–response relationship by interpolation (Fig. 3.3).

3.3   Non-monotonic Dose–Response Curves

Q. What are non-monotonic dose–response curves?

For natural or endogenous chemicals that are required for normal physiological function and survival (e.g., vitamins and essential trace elements such as chromium, cobalt, zinc, manganese, and selenium), the "graded" dose–response relationship in an individual over the entire dose range can be U-shaped, known as non-monotonic dose–response curves. As dose increases to surpass the amount required to maintain homeostasis, overdose toxicity can ensue. Thus, adverse effects are seen at both low and high doses (Fig. 3.4).

Explanation: As essential elements for life, nutrient and vitamin concentrations need to

Fig. 3.3 Quantal dose–response relationship showing linear transformation of dose–response data. Percentage response may be effective dose (ED) or toxic dose (TD) or morality (LD). https://doctorlib.info/pharmacology/manual/manual.files/image054.jpg

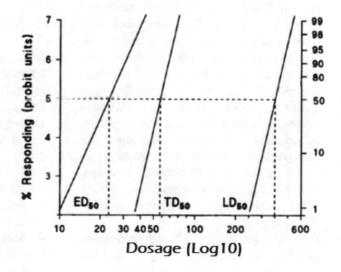

"U"-shaped dose–response curve

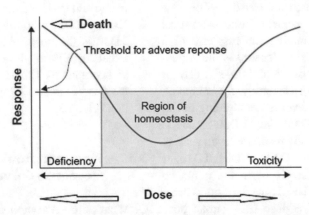

Fig. 3.4 U-shaped dose–response curve for essential metals and vitamins. Vitamins and essential metals are essential for life, and their lack can cause adverse responses (plotted on the vertical axis), as can their excess, giving rise to a U-shaped dose-dependent curve. The colored-shaded region represents the "region of homeostasis"—the dose range that results in neither deficiency nor toxicity

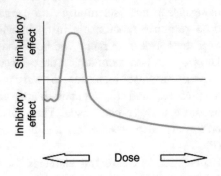

Fig. 3.5 A low dose of a chemical agent may trigger from an organism the opposite response to a very high dose

be maintained within a specific range that allows for homeostasis. Doses or concentrations outside of this range can lead to *deficiency* (observed at very low doses when concentrations are below daily minimum requirements) or *toxicity* (observed at high, excessive doses). Often, the biological adverse responses that occur during periods of deficiency or toxicity will differ. One example that illustrates the importance of proper maintenance of nutrient concentrations and homeostasis is manganese.

Q. What is hormesis dose–response phenomenon?
In toxicology, hormesis is a dose–response phenomenon characterized by a low-dose stimulation, high-dose inhibition, resulting in either a J-shaped or an inverted U-shaped dose–response (Fig. 3.5).

Q. What are the conditions that lead to tolerance?
(a) Requires previous exposure to the chemical
(b) Can result from decreased chemical reaching its target
(c) Can result from reduced responsiveness of the tissue
(d) Results from the induction of protective mechanisms

3.4   Interaction of Chemicals

Q. What do you mean by drug or chemical interaction?
A drug interaction is a reaction between two (or more) drugs or between a drug and a food, beverage, or supplement. Taking a drug while having certain medical conditions can also cause a drug interaction. A drug interaction can make a drug less effective, increase the action of a drug, or cause unwanted side effects.

Q. What is a drug/chemical affinity?
Affinity is the ability of a xenobiotic to combine with its receptors. A ligand of low affinity requires a higher concentration to produce

the same effect than ligand of high affinity. Agonists, partial agonist, antagonist, and inverse agonist have same or similar affinity for the receptor.

Q. What is an inverse agonist?

Inverse agonist is a compound that interacts with the same receptor as the agonist, but it produces a response just opposite to that of the agonist.

Q. What will be the response if two drugs/xenobiotics are used simultaneously?

When two or more xenobiotics are used together, the pharmacological/toxicological response is not necessarily the same of two agents used individually. This is because one agent may interfere with the action of another agent called xenobiotic/drug interaction.

Q. What is additive or summation effect?

Additive or summation effect occurs when the combined responses of two chemicals is equal to the sum of the responses to each chemical given alone (e.g., 2 + 2 = 4). For example, when two organophosphorus insecticides are given together, inhibition of acetylcholinesterase enzymes (AChE) is usually additive, based on the relative ability of each one to inhibit AChE (Fig. 3.6) i.e. when two chemicals with similar mechanisms are given together, they typically produce additive or summation effects.

Q. What is synergistic or potentiation effect?

Synergistic or potentiation effect is observed when the combined responses of two chemicals are much greater than the sum of the response to each chemical when given alone (e.g., 4 + 4 = 10). For example, both carbon tetrachloride and ethanol are hepatotoxic compounds, but together they produce much more liver injury than expected based on the extent of damage at a given dose when administered alone (Fig. 3.7) i.e. if the effect of two chemicals exceeds the sum of their individual effects. Synergistic or potentiation requires that the chemicals act at different receptors or effector systems.

Q. What are the possible mechanisms of antagonism?

There are several mechanisms of antagonism:

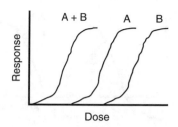

Fig. 3.6 *Additive or summation* effect. When two chemicals with similar mechanisms are given together, they typically produce additive or summation effects

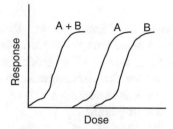

Fig. 3.7 *Synergistic* or potentiation effect. When the effect of two drugs exceeds the sum of their individual effects. Synergistic or potentiation requires that the chemicals act at different receptors or effector systems

(a) Functional antagonism
(b) Chemical antagonism
(c) Receptor antagonism
(d) Dispositional antagonism:

Q. What is antagonism effect?

Antagonism occurs when two chemicals administered together interfere with each other's actions or one interferes with the action of the other (e.g., 4 + 6 = 8; 4 + (−4) = 0; 4 + 0 = 1). Antagonism of the toxic effects of chemicals is often desirable in identifying important mechanisms of toxicity as well as in developing antidotes (Fig. 3.8).

Q. What is receptor antagonism?

Receptor antagonism occurs when two chemicals that bind to the same receptor produce less of an effect when given together relative to the addition of their separate effects (e.g., 3 + 6 = 8) or when one chemical antagonizes the effect of the second chemical (e.g., 0 + 3 = 1). Receptor antagonists are often termed blockers. This concept is exploited in the clinical treatment of poisonings. Treatment of organophosphorus insecticide poisoning with atropine is another example of an antagonism of toxicity by blocking a

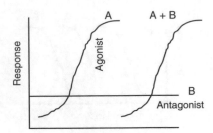

Fig. 3.8 The toxic effect of a chemical, A, agonist, can be reduced when given with another chemical, B, the antagonist

physiological "ligand–receptor interaction." In this example, atropine binds to the acetylcholine receptor and thus blocks the excess acetylcholine that accumulates after inhibition of the cholinesterase

Q. What is a drug affinity?

Affinity is the ability of a xenobiotic to combine with its receptors. A ligand of low affinity requires a higher concentration to produce the same effect than ligand of high affinity. Agonists, partial agonist, antagonist, and inverse agonist have same or similar affinity for the receptor.

Q. What do you mean by intrinsic activity?

Intrinsic activity is defined as a proportionately constant ability of the agonist to activate the receptor as compared to the maximally active compound in the series being studied. It is maximum of unity for full agonist and minimum or zero for antagonist.

Q. What is an agonist?

Agonist (full agonist) is an agent that interacts with a specific cellular constituent (i.e., receptor) and elicits an observable positive response.

Q. What is a partial agonist?

Partial agonist is an agent that acts on the same receptor as other agonists in a group of endogenous ligands or xenobiotics, but regardless of its dose, it cannot produce the same maximal biological response as a full agonist.

Q. What is the difference between synergism and potentiation?

The difference between the two concepts is that synergism is the interaction of two or more substances, while potentiation is about a singular substance and how it may act when in a synergy relationship.

Q. Why are toxins often selective to tissues, give suitable examples?

Toxins are often selective to certain tissues because of the following reasons:

(a) Preferential accumulation: Toxicant may accumulate in only certain tissues and cause toxicity to that particular tissue, e.g., Cd in the kidney, paraquat in the lung.

(b) Selective metabolic activation: Enzymes needed to convert a compound to the active form may be present in highest quantities in a particular organ, e.g., CCl4, nitrosamines in the liver.

(c) Characteristics of tissue repair: Some tissues may be protected from toxicity by actively repairing toxic damage; some tissues may be susceptible because they lack sufficient repair capabilities, e.g., nitrosamines in the liver.

(d) Specific receptors and/or functions: Toxicant may interact with receptors in a given tissue, e.g., curare—a receptor-specific neuromuscular blocker.

(e) Physiological sensitivity: The nervous system is extremely sensitive to agents that block utilization of oxygen, e.g., nitrite, oxidizes hemoglobin (methemoglobinemia); cyanide, inhibits cytochrome oxidase (cells not able to utilize oxygen); and barbiturates, interfere with sensors for oxygen and carbon dioxide content in the blood.

Q. What are the main target organs most frequently affected by toxicants?

(a) Central nervous system
(b) Circulatory system (blood, blood-forming system)
(c) Visceral organs (liver, kidneys, lung)
(d) Muscle and bone

Q. Why effect or response is observed after administration of any chemical? Give primary assumptions.

Primary assumptions include:

(a) There is a molecular site (or receptor) with which the chemical interacts to produce a response.

(b) Production of response is related to the concentration of the compound at the active site.

(c) The concentration of the compound at the active site is related to the dose administered.

Q. What is tolerance?

Repeated exposure to a chemical can reduce its pharmacologic and/or toxicologic responses, a process called *tolerance*. Cross-tolerance occurs when structurally related chemicals cause diminished responses. Typically, days or weeks of repeated exposure are required for tolerance to occur. Depending upon the chemical and biological effects, there may be multiple mechanisms that cause tolerance: *it may be dispositional tolerance which* occurs when the amount of chemical reaching the site of action decreases over time, leading to the reduced responsiveness of the tissue to stimulation, e.g., phenobarbital.or *Chemical or cellular tolerance* may result from a lower availability of receptors and/or mediators (e.g., neurotransmitters). Drugs of abuse such as morphine interact with the opioid receptor; with repeated exposure to morphine, a protein called beta-arrestin-2 binds to the opioid receptor leading to desensitization and tolerance.

3.5 Evaluating the Dose–Response Relationship

Q. Describe different variables of dose–response curve

The dose–response curve has four characteristic variables:
(a) Efficacy
(b) Potency
(c) Slope
(d) Biological variation

Q. What is the difference between therapeutic index and margin of safety?

The therapeutic index is the ratio of the TD50 (or LD50), and the ED50 the margin of safety

(a more conservative estimate) is the ratio of the LD1 and the ED99.

$$\text{Therapeutic index}\,(\text{TI}) = \text{LD50}\,/\,\text{ED50}$$

where LD50 = dose that is lethal for 50% of the population and ED50 = dose that is effective for 50% of the population.

Therapeutic index measure is commonly used for evaluating the safety and usefulness of therapeutic agents. The higher the index, the safer is the drug.

Q. What is a therapeutic ratio?

Therapeutic ratio may be defined as the ratio of the lethal dose-25 (LD25) and the effective dose 75 (ED75).

$$\text{Therapeutic ratio}\,(\text{TR}) = \text{LD25}\,/\,\text{ED75}$$

where LD25 = dose that is lethal for 25% of the population and ED75 = dose that is effective for 75% of the population.

Therapeutic ratio is considered a better index of safety of a compound as it includes steepness of curve also. In toxicity cases, a flatter curve is considered more toxic or hyper-reactive groups are at a much more risk than hypo-reactive or normal group. Shallower curves usually have low therapeutic ratios.

Q. What is a chronicity factor?

Chronicity factor is the ratio of the acute LD50 (one dose) to chronic LD50 doses.

Chronicity factor = acute LD50/chronic LD50.

Chronicity factor is used to assess the cumulative action of a toxicant. Compounds with cumulative effects have a higher chronicity factor.

Q. What is a risk ratio?

The ratio between the inherent toxicity and the exposure level gives the risk ratio. Risk ratio indicates the risk of a compound. Substances of higher inherent toxicity may pose little risk as access of exposure of individuals to such agents is limited. Compounds of low toxicity may be dangerous if used extensively.

Q. What is potency?
Potency is the dose of drug/toxicant required to produce a specific effect of given intensity as compared to a standard reference. It is a comparative rather than an absolute expression of drug activity. Drug potency depends on both affinity and efficacy. The more potent compound is on the left because less compound is needed to produce an equivalent response compared to the compound depicted on the right (Figs. 3.9 and 3.10).

Q. What is efficacy?
The maximal effect or response produced by an agent is called its maximal efficacy or efficacy. The following illustrations show difference between two chemicals (Fig. 3.9).

Q. What is the difference between potency and efficacy?
Potency is the relationship between the dose of a drug and the therapeutic effect. It refers to the drug's strength. When comparing two drugs that work equally, the one with the lower dose has a higher potency. They may have equal efficacy (Fig. 3.10).

Q. What is slope?
The slope of a line is a number that measures its "steepness." It is the change in y for a unit change in x along the line. It also gives the relationship between the receptor/target site and the agent (Figs. 3.9 and 3.10).

Q. What is biological variation?
Biological variation or variance can be defined as the appearance of differences in the magnitude of response among individuals in the same population given the same dose of a compound.

Q. What is a margin of safety?
The main goals of drug development are effectiveness and safety. Because all drugs can be harmful as well as useful, safety is relative. The difference between the usual effective dose and the dose that causes severe or life-threatening side effects is called the margin of safety (Fig. 3.11).

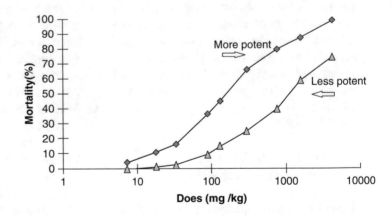

Fig. 3.9 Comparison of potency of drug/toxicant

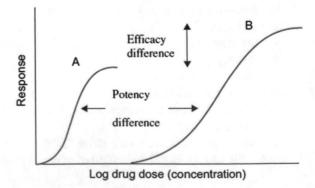

Fig. 3.10 Typical sigmoid log dose–response curves for two drugs/toxicants. Drug A is more potent than drug B; drug B is more efficacious than drug A

Fig. 3.11 The margin of safety of a drug may be determined by comparing the 99% dose–response curve for the efficacy with the curve for a toxic or lethal effect

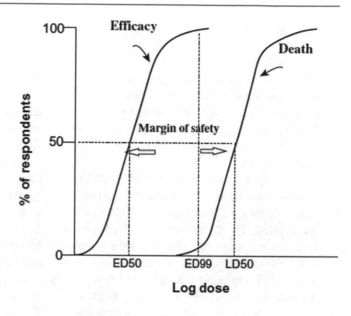

For example:

safety margin = LD1 / ED99

where LD1 = dose that is lethal for 1% of the population and ED99 = dose that is effective for 99% of the population.

Safety margin is a more conservative estimate than therapeutic index as values are derived from extremes of the respective dose–response curves.

3.6   Modifying Factors

Q. Enumerate at least four group of factors that can affect toxicity.
  (a) Host factors (biological factors)
  (b) Factors related to toxicant or associated with xenobiotics
  (c) Environmental factors
  (d) Individual or non-individual factors

Q. What are biological factors that affect toxicity?
  (a) Host (species, age, nutrition, health status)
  (b) Individual
  (c) Environment (housing, ventilation, temp, soil pH, precipitation)

Q. What are species related factors that affect toxicity?
  (a) Sex
  (b) Breed
  (c) Excretion pathways,
  (d) Anatomy/physiology of GI tract
  (e) Respiratory tract
  (f) Target receptor density/subtypes

Q. Discuss briefly the size and age of an individual that affect toxicity. Give suitable examples.

Large individuals can tolerate a larger dose than individuals of small. The metabolism and activity are proportional to the surface area of the body. Life stage, and in turn age, is an important factor that can alter susceptibility to toxicity. Metabolic processes that aid in xenobiotic clearance are often altered at juvenile and advancing ages. For example, newborns have relatively low gastric emptying, gastrointestinal motility, and expression of the metabolic enzymes including CYP2D6, CYP2E1, and CYP3A3. Reduced metabolic capacity can decrease the clearance of some chemicals and increase the risk of toxicity. For example, juvenile rodents exhibit a heightened susceptibility to the insecticides parathion and chlorpyrifos as a result of delayed expression of carboxylesterase enzymes that detoxify organophosphate metabolites. Conversely, the inability of juveniles to bioactivate some chemicals such as acetaminophen to their toxic intermediates appears to protect against liver injury.

Q. Discuss briefly species, breeds, and strains of an individual that affect toxicity. Give suitable examples.

Various species and various strains within species react differently to a particular toxicant because of variations in absorption, metabolism, or elimination. Functional differences in species may also affect the likelihood of toxicosis, e.g., species unable to vomit can be intoxicated with a lower dose of some agents. Such differences are most common and of greatest magnitude when functions which are phylogenetically divergent between species, such as digestive functions (ruminant vs. non-ruminant, carnivore vs. herbivore, etc.), are involved after exposure to toxicants. Interspecies differences also exist in toxic response, but these are generally more limited, except when a particular targeted function has evolved, as is the case for reproductive physiology (mammals vs. birds vs. fishes; annual vs. seasonal reproductive cycle in mammals; etc.). Interspecies difference due to metabolism is a major factor accounting for species differences in pharma kinetic (PK) and also in pharmacodynamics (PD). Recent and future advances in molecular biology and pharmacogenomics will enable a more comprehensive view of interspecies differences and also between breeds with existing polymorphism. Finally, the main message of this chapter is that differences between species are not only numerous but also often unpredictable so that no generalizations are possible. Instead, each toxicant must be investigated on a species-by-species basis to guarantee its effective and safe use, thus ensuring the well-being of animals and safeguarding of the environment and human consumption of animal products. Well-established examples include rabbit can survive even after eating *Atropa belladonna* (belladonna leaves) because they contain the enzyme atropinase, which destroys atropine. Similarly, some breeds of animals are more susceptible to the toxic effects of chemicals. For example, in Koolies, vermectin easily crosses blood–brain barrier and causes neurological symptom. Mink (species) animal is highly sensitive for polychlorinated biphenyls (PCBs) than other species.

Greyhounds are more susceptible to the toxic effects of barbiturates (used as anesthetics) as they mainly distribute to adipose tissue, since greyhounds have little body fat resulting in higher circulating concentration of barbiturates causing toxicity.

Q. Is there any difference in toxicity due to sex of the species?

The sex of an animal often has an influence on the toxicity of chemical agent. The variation in toxicity due to sex is well known; the chemical agents or drugs must be used with special care during pregnancy because they could lead to teratogenic effects in females, and the differences are shown to be under direct endocrine influence. During lactation, it is important to remember that some chemicals or drugs may be excreted in milk and may even act on the offspring. Thus, it is desirable to measure acute toxicity on both male and female animals of any species.

Q. What are the factors associated with toxicants that affect the outcome of response?

   (a) Physical state and chemical properties of the toxicant

   (b) Routes and rates of toxicant administration

   (c) Previous or coincident exposure to other drugs/chemicals (drug–drug/chemical interactions)

   (d) Tolerance of individuals

Q. How do physical state and chemical properties of toxicants affect toxicity?

The physical state and chemical properties of the toxicant such as:

(1) Solubility in water, (2) solubility in vegetable oils, (3) the suspending medium, (4) the chemical stability of the chemical agent, (5) the particle size, (6) rates of disintegration of

formulations of chemicals, (7) the crystal form, and (8) the grittiness of inert substances given in bulk amounts

For example, fine particles are more readily absorbed than coarse ones (in the case of poisons bearing irritating properties, e.g., α-naphthylthiourea, zinc phosphide). Solvents and other substances included in commercial preparations may also affect the overall toxicity of the active principle(s). Nonpolar solvents may considerably increase the absorption rate of lipophilic poisons, especially when considering the exposure by the dermal route.

Q. How do routes and rate of administration of chemicals affect the toxicity?

Generally, toxicity is the highest by the route that carries the compound to the bloodstream most rapidly. For most xenobiotics, parenteral routes of exposure entail a prompt and complete bioavailability than the oral one and therefore often result in a lower LD50.

Q. How does previous or coincident exposure to other chemicals (drug–drug interactions) affect the toxicity?

A variety of chemicals (drugs, plant toxins, pesticides, environmental pollutants) are capable of increasing (enzyme inducers) or decreasing (enzyme inhibitors) the expression and the activity of hepatic and extrahepatic phase I and phase II enzyme systems participating in the biotransformation reactions, hence modulating the toxicity of several xenobiotics. Thus administration of two or more chemicals of different structures when administered simultaneously may lead to additive effect, "summation" or negative summation, or "antagonism" or "potentiation."

Q. How does repeated administration of drug affect the response of a drug?

It is well known that the toxic reaction of an animal to a given dose of a drug may decrease, remain unchanged, or increase on subsequent administration of that dose. A decrease in toxic response is usually called "tolerance" and, an increase in toxic response, "hypersusceptibility." The enzyme induction or the increased activity of enzymes concerned with detoxification and elimination of drug is a common mechanism for the development of tolerance to a drug on repeated administration. For example, repeated administration of chlorpromazine depresses the central nervous system (CNS) of normal albino rats and lessens their loco motor activity.

Q. How do feed and feeding affect the results of toxicity?

The composition of the feed or food can affect the results of toxicity tests. For example, high-fat diets can sensitize animals to, while high carbohydrate and high protein diets provide protection from, the hepatotoxic effects of chloroform.

Q. Discuss in brief environmental conditions that effect toxicity.

The environment can affect the toxic response to chemicals given to animals or human beings. There arc three basic factors in the environment of laboratory animals used in toxicity testing, namely:

(a) The presence of other species of animals, usually human being
(b) The presence of other animals of the same species
(c) Physical environment

Several physical factors such as light, temperature, and relative humidity can influence the LD50 of several chemicals. For example, high ambient temperatures are reported to enhance the toxicity of chlorophenols and nitrophenols that cause an increased production of heat by uncoupling mitochondrial oxidative phosphorylation. Conversely, cold temperatures are predisposing factors for α-chloralose, a rodenticide/avicide formerly used as an anesthetic agent, which may induce a life-threatening hypothermia especially in poisoned cats by acting on hypothalamic thermoreceptors.

Q. How do changes in the internal environment affect toxicity?

Several physiological factors, such as physical activity, stress conditions, hormonal state of animals, and degenerative changes in internal organs, are known to influence the toxicity of any compound. For example, some compounds may induce increased synthesis of liver microsomal enzymes and influence the metabolism of another. The inhibition of drug or chemical agent metabolism, displacement of protein binding of a chemical, or inhibition of its renal clearance can also be accomplished by chemical agents.

Q. How do habitually used drugs affect the sensitivity of man to toxic doses of chemicals?
The habitual use of certain psychoactive drugs, and particularly excessive use, of these chemicals could affect the sensitivity of man to toxic doses of drugs and other chemicals.

3.7 Selective Toxicity

Q. What is selective toxicity?
Selective toxicity means that a chemical produces injury to kind of living matter (such as a cell or organism) without harming another form of life even though the two may exist in intimate contact. In agriculture, for example, there are fungi, insects, and even competitive plants that injure the crop, and thus selective pesticides are needed. Similarly, animal husbandry and human medicine require pharmaceuticals, such as antibiotics, that are selectively toxic to the infectious microbe but do not produce damage to the host.

Q. What is circadian rhythm?
Circadian rhythm is a 24-hour cycle that regulates a number of molecular and physiological processes. Within the 24-hour cycle, there are diurnal (light cycle), nocturnal (dark cycle), and crepuscular (transition) periods. The circadian clock consists of a cellular clock with specific genes that oscillate in expression. Timing in the circadian system is affected by a number of factors including light, activity, food consumption, and social cues. While most changes in physiological processes during the 24-hour period are not readily apparent, they can still impact susceptibility to toxicity.

3.8 Descriptive Animal Toxicity Tests

Q. What are the main principles under lie all descriptive animal toxicity?
There are two basic principles underlie all descriptive animal toxicity. The first is that the effects produced by a compound in laboratory animals, when properly qualified, are applicable to humans. The second principle is that exposure of experimental animals to toxic agents in high doses is a necessary and valid method of discovering possible hazards in humans because the incidence of an effect in a population is greater as the dose or exposure increases.

Q. What type of information one can draw from acute animal toxicity tests?
1. Give a quantitative estimate of acute toxicity (LD50).
2. Identify target organs and other clinical manifestations of acute toxicity.
3. Identify species differences and susceptible species.
4. Establish the reversibility of the toxic response.
5. Provide dose-ranging guidance or other studies.

Q. Why tests for acute dermal or acute inhalation exposure are necessary?
Acute dermal or acute inhalation exposure tests are necessary when there is a reasonable likelihood of substantial exposure to the material by dermal or inhalation exposure. When animals are exposed acutely to chemicals in the air they breathe or the water they (fish) live in, the lethal concentration 50 (LC50) is usually determined for a known time of exposure.

Q. Which animal species is used for acute dermal toxicity?
The acute dermal toxicity test is usually performed in rabbits. The site of application is shaved, and the substance is applied and covered for 24 h and then removed. The skin is cleaned and the animals observed or 14 days to calculate LD50.

Q. Which test is used for the dermal irritation?
For the dermal irritation test (Draize test), the skin of rabbits is shaved, the chemical applied to one intact and two abraded sites and covered for 4 h. The degree of skin irritation is scored for erythema (redness), eschar (scab), edema (swelling) formation, and corrosive action. These dermal irritation observations are repeated at various intervals after the covered patch has been removed.

Q. Which test is used for the eye irritation?
To determine the degree of eye irritation, the chemical is instilled into one eye of each test rabbit. The contralateral eye is used as the control. The eyes of the rabbits are then examined at various times after application.

Q. Which alternative in vitro models are used for the evaluation of cutaneous and ocular toxicity of substances?
Alternative in vitro models, including epidermal keratinocyte and corneal epithelial cell culture models, have been developed or evaluating cutaneous and ocular toxicity of substances.

Q. Which test is used to test the sensitization of a chemical?
Information about the potential of a chemical to sensitize skin is needed in addition to irritation testing or all materials that may repeatedly come into contact with the skin. In general, the test chemical is administered to the shaved skin of guinea pigs topically, intradermally, or both, over a period of 2–4 weeks. About 2–3 weeks after the last treatment, the animals are challenged with a nonirritating concentration of the test substance, and the development of erythema is evaluated.

Q. Why subacute toxicity tests are performed (repeated-dose study) in animals?
Subacute toxicity tests are performed to obtain information on the toxicity of a chemical after repeated administration for typically 14 days and as an aid to establish doses for subchronic studies.

Q. Why subchronic study is performed in animals?
The principal goals of the subchronic study are to establish a "lowest observed adverse effect level" (LOAEL) and a NOAEL and to further identify and characterize the specific organ or organs affected by the test compound after repeated administration. A subchronic study is usually conducted in two species (rat and dog for FDA; mouse and rat for EPA) by the route of intended exposure. At least three doses are employed (a high dose that produces toxicity but less than 10% fatalities, a low dose that produces no apparent toxic effects, and an intermediate dose). Animals should be observed once or twice daily for signs of toxicity. The gross and microscopic conditions of the organs and tissues are recorded and evaluated. Hematology, blood chemistry, and urinalysis measurements are usually done before, in the middle of, and at the termination of exposure.

Q. Why chronic toxicity study is performed in animals?
The period of exposure chronic toxicity is usually for 6 months to 2 years. These tests are often designed to assess both the cumulative toxicity and the carcinogenic potential of chemicals. Both gross and microscopic pathological examinations are made not only on animals that survive the chronic exposure but also on those that die prematurely.

3.9   Other Tests

Tests for chemical carcinogenesis are discussed in Chap. 8, for genetic toxicology in Chap. 9, and for development toxicity in Chap. 10. Information on methods, concepts, and problems associated with inhalation toxicology, neurotoxicity, and behavioral toxicology can be found in other relevant chapters. Immunotoxicity assessment is mentioned in Chap. 7.

3.10   Toxicogenomics

Q. What is toxicogenomics?
Toxicogenomics defines the interaction between genes and toxicants in toxicity etiology. Transcript, protein, and metabolite

profiling is combined with conventional toxicology.

Q. What is genomics?

The identification and characterization of various genetic variants will aid understanding of inter-individual differences in susceptibility to chemicals or other environmental factors and the complex interactions between the human genome and the environment. How chemicals affect genomic DNA, mRNA, small interfering RNA (siRNA), etc. is of particular importance to toxicogenomics.

Q. What is epigenetics?

Toxicants may also act on areas "above or in addition" to genes. Epigenetics concerns a mitotically or meiotically heritable change in gene expression that occurs independently of an alteration in DNA sequence. Changes in DNA methylation or histone acetylation may suppress, silence, or activate gene expression without altering the DNA sequence.

4   Sample MCQ's

(Choose the correct statement; it may be one, two, or none.)

Q.1. Which of the following toxicity can occur due to single exposure?

   A. Acute toxicity
   B. Subacute toxicity
   C. Subchronic toxicity
   D. Chronic toxicity

Q.2. If two organophosphate insecticides are absorbed into an organism, the result will be_____

   A. Additive effect
   B. Synergy effect
   C. Potentiation
   D. Substraction effect

Q.3. If ethanol and carbon tetrachloride are chronically absorbed into an organism, the effect on the liver would be _____

   A. Additive effect
   B. Synergy
   C. Potentiation
   D. Substraction effect

Q.4. If propyl alcohol and carbon tetrachloride are chronically absorbed into an organism, the effect on the liver would be _____

   A. Additive effect
   B. Synergy
   C. Potentiation
   D. Substraction effect

Q.5. The treatment of strychnine-induced convulsions by diazepam is an example of _____

   A. Chemical antagonism
   B. Dispositional antagonism
   C. Receptor antagonism
   D. Functional antagonism

Q.6. The use of antitoxin in the treatment of snakebite is an example of _____

   A. Dispositional antagonism
   B. Chemical antagonism
   C. Receptor antagonism
   D. Functional antagonism

Q.7. The use of charcoal to prevent the absorption of diazepam is an example of _____

   A. Dispositional antagonism
   B. Chemical antagonism
   C. Receptor antagonism
   D. Functional antagonism

Q.8. The use of tamoxifen in certain breast cancer is an example of _____

   A. Dispositional antagonism
   B. Chemical antagonism
   C. Receptor antagonism
   D. Functional antagonism

Q.9. Chemicals known to produce dispositional tolerances are _____

A. Benzene and xylene
B. Trichloroethylene and methylene chloride
C. Paraquat and diquat
D. Carbon tetrachloride and cadmium

Q.10. The most rapid exposure to a chemical would occur through which of the following routes_____

A. Oral
B. Subcutaneous
C. Inhalation
D. Intramuscular

Q.11. A chemical that is toxic to the brain but which is detoxified in the liver would be expected to be _____

A. More toxic orally than intramuscularly
B. More toxic rectally than intravenously
C. More toxic via inhalation than orally
D. More toxic on the skin than intravenously

Q.12. The LD50 is calculated from _____

A. A quantal dose–response curve
B. A hormesis dose–response curve
C. A graded dose–response curve
D. A log–log dose–response curve

Q.13. A U-shaped graded toxicity dose–response curve is seen in humans with_____

A. Pesticides
B. Sedatives
C. Opiates
D. Vitamins

Q.14. The TD1/ED99 is called-

A. Margin of safety
B. Therapeutic index

C. Potency ratio
D. Efficacy ratio

Q.15. All of the following are reasons for selective toxicity except_____

A. Transport differences between cell
B. Biochemical differences between cell
C. Cytology of male neurons versus female neurons
D. Cytology of plant cells versus animal cells

Answers
1. A.   2. A.   3. B.   4. C.   5. D.   6. B.
7. A.   8. C.   9. D.   10. C.   11. C.   12. A.
13. D.   14. A.   15. C.

Further Reading

Fruncillo RJ (2011) 2,000 Toxicology board review questions. Xlibris, Publishers, Bloomington
Gupta PK (2010) In: Gupta PK (ed) Basis of organ and reproduction toxicity, vol 1, 2nd reprint edn. PharmaMed Press, Hyderabad
Gupta PK (2014) Essential concepts in toxicology. Published by PharmaMed Press (A unit of BSP Books Pvt. Ltd), Hyderabad
Gupta PK (2016) Fundamentals of toxicology: essential concepts and applications, 1st edn. BSP/Elsevier, Boston
Gupta PK (2018) Illustrative toxicology, 1st edn. Elsevier, San Diego
Gupta PK (2019a) Concepts and applications in veterinary toxicology: an interactive guide. Springer-Nature, Cham
Gupta RC (ed) (2019b) Veterinary toxicology: basic and clinical principles, 3rd edn. Academic Press/Elsevier, San Diego
Gupta PK (2020) Principles of toxicology. In: Brain storming questions in toxicology. Francis and Taylor CRC Press, Boca Raton
Klaassen CD, Watkins JB III (eds) (2015) Casarett & Doull's essentials of toxicology, 3rd edn. McGraw-Hill, New York

Mechanism of Toxicity

4

Abstract

This chapter deals with various aspects of mechanism of action of chemical or physical agents, their interaction with living organisms, and how they trigger perturbations in cell function and/or structure or that may initiate repair mechanisms at the molecular, cellular, and/or tissue levels including necrosis and apoptosis of different xenobiotics. The most important aspect is apoptosis, or programmed cell death is a tightly controlled. This process is completely organized whereby individual cells break into small fragments that are phagocytosed by adjacent cells or macrophages without producing an inflammatory response. Knowledge of the mechanism of toxicity of a substance enhances the ability to prevent toxicity and design more desirable chemicals; it constitutes the basis for therapy upon overexposure, and frequently enables a further understanding of fundamental biological processes. Therefore, this chapter briefly highlights the overview, key points, and relevant text that are in the format of problem-solving study questions followed by multiple-choice questions (MCQs) along with their answers as applicable to mechanism of toxicity.

Keywords

Mechanism of toxicity · Necrosis · Apoptosis · Toxicity · Cytotoxicity · Cellular dysfunction · Cell death · Questions and answers · MCQs

1 Introduction

Mechanism of toxicity of a substance enhances the ability to prevent toxicity and design more desirable chemicals. It also constitutes the basis for therapy upon overexposure and frequently enables a further understanding of fundamental biological processes. The chapter deals with the overview, key points, and relevant text that are in the format of problem-solving study questions followed by multiple-choice questions (MCQ's) along with their answers as applicable to mechanism of toxicity.

2 Overview

A mode of toxic action is a common set of physiological and behavioral signs that characterize a type of adverse biological response. A mode of action should not be confused with mechanism of action, which refers to the biochemical processes underlying a given mode of action. Modes of toxic action are important, widely used tools in ecotoxicology and aquatic toxicology because they classify toxicants or pollutants according to their type of toxic action. Knowledge of the mechanism of toxicity of a substance enhances the ability to prevent toxicity and design more desirable chemicals; it constitutes the basis for therapy upon overexposure and frequently enables a further understanding of fundamental biological processes. The cellular mechanisms that contribute to the manifestation of toxicities are overviewed by relating a series of events that begins with exposure, involves a multitude of interactions between the invading toxicant and the organism, and culminates in a toxic effect.

Key Points

- Mechanism of toxicity is the study of how chemical or physical agents interact with living organisms that may trigger perturbations in cell function and/or structure or that may initiate repair mechanisms at the molecular, cellular, and/or tissue levels.
- Apoptosis, or programmed cell death, is a tightly controlled, organized process whereby individual cells break into small fragments that are phagocytosed by adjacent cells or macrophages without producing an inflammatory response.
- Sustained elevation of intracellular Ca2+ is harmful because it can result in (1) depletion of energy reserves by inhibiting the ATPase used in oxidative phosphorylation, (2) dysfunction of micro-aments, (3) activation of hydrolytic enzymes, and (4) generation of reactive oxygen and nitrogen species (ROS and RNS).
- Cell injury progresses toward cell necrosis (death) if molecular repair mechanisms are inefficient or the molecular

damage is not readily reversible cell proliferation.
- Chemical carcinogenesis involves insufficient function of various repair mechanisms, including (1) failure of DNA repair, (2) failure of apoptosis (programmed cell death), and (3) failure to terminate.

3   Problem-Solving Study Questions

3.1   Mode of Action

Q. What is mode of toxic actions?
Modes of toxic action. A mode of toxic action is a common set of physiological and behavioral signs that characterize a type of adverse biological response. A mode of action should not be confused with mechanism of action, which refers to the biochemical processes underlying a given mode of action.

Q. List the variety of processes of absorption including their characteristics.
(a) Diffusion: molecules move from areas of high concentration to low concentration;
(b) Facilitated diffusion: require specialized carrier proteins; no high-energy phosphate bonds are required.
(c) Active transport: ATP is required in conjunction with special carrier proteins to move molecules through a membrane against a concentration gradient.
(d) Endocytosis: particles and large molecules that might otherwise be restricted from crossing a plasma membrane can be brought in or removed by this process.

Q. How do toxic substances enter the body?
There are several ways in which toxic substances can enter the body. They may enter through the lungs by inhalation, through the skin, mucous membranes or eyes by absorption, or through the gastrointestinal tract by ingestion.

Q. What are the major functions of the skin?
The skin can help to:
(a) Regulate body temperature through sweat glands.
(b) Provide a physical barrier to dehydration, microbial invasion, and some chemical insults.
(c) Excrete salts, water, and organic compounds.
(d) Serve as a sensory organ for touch, temperature, pressure, and pain.
(e) Provide some important components of immunity.

Q. What are the three major mechanisms for the harmful effects of environmental toxins?
(a) The toxins influence on enzymes.
(b) Direct chemical combination of the toxin with a cell constituent.
(c) Secondary action as a result of the toxins presence in the system.

Q. Name two major types of modes of toxic actions.
(a) Nonspecific: nonspecific acting toxicants are those that produce narcosis.
(b) Specific: specific acting toxicants are those that are nonnarcotic and that produce a specific action at a specific target site.

Q. What are the different specific modes of toxic actions?
There are several modes of actions. Some of them include:
• Uncouplers of oxidative phosphorylation: The action involves toxicants that uncouple the two processes that occur in oxidative phosphorylation: electron transfer and adenosine triphosphate (ATP) production.
• Acetylcholinesterase (AChE) inhibitors: AChE is an enzyme associated with nerve synapses that is designed to regulate nerve impulses by breaking down the neurotransmitter acetylcholine (ACh). When toxicants bind to AChE, they inhibit the breakdown of ACh. This results in continued nerve impulses across the synapses, which eventually cause nerve system damage. Examples of AChE inhibitors are organophosphates and carbamates.

• Irritants: These are chemicals that cause an inflammatory effect on living tissue by chemical action at the site of contact. The resulting effect of irritants is an increase in the volume of cells due to a change in size (hypertrophy) or an increase in the number of cells (hyperplasia). Examples of irritants are benzaldehyde, acrolein, zinc sulfate, and chlorine.
• Central nervous system (CNS) seizure agents: CNS seizure agents inhibit cellular signaling by acting as receptor antagonists. They result in the inhibition of biological responses. Examples of CNS seizure agents are organochlorine pesticides.
• Respiratory blockers: These are toxicants that affect respiration by interfering with the electron transport chain in the mitochondria. Examples of respiratory blockers are rotenone and cyanide.

3.2 Steps Involved in Cellular Toxicity

Q. What are the steps involved in the process of mechanisms of toxicity?
(a) Delivery: Site of exposure to the target
(b) Reaction of the ultimate toxicant with the target molecule
(c) Cellular dysfunction and resultant toxicity
(d) Repair or disrepair (Fig. 4.1)

Q. What are the chemical factors that cause cellular dysfunction?
• Chemicals that cause DNA adducts can lead to DNA mutations which can activate cell death pathways; if mutations activate oncogenes or inactivate tumor suppressors, it can lead to uncontrolled cell proliferation and cancer (e.g., benzopyrene).
• Chemicals that cause protein adducts can lead to protein dysfunction which can activate cell death pathways; protein adducts can also lead to autoimmunity; if protein adducts activate oncogenes or inactivate tumor suppressors, it can lead to uncontrolled cell proliferation and cancer (e.g., diclofenac glucuronidation metabolite).

Fig. 4.1 Mechanisms of toxicity. Nature. berkeley.edu/Bdnomura/ pdf/ Lecture6Mechanisms3. pdf

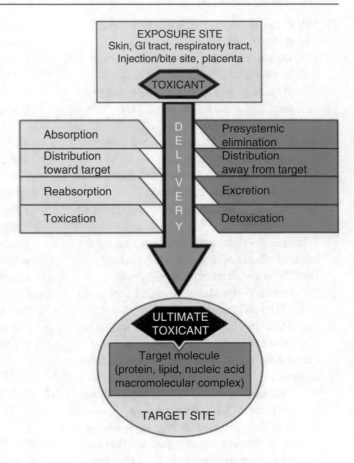

- Chemicals that cause oxidative stress can oxidize DNA or proteins leading to DNA mutations or protein dysfunction and all of the above (e.g., benzene, CCl4).
- Chemicals that specifically interact with protein targets chemicals that activate or inactivate ion channels can cause widespread cellular dysfunction and cause cell death and many physiological symptoms. For example,—Na1, Ca21, and K1 levels are extremely important in neurotransmission, muscle contraction, and nearly every cellular function (e.g., tetrodotoxin closes voltage-gated Na1 channels).
- Chemicals that inhibit cellular respiration—inhibitors of proteins or enzymes involved in oxygen consumption, fuel utilization, and ATP production will cause energy depletion and cell death (e.g., cyanide inhibits cytochrome c oxidase).

- Chemicals that inhibit the production of cellular building blocks, e.g., nucleotides, lipids, and amino acids (e.g., amanitin from death cap mushrooms), and that alter ion channels and metabolism (e.g., sarin inhibits AChE and elevates ACh levels to active signaling pathways and ion channels).
  All of the above can also cause inflammation which can lead to cellular dysfunction.

3.3   Cell Deaths and Apoptosis

Q. What are two forms of cell deaths?
  (a) Necrosis: unprogrammed cell death (dangerous)
  (b) Apoptosis: one of the main forms of programmed cell death (not as dangerous to organism as necrosis)

Q. What is necrosis?

Necrosis is unprogrammed cell death (dangerous) and is caused by factors external to the cell or tissue, such as infection, toxins, or trauma which result in the unregulated digestion of cell components. Cell commits homicide by necrosis. Necrosis of the apex of the pedal bone is extremely common in yearling beef calves after transportation over long distances (Fig. 4.2).

Necrosis may be:

(i) Passive form of cell death induced by accidental damage of tissue does not involve the activation of any specific cellular program.

(ii) Early loss of plasma membrane integrity and swelling of the cell body followed by bursting of cell.

(iii) Mitochondria and various cellular processes contain substances that can be damaging to surrounding cells and are released upon bursting and cause inflammation.

(iv) Cells necrotize in response to tissue damage (injury by chemicals and viruses, infection, cancer, inflammation, ischemia (death due to blockage of blood to tissue)).

Q. What is apoptosis?

Apoptosis is the term used to describe the generally normal death of the cell in living organisms. Since new cells regenerate, cell death is a normal and constant process in the body.

Q. What are the different stages of apoptosis?

Apoptosis has several distinct stages. In the first stage, the cell starts to become round as a result of the protein in the cell being eaten by enzymes that become active. Next, the DNA in the nucleus starts to come apart and shrink down. The membrane surrounding the nucleus begins to degrade and ultimately no longer forms the usual layer. Cell commits suicide by apoptosis.

Q. What are the possible toxic mechanisms for chemicals?

(a) Produce reversible or irreversible bodily injury.

(b) Have the capacity to cause tumors, neoplastic effects, or cancer.

(c) Cause reproductive errors including mutations and teratogenic effects.

(d) Produce irritation and sensitization of mucous membranes.

(e) Cause a reduction in motivation, mental alertness, or capability.

(f) Alter behavior or cause death of the organism.

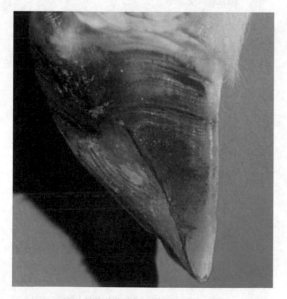

Fig. 4.2 Toe necrosis syndrome, distal phalanx necrosis. https://www.merckvetmanual.com/-/media/manual/veterinary/images/toe_necrosis_syndrome_distal_phalanx_necrosis_high.jpg?la=en&thn=0&mw=350

3.4 Hypersensitivity Reactions

Q. List the four major types of hypersensitivity reactions:

(a) Cytotoxic

(b) Cell-mediated

(c) Immune complex

(d) Anaphylactic

Q. What is the difference between mode of action and mechanism of toxicity?

A mode of action should not be confused with mechanism of action, which refers to the biochemical processes underlying a given mode of action. Modes of toxic action are important, widely used tools in ecotoxicology and aquatic toxicology because they classify toxicants or pollutants according to their type of toxic action.

Q. What is cytotoxicity

Cytotoxicity is the quality of being toxic to cells. Treating cells with the cytotoxic compound can result in a variety of cell fates. The cells may undergo necrosis, in which they lose membrane integrity and die rapidly as a result of cell lysis. The cells can stop actively growing and dividing (a decrease in cell viability), or the cells can activate a genetic program of controlled cell death (apoptosis). Examples of toxic agents are an immune cell or some types of venom, e.g., from the puff adder (*Bitis arietans*) or brown recluse spider (*Loxosceles reclusa*).

Q. What is anaphylaxis?

Anaphylaxis is a serious allergic reaction that is rapid in onset and may cause death. It typically causes more than one of the following: an itchy rash, throat or tongue swelling, shortness of breath, vomiting, lightheaded ness, and low blood pressure. These symptoms typically come on over minutes to hours. Common causes include insect bites and stings, foods, and medications.

5.0 Sample MCQ's (choose the correct statement, it may be one, two, more, or none).

Q.1. A possible reason for the selective embryo-fetal toxicity of DES is --.

   A. Higher concentration of free DES in embryo/fetal compared to adults
   B. Binding to retinoic acid receptors
   C. Lack of placental drug metabolism
   D. All of the above

Q.2. The liver and kidney are major target organs of toxicity because------.

   A. They both receive a high percentage of cardiac output.
   B. They both have substantial xenobiotic-metabolizing capacity.
   C. They both have transport systems that can concentrate xenobiotics.

   D. All of the above.

Q.3. Acyl glucuronides are particularly toxic to the liver because ---.

   A. They selectively interact with macrophages releasing active oxygen.
   B. Active transport systems in the hepatocyte and bile duct system can greatly upconcentrate them.
   C. They are resistant to glucuronidase.
   D. They are suitable inhibitors of UGT2B7.

Q.4. The selective renal toxicity of cephaloridine over cephalothin is due to -----

   A. Selective uptake by the organic cation transporter
   B. Selective inhibition of P-glycoprotein
   C. Selective uptake by the organic anion transporter
   D. Significantly less plasma protein binding of cephaloridine

Q.5. All of the following are of alpha-amanitin *except* …

   A. It is less orally available than phalloidin.
   B. It inhibits RNA polymerase II.
   C. It is transported into the hepatocyte by a bile acid transporter.
   D. It is a mushroom toxin.

Q.6. All of the following are true of the toxic mechanism of paraquat *except* ---.

   A. Lungs accumulate paraquat in an energy-dependent manner.
   B. Its energy into the lungs is assumed to be via the polyamine transport system.
   C. Similar molecules with smaller distances between nitrogen atoms do not enter lungs as readily.
   D. Cytotoxicity to alveolar cells is caused by interference with calcium channels.

Q.7. Enzyme induction of phenobarbital is mediated through ---

A. Aryl hydrocarbon receptor
B. PPAR-alpha receptor
C. Constitutively active receptor (CAR)
D. Estrogen receptor

Q.8. CAR is downregulated by -----

A. Hypericum extracts
B. Acetaminophen
C. Aspirin
D. Proinflammatory cytokines

Q.9. The pregnane X receptor ----

A. Is a cytosolic receptor
B. Is involved in induction of CYP3A4
C. Is primarily expressed in the skin
D. All of the above

Q.10. Downregulation of receptors is due to continuous exposure of------

A. Antagonist
B. Agonist
C. Inverse agonist
D. All the above

Q.11. Amphipathic xenobiotics that can become trapped in lysosomes and cause phospholipidosis include all of the following *except* ------.

A. Ethylene glycol
B. Amiodarone
C. Amitriptyline
D. Fluoxetine

Q.12. Which of the following parent toxicant-electrophilic metabolite pairs is incorrect?

A. Halothane – phosgene
B. Bromobenzene – bromobenzene 3, 4-oxide

C. Benzene – muconic aldehyde
D. Allyl alcohol – acrolein

Q.13. All of the following are capable of accepting the electrons from reductases and forming radicals *except* ----------

A. Paraquat
B. Doxorubicin
C. n-hexane
D. Nitrofurantoin

Q.14. An example of the formation of an electrophilic toxicant from an inorganic chemical is ---

A. CO to CO_2
B. AsO_4
C. NO to NO_2
D. Hydroxide ion to water

Q.15. The general mechanism for detoxification of electrophiles is -----

A. Conjugation with glucuronic acid
B. Conjugation with acetyl CoA
C. Conjugation with glutathione
D. Conjugation with sulfate

Q.16. The most common nucleophilic detoxification reaction that amines undergo is ----

A. Acetylation
B. Sulfation
C. Methylation
D. Amino acid conjugation

Q.17. Detoxification mechanisms fail because ---

A. Toxicants may overwhelm the detoxification process.
B. A reactive toxicant may inactivate a detoxicating enzyme.
C. Detoxication may produce toxic by-product.
D. All of the above.

Q.18. Receptors for which agonist binds but unable to elicit chemical response are ----

A. Spare receptors
B. Orphan receptors
C. Silent receptors
D. None

Q.19. Hydroxyl radical can be produced by all of the following *except* ----

A. The action of nitric oxide synthase on water
B. Interaction of ionizing radiation and water
C. Reductive homolytic fission of hydrogen peroxide
D. Interaction of silica with surface iron ions in lung tissue

Q.20. If an electrophile is covalently bound to a protein that does not play a critical function, the result is considered a -----.

A. Toxication reaction
B. Detoxication reaction
C. MNA adduct formation
D. Fenton reaction

Answers
1. A.   2. D   3. B.   3. C.   4. A.   6. D.
7. C.   8. D.   9. B.   10. B.   11. A.
12. A.   13. C.   13. B.   14. C.   16. A.
17. D.   18. C.   19. A.   20. B.

Further Reading

Boelsterli UA (2007) Mechanistic toxicology. In: The molecular basis of how chemicals disrupt biological targets, 2nd edn. CRC Press, Taylor and Francis, Boca Raton

Zoltán G (2015) Mechanisms of toxicity. In: Klaassen CD, Watkins JB (eds) Casarett & Doull's essentials of toxicology, 3rd edn. McGraw-Hill, New York, pp 21–48

Gupta PK (2016) Fundamentals of toxicology: essential concepts and applications, 1st edn. BSP/Elsevier, San Diego

Gupta PK (2018) Illustrative toxicology, 1st edn. Elsevier, San Diego

Gupta PK (2019) Concepts and applications in veterinary toxicology: an interactive guide. Springer-Nature, Switzerland

Gupta PK (2020) Brainstorming questions in toxicology. Francis and Taylor CRC Press, Boca Raton

Fruncillo RJ (2011) 2,000 Toxicology board review questions. Xlibris Publishers, Bloomington

Part II
Disposition and Kinetics

Disposition of Toxicants

5

Abstract

This chapter deals with the study of absorption, distribution, metabolism/biotransformation, and excretion (ADME) of xenobiotics and the study of toxicokinetics of toxicants/ xenobiotics in relation to time in animals. The disposition of a chemical determines its concentration at the site of action such that the concerted actions of absorption, distribution, and elimination also determine the potential for adverse events to occur. Metabolism or biotransformation of toxicants by the body is an "attempt to detoxify." There are two phases of metabolism. Phase I includes oxidation, reduction, and hydrolysis mechanisms. These reactions, catalyzed by hepatic enzymes, generally convert foreign compounds to derivatives for Phase II reactions. This chapter briefly focuses on the overview, key points, and relevant text that are in the format of problem-solving study questions followed by multiple-choice questions (MCQs) along with their answers.

Keywords

Absorption · Disposition · Biotransformation · Metabolism · Excretion · Redistribution · ADME · Questions · MCQ's

1 Introduction

Disposition of any compound is a fundamental factor that contributes to its potential for toxicity. The process of D disposition includes absorption, distribution, metabolism, and excretion (ADME) of toxicants in the body. In addition, a range of factors which includes age, strain, species, sex, etc. may influence ADME and other aspects of susceptibility to hazards related to a given toxicant. Included among many, these are maturity at birth, time to sexual maturity, and life span of various species of animals. This chapter briefly describes the overview, key points, and relevant text that is in the format of problem-solving study questions followed by multiple-choice questions (MCQ's) along with their answers.

2 Overview

The disposition of a chemical or xenobiotic is defined as the composite actions of its absorption, distribution, biotransformation, and elimination. Moreover, the disposition of any compound is a fundamental factor that contributes to its potential for toxicity. Specifically, the toxicity of a substance is directly dependent on the dose, where "dose" is defined as the amount that ultimately reaches the site or sites of action

P K Gupta, *Problem Solving Questions in Toxicology*, https://doi.org/10.1007/978-3-030-50409-0_5

(tissue, cell, or molecular target). Therefore, the disposition of a chemical determines its concentration at the site of action such that the concerted actions of absorption, distribution, and elimination also determine the potential for adverse events to occur. Metabolism or biotransformation of toxicants by the body is an "attempt to detoxify." In some instances, metabolized xenobiotic agents are more toxic than the original compound. This is referred to as lethal synthesis. Metabolism of many organophosphorus insecticides produces metabolites more toxic than the initial (or parent) compounds (e.g., parathion to paroxan). There are two phases of metabolism. Metabolism of xenobiotic agents seldom follows a single pathway. Usually, a fraction is excreted unchanged, and the rest is excreted or stored as metabolites. Significant differences in metabolic mechanisms exist between species. For example, because cats lack forms of glucuronyl transferase, their ability to conjugate compounds such as morphine and phenols is compromised. Increased tolerance to subsequent exposures of a toxicant, in some instances, is due to enzyme induction initiated by the previous exposure. Excretion of most toxicants and their metabolites is by way of the kidneys. Some excretion occurs in the digestive tract and some via milk. Many polar and high-molecular-weight compounds are excreted into the bile. An enterohepatic cycle occurs when these compounds are excreted from the liver via bile, reabsorbed from the intestine, and returned to the liver. Different body compartments will likely have different elimination rates.

Key Points

- The acronym ADME stands for absorption, distribution, metabolism (biotransformation), and elimination. The acronym is sometimes extended to include toxicant transport (ADME-T) or toxicant toxicity (ADME-Tox).
- Absorption is the transfer of a chemical from the site of exposure, usually an

external or internal body surface, into the systemic circulation.
- After absorption, toxicants are removed from the systemic circulation.
- Biotransformation is the metabolic conversion of endogenous and xenobiotic chemicals to more water-soluble compounds and is accomplished by a limited number of enzymes with broad substrate specificities. The enzymes that catalyze xenobiotic biotransformation are often called toxicant-metabolizing enzymes.
- Excretion is the removal of xenobiotics from the blood and their return to the external environment via urine, feces, exhalation, etc.
- Glutathione Phase I reactions involve hydrolysis, reduction, and oxidation. These reactions expose or introduce a functional group (-OH, -NH2, -SH, or -COOH) and usually result in only a small increase in hydrophilicity.
- Phase II biotransformation reactions include glucuronidation, sulfonation (more commonly called sulfation), acetylation, methylation, and conjugation (mercapturic acid synthesis), which usually result in increased hydrophilicity and elimination.

---

3   Problem-Solving Study Questions

Q. What are the inter-related processes of absorption, distribution, biotransformation, and elimination?

Absorption, distribution, biotransformation, and elimination are inter-related processes (Fig. 5.1). After the substance is absorbed, it is distributed through the blood, lymph circulation, and extracellular fluids into organs or other storage sites and may be metabolized. Then, the substance or its metabolites are eliminated through the body's waste products.

Fig. 5.1 Absorption, distribution, metabolism, and elimination. (Image Source: NLM) https://toxtutor.nlm.nih.gov/img/adme.png

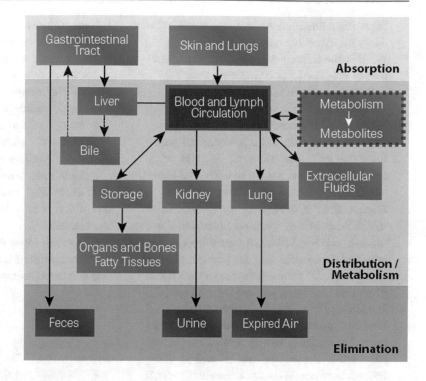

3.1   Absorption

Q. What are the primary routes of exposure for toxic substances?

Following are the routes of exposure

(a) Oral

(b) Respiratory

(c) Dermal

(d) Parenteral

Explanation: Oral or gastrointestinal (GI), respiratory, and dermal systems are lined with epithelia that present significant barriers to the entry of foreign substances due to tight junctions between their cells or continuous lipid layers in the case of the skin. The onset, duration, and intensity of a substance's toxic effects are therefore dependent on the toxicant's ability to permeate lipid cell membranes directly and its interactions with transporter proteins. Dermal penetration is unique in the sense that the outer epithelial cellular layers (corneocytes) are non-viable and do not contain transporter proteins. Absorption, in this case, is therefore dependent on the ability of toxicants to penetrate

the intercellular lipid matrix found between corneocytes.

The plasma membranes surrounding all these cells are remarkably similar (such as the stratified epithelium of the skin, the thin cell layers of the lungs or the GI tract, capillary endothelium, and ultimately the cells of the target organ). The plasma membranes surrounding all these cells are remarkably similar.

Q. Which common toxicants are absorbed through the lungs?

Toxicants absorbed by the lungs are usually gases, vapors or volatile or volatilizable liquids, and aerosols.

Q. What are the major characteristics that affect absorption after exposure to aerosols?

Major characteristics that affect absorption after exposure to aerosols are the aerosol size and water solubility of any chemical present in the aerosol.

Q. Why absorption of toxicants through the skin is limited?

Skin is the largest body organ and provides a relatively good barrier or separating organisms from their environment because it has relatively impermeable nature.

Q. What is the influence of route of administration of drug/toxicant on bioavailability?
- It is generally in the following order:
  IV > oral route > topical route

Q. What is plasma membrane?

The biological cell has a fundamental structure, the cell membrane or, as it is often called, the plasma membrane. The thickness of the membranes is of the order of 100 Å.

Explanation: The majority of chemicals to which most of the population is exposed are organic acids or bases. An acid with a low pKa is a strong acid, and one with a high pKa is a weak acid. Conversely, a base with a low pKa is a weak base, and one with a high pKa is a strong base. The weak acids are absorbed readily from the stomach because they all are almost completely non-ionized at the gastric pH. Weak bases are not absorbed well; indeed, they would tend to accumulate within the stomach at the expense of the chemical agent in the bloodstream. Naturally, in the more alkaline intestine, bases would be absorbed better, acids more poorly.

The concentration of a chemical that is in ionized or in non-ionized form depends on both pKa of the chemical and the pH of the solution in which it is dissolved. The relationship may be derived by mathematical transformation of Henderson Hasselbalch equation:

For weak acidic compound

$$pKa - pH = \log \frac{Conc.\,of\ unionized\ compound}{Conc.\,of\ ionized\ compound}$$

$$\%\,ionized\ compound = \frac{100}{1 + antilog\,(pKa - pH)}$$

For weak basic compound

$$pH - pKa = \log \frac{Conc.\,of\ unionized\ compound}{Conc.\,of\ ionized\ compound}$$

$$\%\,ionized\ compound = \frac{100}{1 + antilog\,(pH - pKa)}$$

It is therefore assumed that the gastric mucosal wall acts as a simple lipoid barrier which is permeable only to the lipid-soluble, non-dissociated form of the acid. Thus, in plasma, the ratio of non-ionized to ionized drug is 1:1000; in gastric juice, the ratio is 1:0.001. The total concentration ratio between the plasma and the gastric sides of the barrier is therefore 1000:1. For a weak base with a pKa of 3.4, the ratio is reversed.

Q. Discuss briefly translocation of xenobiotics and their mechanism of transport across membranes.

Translocations may take place through different mechanisms such as passive process or active process as given in Table 5.1.

Table 5.1 Transfer of molecules across biological membranes

Transfer process	Mechanism	Substrate specificity
Passive diffusion	Diffusion through lipoidal membrane down a concentration gradient	None, most foreign compounds
Filtration	Diffusion through aqueous pores in the membrane down to concentration gradient	Hydrophilic molecules and ions of the molecular weight, e.g., water, urea
Facilitated diffusion	Carrier transport through membrane down a concentration gradient. Saturated by excess substrate	Narrow, mainly for molecules concerned with process of intermediary metabolism, e.g., sugars and amino acids
Active transport	Carrier transport through membrane against a concentration gradient requires metabolic energy. Saturated by excess substrate	Narrow, mainly for molecules concerned with process of intermediary metabolism, e.g., sugars and amino acids
Pinocytosis	Invaginations of the membrane absorbs extracellular material	Uncertain

3.2 Distribution

Q. Describe factors that determine a compound's rate and extent of distribution.

Factors that influence distribution include:

(a) Molecular size, i.e., physicochemical properties of compound

(b) Lipophilicity

(c) Plasma protein and tissue binding

(d) Blood flow and organ size

(e) Special compartmental and barriers, e.g., blood–brain barrier, blood–cerebrospinal barrier, placental barrier, and other barriers

(f) Availability of special transport system

(g) The ability to interact with transmembrane transporter proteins

(h) Disease state, etc.

Explanation: After absorption into the bloodstream, the chemicals penetrate in the various fluid compartments—(i) plasma, (ii) interstitial fluid, (iii) transcellular fluid, and (iv) cellular fluids. The non-ionized lipid/soluble fractions penetrate most readily. Some chemicals may accumulate in various areas as a result of binding or due to their affinity for fat.

Q. Describe important blood–organ barriers for transport of xenobiotics.

For transport of xenobiotics, the effective tight junction occurs at the level of capillary endothelium, e.g., brain, placenta, and thymus barriers. These barriers are called blood–organ barriers. In blood–bile barriers, the blood has direct access to the membranes of the hepatocytes. Tight junctions formed by adjacent hepatocytes constitute the physical barrier immediately interposed between blood and bile. Some of the so called blood–organ barriers do not directly involve the blood. For example, in blood–urine barrier, tight junction occurs near the luminal surface of bladder epithelial cells and in the blood–testes barriers within the seminiferous tubules. Thus blood–testes barrier resembles the blood–urine barriers more than the blood–brain barriers with which it is often compared. A few important barriers are:

(a) Blood–brain barrier

(b) Placental barrier

(c) Blood–testes barrier

Q. Describe in brief different factors that affect distribution and tissue retention of drugs.

The following factors affect the distribution and retention of drugs:

(a) Blood flow

(b) Volume of distribution

(c) Enzyme induction

(d) Chemical interaction

(e) Age and sex differences

(f) Genetic factors

(g) Binding with proteins

(h) Storage in various body tissues including brain and fat

Q. What are transporters?

Transporters, also called transporter proteins, play an important role in the processes of absorption, distribution, metabolism, and elimination (ADME). They are important to pharmacological, toxicological, clinical, and physiological applications.

Explanation: In the liver, transmembrane transporters, together with drug metabolizing enzymes, are important in drug metabolism and drug clearance by the liver. Xenobiotics, endogenous metabolites, bile salts, and cytokines affect the levels (or "expression") of these transporters in the liver. Adverse reactions in the liver to a xenobiotic such as a drug could be caused by genetic or disease-induced variations of transporter expression or drug–drug interactions at the level of these transporters.

In the kidneys, renal proximal tubules are targets for toxicity partly because of the expression of transporters that mediate the secretion and reabsorption of xenobiotics. Changes in transporter expression and/or function could enhance the accumulation of toxicants and make the kidneys more susceptible to injury, for example, when xenobiotic uptake by carrier proteins is increased or the efflux of toxicants and their metabolites is reduced. The list of nephrotoxic chemicals is a long one, and selected ones include:

(i) Environmental contaminants such as some hydrocarbon solvents, some heavy metals, and the fungal toxin ochratoxin.

(ii) Some antibiotics

(iii) Some antiviral drugs

(iv) Some chemotherapeutic drugs

The competition of xenobiotics for transporter-related excretion and genetic polymorphisms affecting transporter function affects the likelihood of nephrotoxicity.

Because of concerns that such changes to transporter expression and function can adversely affect clinical outcomes and physiological regulation, increased drug transporter activity is important to study and understand. There is clinical and laboratory research including in vitro, ex vivo, and in vivo studies that show how powerful drug–drug interactions can be.

For example, drugs might compete with each other for binding to a transporter, which can lead to changes in serum and tissue drug levels and possible side effects.

This is one possible explanation for the rare occurrence of potentially severe toxicity when the drug methotrexate and nonsteroidal anti-inflammatory drugs are given at the same time.

The drug probenecid, which competitively inhibits some transporters, has been used to increase the half-life of antibiotics such as penicillin and antiviral drugs and improve their therapeutic value.

3.3   Excretion

Q. What is excretion?

Excretion is a process by which metabolic waste is eliminated from an organism. In vertebrates this is primarily carried out by the lungs, kidneys, and skin. This is in contrast with secretion, where the substance may have specific tasks after leaving the cell. Excretion is an essential process in all forms of life.

Q. What are excretion and secretions?

"Excretion" is the removal of material from a living thing, while "secretion" is the movement of material from one point to another. For an example of excretion, humans excrete such materials as tears, feces, urine, carbon dioxide, and sweat, while secretion, on the other hand, includes enzymes, hormones, or saliva.

Q. What is secretion in the kidney?

Tubular secretion is the transfer of materials from peritubular capillaries to the renal tubular lumen; it is the opposite process of reabsorption. This secretion is caused mainly by active transport and passive diffusion. Usually only a few substances are secreted and are typically waste products.

Q. What are the factors that are responsible for biliary excretion?

(a)   Enterohepatic recirculation

(b)   Glucuronide conjugates

Q. Which are the principal organs of excretion?

• The principal organ of excretion is renal (kidney). Organs other than kidneys is known as extra-renal or non-renal excretion.

The biliary route of excretion plays a major role in the elimination of anions, cations, and non-ionized molecules containing both polar and lipophilic groups. The biliary excretion of foreign compounds varies with species and is generally highest in the dog and rat. The hepatic excretory system is not fully developed in the infants and is additional reason for some compounds being more toxic in infants than in the adults. More information is required to see if increased toxicity of some compounds in the infants is due to this reason.

In addition to renal excretion, there are non-renal or extra renal excretion through GI tract, expired air, sweat, saliva, milk, vaginal secretions, and other route such as lachrymal fluid, intestinal fluid, tracheobronchial secretions, etc.

3.4   Biotransformation

Q. What are the functions of biotransformation. Give suitable examples.

Biotransformation performs the following functions:

(a) It causes conversion of an active compound to less active called inactivation or detoxification. Examples are phenobarbitone to p-hydroxyphenobarbitone and DDT to metabolite products DDE and DDA.

(b) It causes conversion of an active compound to more active metabolite(s) called bioactivation. Examples are malathion to malaoxon or parathion to paraoxon and acetonitrile to cyanide.

(c) It causes conversion of an inactive compound (i.e., pro-drug or precursor compound) to active metabolite(s) called activation. Examples are phenacetin to paracetamol and thiocyanates to cyanide.

(d) It causes conversion of an active compound to equally active metabolite(s) (no change in the activity). Examples are dichrotophos to monochrotophos and digitoxin to digoxin.

(e) It causes conversion of an active compound to active metabolite(s) having entirely pharmacological/toxicological activity (change in activity). Examples are Iproniazid (antidepressant) to isoniazid (antitubercular) and Aflatoxin B1 (hepatotoxin) to aflatoxin M1 (carcinogen).

Q. What are xenobiotic metabolizing enzymes? These enzymes can be divided into two main groups;

(a) Microsomal enzymes
(b) Non-microsomal enzymes

Microsomal enzymes: These enzymes are present in the endoplasmic reticulum (ER) (especially smooth) of liver and other tissues.

Non-microsomal enzymes: Enzymes occurring in organelles/sites other than microsomes are called non-microsomal enzymes. These are usually present in the cytoplasm, plasma, and mitochondria.

Q. Describe briefly fine pathways of biotransformation.

The major transformation reactions for xenobiotics are divided into two phases known as Phase I and Phase II.

(a) Phase I reactions (non-synthetic or non-conjugative phase)

Phase I reactions modify the compound's structure by adding a functional group. This allows the substance to interact with a reactive group, such as -OH, SH, -NH2, or -COOH. Most of these reactions involve different types of microsomal enzymes, except a few where reactions involve non-microsomal enzymes. Phase I reactions usually yield products with decreased activity. However, some may give rise to products with similar or even greater activity.

Oxidation: It is the most common reaction and may take place in a number of ways such as hydroxylation, deamination, desulfurization, dealkylation or sulfoxide formation, etc. In the biotransformation of lipophilic xenobiotics, microsomal oxidation is the most prominent reaction where microsomal enzymes associated with smooth endoplasmic reticulum of hepatocytes are involved and the enzyme cytochrome P450, a hemeprotein, which is a part of an enzyme system termed as mixed function oxidase (MFO) system, plays an important role.

• The other enzyme systems of Phase I biotransformation are involved in metabolism when the appropriate functional groups are available, e.g., alcohol dehydrogenase is involved in the biotransformation of alcohols and aldehydes, and monomine oxidase is a flavin adenine dinucleotide (FAD)-containing enzyme that catalyzes the oxidative deamination. Epoxide hydrolases are enzymes that add water across epoxide bonds to form diols. A number of carbroxyl esterases are responsible for biotransformation of certain compounds including organophosphates. The extent to which these metabolic reactions take place appears to vary with the species.

Reduction: Reduction is acceptance of one or more electrons(s) or their equivalent from another substrate. Biotransformation by reduction is also capable of generating polar functional groups such as hydroxyl and amino groups which can undergo further biotransformation or conjugation. Many reductive reactions are exact opposite of oxidative reactions.

Hydrolysis: It is the process of cleaving of a foreign compound by the addition of water. It occurs both in the cytoplasm and smooth endoplasmic reticulum. It is an important metabolic pathway for compounds with an ester linkage (-CO, O-) or an amide (-CO, HN-) bond. The cleavage of esters or amides generates nucleophilic compounds which undergo conjugation.

(b) Phase II reactions or conjugation/synthetic reactions

Phase II reactions (conjugation/synthetic reactions) includes reactions that catalyzes conjugation of xenobiotics or their Phase I metabolites with endogenous substances with a water-soluble molecule. In Phase II, most of the reactions involve non-microsomal process (except a few that involve microsomal enzyme). Due to biotransformation, the water solubility of a compound is typically increased.

Synthetic reactions may take place when a xenobiotic or with a polar metabolite of Phase I metabolism containing -OH, -COOH, -NH2, or -SH group that undergoes further transformation to generate nontoxic products of high polarity which are highly water soluble and readily excretable by combining with some hydrophilic endogenous moieties. Conjugating agents are glucuronic acid, acetyl, sulfate, glycine, cysteine, methionine, and glutathione which conjugate with different functional groups of xenobiotics.

Most of the Phase II biotransforming enzymes are located in the cytosol with the exception of uridine diphosphate glucuronyl transferase (UDPGT) which is a microsomal enzyme.

Q. What do you understand by induction or inhibition of metabolizing enzymes?

(a) Induction of enzymes

Several drugs and chemicals have ability to increase the metabolizing activity of enzymes called enzyme induction. Microsomal enzyme induction by drugs and chemicals usually requires repetitive administration of the inducing agent over a period of several days, and the induction, once started, may continue for several days. Metabolizing enzyme induction has great clinical importance because it affects the plasma half-life and duration of action of xenobiotics.

(b) Inhibition of enzymes

Contrary to metabolizing enzyme induction, several drugs and chemicals have ability to decrease the metabolizing activity of certain enzymes called enzyme inhibition. Enzyme inhibition can be either non-specific of chromosomal enzymes or specific of some non-microsomal enzymes (e.g., monoamine oxidase, cholinesterase, and aldehyde dehydrogenase). The inhibition of hepatic microsomal enzymes mainly occurs due to administration of hepatotoxic agents, which cause either rise in the rate of enzyme degradation (e.g., carbon tetrachloride and carbon disulfide) or fall in the rate of enzyme synthesis (e.g., puromycin and dactinomycin). Enzyme inhibition may also produce undesirable xenobiotic interactions.

Q. In which tissue microsomal enzymes are present?

- These enzymes are present in the endoplasmic reticulum (ER) (especially smooth) of liver and other tissues.

Q. In which tissue non-microsomal enzymes are present?

- Enzymes occurring in organelles/sites other than microsomes are called non-microsomal enzymes. These are usually present in the cytoplasm, plasma, and mitochondria.

Q. In which main tissue/organ biotransformation of toxicants occurs?

- Liver

Q. What are the factors that are responsible for renal reabsorption of toxicants?

(a) Lipid solubility

(b) Weak acids/bases

(c) Urine pH

Q. Name the solute carrier proteins (SLC) family.
   (a) OATs (organic anion transporters)
   (b) OCTs (organic cation transporters)
   (c) OATPs (organic anion transporter polypeptides)
Q. Name main sites for biotransformation.
   (a) Liver
   (b) Lung
   (c) Kidney
   (d) Also skin, intestine, testes, placenta
Q. What is the outcome of biotransformations?
   (a) Detoxification (inactivation)
   (b) Bioactivation
   (c) Facilitate excretion
Q. What type of Phase I biotransformation reactions are?
   (a) Simple degradation reactions
   (b) ATP-dependent, add or expose a functional group such as -hydroxyl, carboxyl and amino
Q. Write Phase I biotransformation reactions.
   (a) Oxidative
   (b) Reductive
   (c) Hydrolytic reactions
Q. During Phase I reactions: uses what enzymes?
   • Cytochrome P450
Q. During oxidation biotransformation (Phase I) cytochrome b contains what?
   • Fe-containing heme proteins
Q. Where cytochrome P450 enzymes are located?
   • ER membrane (multiple isoforms) (broad range of substrates)
Q. What happens (reactions) during biotransformation Phase II?
   (a) Conjugation reactions that are ATP dependent (alteration of chemicals)
   (b) Renders nonpolar compounds to polar
   (c) Promote excretion (larger, charged, water soluble)
Q. Name Phase II conjugation reactions and their location
   (a) Glucuronidation (ER)
   (b) Sulfation (cytosol)
   (c) Acetylation (cytosol)
   (d) Methylation (cytosol and ER)
   (e) Glutathione conjugation (cytosol and ER)
Q. Out of bound or unbound toxicant which one is active?
   • Unbound
Q. Name the proteins to which plasma can bind.
   • Albumin alpha glycoproteins
Q. What is the problem with highly bound toxicants?
   • Slowly eliminated, so linger longer
Q. What is the meaning of kernicterus?
   • Kernicterus is a bilirubin-induced brain dysfunction. Bilirubin is a highly neurotoxic substance that may become elevated in the serum, a condition known as hyperbilirubinemia.

3.5 Bioactivation

Q. Describe briefly bioactivation.
Formation of harmful or highly reactive metabolic from relatively inert/nontoxic chemical compounds is called bioactivation or toxication. The bioactive metabolites often interact with the body tissues to precipitate one or more forms of toxicities such as carcinogenesis, teratogenesis, tissue necrosis, etc. The bioactivation reactions are generally catalyzed by cytochrome P450-dependent monooxygenase systems, but some other enzymes like those in intestinal flora are also involved in some cases. The reactive metabolites primarily belong to three main categories—electrophiles, free radicals, and nucleophiles. The formation of electrophiles and free radicals from relatively harmless substances/xenobiotics account for most toxicities.

3.6 Electrophiles, Free Radicals, and Nucleophiles

Q. Define electrophiles.

   • Electrophiles are molecules which are deficient in electrons pair with a positive charge that allows them to react by sharing electron pairs with electron-rich atoms in nucleophiles. Important electrophiles are epoxides, hydroxyamines, nitroso and azoxy derivatives, nitrenium ions, and elemental sulfur. These eletrophiles form covalent binding to nucleophilic tissue components such as macromolecules (proteins, nucleic acids, and lipids) or low-molecular-weight cellular constituents to precipitate toxicity. Covalent binding to DNA is responsible for carcinogenicity and tumor formation.

Q. Define free radicals
  • Free radicals are molecules which contain one or more unpaired electrons (odd number of electrons) in their outer orbit.

Q. Define nucleophiles.
  • Nucleophiles are molecules with electron-rich atoms. Formation of nucleophiles is a relatively uncommon mechanism for toxicants. Examples of toxicity induced through nucleophiles include formation of cyanides from amygdalin, acrylonitrile, and sodium nitroprusside and generation of carbon monoxide from dihalomethane.

---

4   Sample MCQ's

(Choose the correct statement; it may be one, two, or more or none.)

Q.1. Biotransformation is vital in removing toxins from the circulation. All of the following statements regarding biotransformation are true *except*___

  A. Many toxins must be biotransformed into a more lipid-soluble form before they can be excreted from the body.
  B. The liver is the most active organ in the biotransformation of toxins.
  C. Water solubility is required in order for many toxins to be excreted by the kidney.
  D. The kidney plays a major role in eliminating toxicants from the body.

E. The lungs play a minor role in ridding the body of certain types of toxins.

Q.2. Which of the following statements about active transport across cell membranes is *false*?

  A. Unlike simple or facilitated diffusion, active transport pumps chemicals against an electrochemical or concentration gradient.
  B. Unlike simple diffusion, there is a rate at which active transport becomes saturated and cannot move chemicals any faster.
  C. Active transport requires the expenditure of ATP in order to move chemicals against electrochemical or concentration gradients.
  D. Active transport exhibits a high level of specificity or the compounds that are being moved.
  E. Metabolic inhibitors do not affect the ability to perform active transport.

Q.3. Which of the following might increase the toxicity of a toxin administered orally?

  A. Increased activity of the MDR transporter (p-glycoprotein)
  B. Increased biotransformation of the toxin by gastrointestinal cells
  C. Increased excretion of the toxin by the liver into bile
  D. Increased dilution of the toxin dose
  E. Increased intestinal motility

Q.4. Which of the following most correctly describes the first-pass effect?

  A. The body is most sensitive to a toxin the first time that it passes through the circulation.
  B. Orally administered toxins are partially removed by the GI tract before they reach the systemic circulation.
  C. It only results from increased absorption of toxin by GI cells.

D. It is often referred to as "postsystemic elimination."

E. A majority of the toxin is excreted after the first time the blood is filtered by the kidneys.

Q.5. Which of the following is an important mechanism of removing particulate matter from the alveoli?

A. Coughing
B. Sneezing
C. Blowing one's nose
D. Absorption into the bloodstream, followed by excretion via the kidneys
E. Swallowing

Q.6. For a toxin to be absorbed through the skin, it must pass through multiple layers in order to reach the systemic circulation. Which of the following layers is the most important in slowing the rate of toxin absorption through the skin?

A. Stratum granulosum
B. Stratum spinosum
C. Stratum corneum
D. Stratum basale
E. Dermis

Q.7. A toxin is selectively toxic to the lungs. Which of the following modes of toxin delivery would most likely cause the *least* damage to the lungs?

A. Intravenous
B. Intramuscular
C. Intraperitoneal
D. Subcutaneous
E. Inhalation

Q.8. Which of the following is *not* an important site of toxicant storage in the body?

A. Adipose tissue
B. Bone
C. Plasma proteins

D. Muscle
E. Liver

Q.9. Which of the following regarding the blood–brain barrier is *true*___

A. The brains of adults and newborns are equally susceptible to harmful blood-borne chemicals.
B. The degree of lipid solubility is a primary determinant in whether or not a substance can cross the blood–brain barrier.
C. Astrocytes play a role in increasing the permeability of the blood–brain barrier.
D. Active transport processes increase the concentration of xenobiotics in the brain.
E. The capillary endothelial cells of the CNS possess large fenestrations in their basement membranes.

Q.10. Which of the following will result in *decreased* excretion o toxic compounds by the kidneys?

A. A toxic compound with a molecular weight of 25,000 Da.
B. Increased activity of the multidrug resistance (MDR) protein.
C. Increased activity of the multiresistant drug protein (MRP).
D. Increased activity of the organic cation transporter.
E. Increased hydrophilicity of the toxic compound.

Q.11. Toxicants are most likely to be reabsorbed after being filtered at the glomerulus are___

A. Organic anions
B. Organic cations
C. Natural polar molecules
D. Highly lipid-soluble molecules

Q.12. A high urinary pH would favor the excretion of___

A. Organic acids
B. Organic bases
C. Neutral organic compounds
D. None of the above

Q.13. Diuretics can enhance the renal elimination of compounds that___

A. Are of molecular weight greater than 70 kDa
B. Are ions trapped in the tubular lumen
C. Are highly lipid soluble
D. Are highly protein bound

Q.14. The amount of a volatile liquid excreted by the lungs is___

A. Inversely proportional to its lipid–water partition coefficient
B. Directly proportional to its vapor pressure
C. Directly proportional to its molecular weight
D. Inversely proportional to cardiac output

Q.15. Kernicterus results from___

A. Enzyme induction leading to decreased glucocorticoid levels
B. Excess ingestion of foods containing tyramine
C. Displacement of bilirubin from plasma proteins
D. Malabsorption of fat-soluble vitamins

Q.16. All of the following could influence the GI absorption of xenobiotics except___

A. pH
B. Intestinal microflora
C. Presence of food
D. Time of day

Q.17. The rate of diffusion of a xenobiotic across the GI tract is proportional to all of the following except ___

A. Hepatic blood flow
B. Surface area
C. Permeability
D. Residence time

Q.18. Which of the following is *not* absorbed in the colon?

A. Water
B. Sodium ion
C. Glucose
D. Hydrogen ion

Answers
1. A.   2. E.   3. D.   3. B.   4. E.   6. C.
7. C   8. D.   9. B.   10. D.   11. D.   12. A.
13. B.   13. B.   14. C.   16. D.   17. A.
18. C

Further Reading

Fruncillo RJ (2011) 2,000 Toxicology board review questions. Xlibris, Publishers, Bloomington
Gupta PK (2010) Absorption, distribution, & excretion of xenobiotics. In: Gupta PK (ed) Modern toxicology: basis of organ and reproduction toxicity, vol 1, 2nd reprint edn. PharmaMed Press, Hyderabad, pp 71–92
Gupta PK (2014) Essential concept in toxicology, 1st edn. BSP, Hyderabad
Gupta PK (2016) Fundamental of toxicology: essential concept and applications. Elsevier/BSP, San Diego
Gupta PK (2018) Illustrative toxicology, 1st edn. Elsevier, San Diego
Gupta PK (2019) Concepts and applications in veterinary toxicology: an interactive guide. Springer-Nature, Switzerland
Gupta PK (2020) Brain storming questions in toxicology. Francis and Taylor CRC Press, Boca Raton
Krishnamurti CR (2010) Biotransformation of xenobiotics. In: Gupta PK (ed) Modern toxicology: basis of organ and reproduction toxicity, vol 1, 2nd reprint edn. PharmaMed Press, Hyderabad, pp 95–129
Lehman-McKeeman LD (2015) Absorption, distribution, and excretion of toxicants. In: Klaassen CD, Watkins JB III (eds) Casarett & Doull's essentials of toxicology, 3rd edn. McGraw-Hill, New York, pp 61–78
Parkinson A, Ogilvie BW, Buckley DB, Kazmi F, Czerwinski M, Parkinson O (2015) Biotransformation of xenobiotics. In: Klaassen CD, Watkins JB III (eds) Casarett & Doull's essentials of toxicology, 3rd edn. McGraw-Hill, New York, pp 79–108

Toxicokinetic of Xenobiotics

6

Abstract

Toxicokinetics, which is analogous to pharmacokinetics, is the study of the absorption, distribution, metabolism, and excretion of a xenobiotic under circumstances that produce toxicity. *Toxicodynamics*, which is analogous to pharmacodynamics, is the study of the relationship of toxic concentrations of xenobiotics to clinical effects. Although different, *plasma concentration* and *serum concentration* are terms often used interchangeably. When a reference or calculation is made with regard to a concentration in the body, it is actually a plasma concentration. Frequently, this is not the case for whole-blood determination if the xenobiotic distributes into the erythrocyte, such as lead and most other heavy metals. Overdoses provide many challenges to the mathematical precision of toxicokinetics and toxicodynamics because many of the variables, such as dose, time of ingestion, and presence of vomiting, that affect the result are often unknown. This chapter briefly describes the overview, key points, and relevant text that are in the format of problem-solving study questions followed by multiple-choice questions (MCQs) along with their answers.

Keywords

Toxicokinetics · Xenobiotics · Toxicity · Questions · MCQ's · Models in toxicology · Compartments models · Half-life

1 Introduction

Toxicokinetics is the study of the modeling and mathematical description of the time courses of disposition (absorption, distribution, biotransformation, and excretion) of xenobiotics in the whole organism. This chapter briefly describes the overview, key points, and relevant text that are in the format of problem-solving study questions followed by multiple-choice questions (MCQ's) along with their answers.

2 Overview

A fundamental goal of toxicokinetics is to facilitate the determination of dose delivered to the organism in view of understanding systemic exposure to the toxicant. For a scientifically sound interpretation of toxicology studies and characterization of dose-response relationships, it is preferable to relate adverse responses to the dose delivered to the target organ (or to systemic circulation) in the form of putative toxic moiety. Although different, *plasma concentration* and *serum concentration* are terms often used interchangeably. When a reference or calculation is made with regard to a concentration in the body, it is actually a plasma concentration. Frequently, this is not the case for whole-blood determination if the xenobiotic distributes into the erythrocyte, such as lead and most other heavy metals. The accuracy of calculated dose metrics depends upon the number of data points collected in a toxicokinetic study, whereas their magnitude depends upon the dose administered, exposure route, scenario (single or multiple doses), as well as the rates and extent of ADME influenced by factors such as age and pathophysiological state of the test subject or animal. Overdoses provide many challenges to the mathematical precision of toxicokinetics and toxicodynamics because many of the variables, such as dose, time of ingestion, and presence of vomiting, that affect the result are often unknown.

Key Points

- Toxicokinetics is the study of the modeling and mathematical description of the time courses of disposition (absorption, distribution, biotransformation, and excretion) of xenobiotics in the whole organism.
- The area under the plasma drug concentration-time curve (AUC) is dependent on the rate of elimination of the drug from the body and the dose administered.
- The apparent volume of distribution (Vd) is the space into which an amount of chemical is distributed in the body to result in a given plasma concentration.
- Clearance describes the rate of chemical elimination from the body in terms of

volume of fluid containing chemical that is cleared per unit of time.
- The half-life of elimination (T1/2) is the time required for the blood or plasma chemical concentration to decrease by one-half.

---

3   Problem-Solving Study Questions

Q. What is toxicokinetics?
- Toxicokinetics (often abbreviated as "TK") is the description of what rate a chemical will enter the body and what happens to it once it is in the body.

Q. What is toxicokinetics and toxicodynamics?
- Toxicokinetics describes the ADME of an exogenous compound, while toxicodynamics describes the actions and interactions of the compound within an organism or tissue.

Q. What steps are involved in toxicokinetics?
Four processes are involved in toxicokinetics (Fig. 4.2):
(a) Absorption—the substance enters the body.
(b) Distribution—the substance moves from the site of entry to other areas of the body.
(c) Biotransformation—the body changes (transforms) the substance into new chemicals (metabolites).
(d) Excretion—the substance or its metabolites leave the body.

Q. What do you mean by extravascular administration (EV)?
Drug or toxicant administration by any other route (e.g., oral IM, SC, IP, etc.) than the intravenous route is called EV administration.

Q. Using one-compartment model, show with the help of schematic representation regular and semilog plots of distribution of chemicals after intravenous administration (IV).

In case of IV bolus administration of any chemical, the chemical distributes instantaneously in the body, and the entire dose of the chemical enters the body and is distributed immediately via circulation to all tissues. In such a situation, the xenobiotic concentration drug time curve will be obtained as a straight line on semilogarithmic paper showing monophasic exponential decline (Fig. 6.1).

Q. Using one-compartment model, show with the help of schematic representation the distribution curve of chemicals after oral or extravascular administration (EV).

In contrast to IV bolus (Fig. 6.2) after oral or EV administration (instead of a straight line), there are two exponents (i.e., absorption and elimination phase).

Q. What do you mean by maximum plasma concentration/peak plasma concentration (C_{max} or Cp_{max}).

Maximum plasma concentration/peak plasma concentration is the point of maximum concentration of drug in plasma. The maximum plasma concentration depends on administered dose and rates of absorption (absorption rate constant, K_a) and elimination (elimination rate constant, β). The peak represents the point of time when absorption equals elimination rate of the drug. It is often expressed as $\mu g/ml$ (Fig. 6.3).

Q. What do you mean by area under curve (AUC)?

• Area under curve (AUC) is the total integrated area under the plasma drug concentration-time curve. It expresses the total amount of drug that come into systemic circulation after administration of the drug (Fig. 6.3).

Q. What do you mean by peak effect?

• Peak effect is the maximal or peak pharmacological or toxic effect produced by the drug. It is generally observed at peak plasma concentration (Fig. 6.3).

Q. Define time of maximum concentration/time of peak concentration (t_{max})

• Time of maximum concentration/time of peak concentration is the time required for a drug to reach peak concentration in plasma. The faster is the absorption rate, the lower is the t_{ax}. It is also useful in assessing efficacy of drugs used to treat acute conditions (e.g., pain) which can be treated by a single dose. It is expressed in min/hours (Fig. 6.3).

Q. What is onset of action in relation to response?

• Onset of action: It is the beginning of pharmacological or toxicological effect or response produced by the drug. It occurs when the plasma drug concentration just exceeds the MEC (Fig. 6.3).

Q. Define onset time to response.

• Onset time is the time required for the drug to start producing pharmacological or toxic response. It usually corresponds to the time for the plasma concentration to reach MEC after administration of the drug (Fig. 6.3).

Q. Define duration of action

• Duration of action is the time period for which pharmacological or toxic response is produced by the drug. It usually corresponds

Fig. 6.1 Graph showing one-compartment open model following intravenous (IV) bolus and oral or extravascular (EV) route of a single dose of toxicant. After IV bolus, the curve is a straight line on semilogarithmic paper and shows monophasic decline

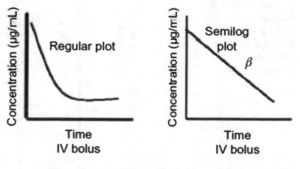

One-Compartment open model

to the duration for which the plasma concentration of drug remains above the MEC level (Fig. 6.3).

3.1 Classic Toxicokinetic Models

Q. What is zero-order process or kinetic?
- Zero-order process/zero-order kinetics or constant-rate kinetics is defined as a toxicokinetic process whose rate is independent of the concentration of the xenobiotic/chemical, i.e., the rate of toxicokinetic process remains constant and cannot be increased further by increasing their concentration of xenobiotic.

Q. What is first-order process or kinetic?
- First-order process (first-order kinetics or linear kinetics) is defined as a toxicokinetic

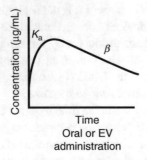

Fig. 6.2 In one-compartment model, after oral or EV administration (instead of a straight line), there are two exponents (i.e., absorption and elimination phase)

process whose rate is directly proportionate to the concentration of the xenobiotic/chemical, i.e., the greater the concentration, the faster is the process.

Q. What is mixed process or mixed-order kinetic?
- Mixed process (mixed-order kinetics, nonlinear kinetic, or dose-dependent kinetics) is defined as a toxicokinetic process whose rate is a mixture of both zero-order and first-order processes. The mixed-order process follows zero-order kinetics at high concentration and the first-order kinetics at lower concentration of the xenobiotic. This type of kinetics is usually observed at increased or multiple doses of some chemicals.

Q. Name three toxicokinetic models that are commonly used.
- (a) Classic toxicokinetics (traditional)
- (b) Noncompartment models/noncompartment analysis
- (c) Physiological models

Q. What are classic toxicokinetic models?
- Classic toxicokinetic modeling (traditional) is the simplest mean of gathering information on absorption, distribution, metabolism, and elimination of a compound and to examine the time course of blood or plasma toxicant concentration over time. In this approach the body represents as a system of one or two

Fig. 6.3 Plasma concentration time profile of drug/toxicant after oral administration of a single dose of a toxicant. K_a, absorption rate constants (absorption phase); Eβ, elimination rate constant (elimination phase)

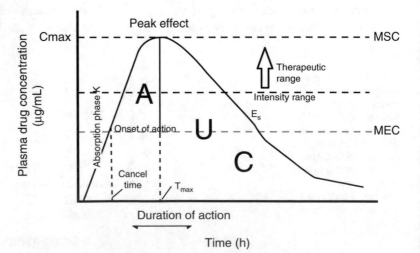

compartments (sometimes more than two compartments) even though the compartments do not have exact correspondence to anatomical structures or physiologic processes.

Q. What are the advantages of classic models?

(a) They do not require information on tissue physiology or anatomic structure.

(b) They are useful in predicting the toxicant concentrations in the blood at different doses.

(c) They are useful in establishing the time course of accumulation of the toxicant, either in its parent form or as biotransformed products during continuous or episodic exposures, in defining concentration-response (vs. dose-response) relationships.

(d) Provide help/guidance in the choice of effective dose and design of dosing regimen in animal toxicity studies.

Q. Define one-compartment open model.

• One-compartment open model is the simplest model, which considers the whole body as a single, kinetically homogeneous unit, in this model, the final distribution equilibrium between the chemical in plasma and other body fluids is attained rapidly and maintained at all times (Fig. 6.4).

Q. Define two-compartment open model.

• Two-compartment open model assumes that the body is composed of two compartments—the central compartment and peripheral compartment. The central compartment (compartment 1) consists of the blood and highly perfused organs like the liver, kidney, lungs, heart, brain, etc.; the less perfused tissues (compartment 2) like the skin, muscles, bone, cartilage, etc. make the peripheral compartment (Fig. 6.4).

Q. What kind of time curve is obtained in two-compartment model?

• In two-compartment open model, after intravenous (IV) bolus or extravascular administration of a single dose of toxicant, the curve is biexponential.

Q. Describe three-compartment open model.

• In three-compartment open model, the body is conceived as consisting of three compartments—one central and two peripheral compartments. The central compartment (compartment 1) comprises of plasma and highly perfused organs, whereas peripheral compartment 2 comprises of moderately (e.g., skin and muscles) and compartment 3 poorly perfused tissues (e.g., bone, teeth, ligaments, hair, and fat). If any chemical is administered by

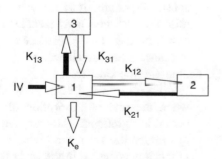
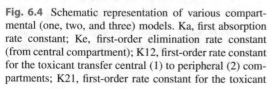
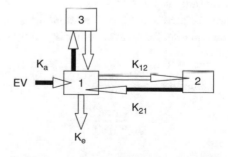

Fig. 6.4 Schematic representation of various compartmental (one, two, and three) models. Ka, first absorption rate constant; Ke, first-order elimination rate constant (from central compartment); K12, first-order rate constant for the toxicant transfer central (1) to peripheral (2) compartments; K21, first-order rate constant for the toxicant transfer peripheral (2) to central (1) compartments; K13, first-order rate constant for the toxicant transfer central (1) to peripheral (3) compartments; K31, first-order rate constant for the toxicant transfer peripheral (3) to central (1) compartments

IV, it is first distributed immediately into the highly perfused tissues (compartment 1), then slowly into the moderately perfused tissues (compartment 2), and thereafter very slowly to the poorly perfused tissues (compartment 3). If plasma level-time profile is plotted on semilogarithmic graph, it gives triexponential appearance (Fig. 6.4).

Q. Define the term half-life.
- Half-life (T1/2) may be defined as the time taken for the concentration of a compound/toxicant in plasma to decline by ½ or 50% of its initial value (or it may be defined as the time required for the body to eliminate half of the chemical). This value is determined during the elimination phase of a chemical; therefore, it is called as elimination half-life.

Q. What is bioavailability?
- After oral or EV routes, often only a fraction of the total dose to which an animal or human is exposed gets absorbed systemically. This fraction is referred to as the bioavailability (F).

Q. How bioavailability is determined?
- Bioavailability is determined by measuring the area under plasma drug concentration versus time curve (AUC) after oral or EV routes. This is compared with AUC measured after IV bolus administration of the same drug.
  If the AUC for both curves are equal, bioavailability is 100% (F = 1).

Q. Describe equation used for bioavailability.
- The equation for bioavailability is given as under:

$$\text{Bioavailability} = \frac{\text{AUC oral.}\beta'}{\text{AUC IV.}\beta} \times 100 \text{ or } F$$
$$= \frac{\text{AUC oral.}\beta'}{\text{AUC IV.}\beta}$$

where β and β' are elimination rate constants after IV bolus and EV routes and F = bioavailability fraction (fraction of the administered dose that enters the systemic circulation.

Bioavailability is a useful parameter, which is used to predict the drug efficacy after different routes of administration.

Q. What is the influence of route of administration of drug/toxicant on bioavailability?
- It is generally in the following order:
  IV > oral route > topical route

Q. Define volume of distribution (V_d).
- The total volume of fluid in which a toxic substance must be dissolved to account for the measured plasma concentrations is known as the apparent volume of distribution (V_d). If a compound is distributed only in the plasma fluid, the V_d is small, and plasma concentrations are high. Conversely, if a compound is distributed to all sites in the body or if it accumulates in a specific tissue such as fat or the bone, the V_d becomes large, and plasma concentrations are low.

Q. How the value of V_d is determined by area method?
- The value of V_d may be determined by area method using the following equation:

$$V_d = \frac{\text{Dose}(D)}{C}$$

Q. Define total body clearance, the term used in kinetic studies of toxicants.
- In toxicology, the clearance is a pharmacokinetic measurement of the volume of plasma that is completely cleared off of a substance per unit time. The usual units are mL/min. The total body clearance will be equal to the renal clearance + hepatic clearance + lung clearance.

Q. Define flip-flop kinetics.
- Flip-flop kinetics refers to a situation when the rate of absorption of a compound is significantly slower than its rate of elimination from the body. The compound's persistence in the body therefore becomes dependent on absorption rather than elimination processes. This sometimes occurs when the route of exposure is dermal.

Q. What is dosage regimen?
- Dosage regimen is defined as the manner in which a drug is administered.
- Irrespective of the route of administration, a dosage regimen is composed of two important variables;
  - (a) The magnitude of each dose (dose size)
  - (b) The frequency with which the dose is repeated (dosing interval).

Q. Define in brief dose size?
- Dose or dose size is a quantitative term estimating the amount of drug, which must be administered to produce a particular biological response, i.e., to achieve a specified target plasma drug concentration.

Q. How the therapeutic dose should be selected?
- As the magnitude of both therapeutic and toxic responses depends on plasma drug concentration, size of dose should be so selected that it produces the peak plasma concentration (C_{max}) or steady-state level within the limits of therapeutic range (between minimum effective concentration and maximum safe concentration). The therapeutic plasma concentration range is obtained by careful clinical evaluation of the response in a sufficient number of appropriately selected individuals (for microbial, the range is based upon the minimum inhibitory concentration for susceptible microorganisms).

Q. What do you mean by dosing interval?
- Dosing interval is the time interval between doses. It ensures maintenance of plasma concentration of a drug within the therapeutic range for entire duration of therapy.

Q. Define minimum effective concentration (MEC)
- Minimum effective concentration (MEC) is the minimum concentration of drug in plasma required to produce the desirable pharmacological/therapeutic response. In case of antimicrobials, the term minimum inhibitory concentration (MIC) is used, which may be defined as the minimum concentration of antimicrobial agent in plasma required to inhibit the growth of microorganisms.

Q. Define maximum safe concentration (MSC) or minimum toxic concentration (MTC).
- Maximum safe concentration (MSC) or minimum toxic concentration (MTC) is the concentration of drug in plasma above which toxic effects are produced. Concentration of drug above MSC is said to be in toxic level. The drug concentration between MEC and MSC represents the therapeutic range.

Q. Define maximum plasma concentration/peak plasma concentration (C_{max} or Cp_{max}).
- Maximum plasma concentration/peak plasma concentration is the point of maximum concentration of drug in plasma. The maximum plasma concentration depends on administered dose and rates of absorption (absorption rate constant, K_a) and elimination (elimination rate constant, β). The peak represents the point of time when absorption equals elimination rate of the drug. It is often expressed as $\mu g/ml$.

Q. Define time of maximum concentration/time of peak concentration (t_{max}).
- Time of maximum concentration/time of peak concentration is the time required for a drug to reach peak concentration in plasma. The faster is the absorption rate, the lower is the t_{max}. It is also useful in assessing efficacy of drugs used to treat acute conditions (e.g., pain) which can be treated by a single dose. It is expressed in hours.

Q. What is elimination t1/2?
- The time it takes for plasma concentration to drop by 50%

3.2 Physiologically Based Toxicokinetic (PBTK) Models

Q. Define PBTK models.
Physiologically based toxicokinetic model is (synonym TK models) an alternative approach to toxicokinetic modeling. It is a physiologically based toxicokinetic (PBTK) model. These models are mathematical stimulation of physiological processes that determine the

rate and extent of xenobiotics/toxicant absorption, distribution, metabolism, and excretion.

Q. What is the difference between physiological models in toxicokinetic studies and classical models?

The primary difference between physiologic compartmental models and classic compartmental models lies in the basis for assigning the rate constants that describe the transport of chemicals into and out of the compartments. In classic kinetics, the rate constants are defined by the data; thus, these models are often referred to as data-based models. In PBTK models, the rate constants represent known or hypothesized biological processes, and these models are commonly referred to as physiologically based toxicokinetic models.

---

4   Sample MCQ's

(Choose the correct statement, it may be one, two, more, or none).

Q.1. The hepatic clearance of a drug with a high hepatic extraction ratio is largely dependent on _____

A. Drug protein binding
B. Hepatic blood flow
C. Drug-metabolizing enzyme activity
D. Intestinal blood flow

Q.2. All of the following are true of saturation kinetics with increasing dose *except* _____

A. Clearance must decrease.
B. Half-life can increase or decrease.
C. Volume of distribution will decrease if there is saturation of serum protein binding.
D. Volume of distribution will decrease if there is saturation of tissue binding.

Q.3. All of the following are true of nonlinear kinetics *except* _____

A. Ratio of metabolites will remain constant with change in dose.
B. Clearance will change with change in dose.
C. AUC will not be dose proportional.
D. Decline of xenobiotic is nonexponential.

Q.4. All of the following are true of first-order kinetics *except* _____

A. Steady-state concentration is proportional to rate of intake.
B. Rate of intake will not change time to steady state.
C. Half-life is inversely proportional to clearance.
D. A change in half-life will not change time to steady state.

Q.5. All of the following are true of first-order kinetics *except* _____

A. The elimination rate constant increases with dose.
B. A semilogarithmic plot of plasma concentration versus time yields a single straight line.
C. The concentration of xenobiotic in plasma decreases by a constant fraction per unit time.
D. The volume of distribution is independent of dose.

Q.6. After _____, 93.8% of a dose of drug is eliminated

A. Three half-lives
B. Four half-lives
C. Five half-lives
D. Six half-lives

Q.7. All of the following are components of the central compartment *except* _____

A. Liver
B. Lungs
C. Bone
D. Kidney

Q.8. Which of the following has the largest value of distribution?

A. Chloroquine
B. Ethyl alcohol
C. Albumin
D. Ethylene glycol

Q.9. The common units used to express total clearance of a toxicant are _____

A. mg/mL
B. mg/min
C. mL/ min
D. mg/min/mL

Q.10. In first-order kinetics _____

A. A constant amount of toxicant is removed over unit time.
B. AUC is not proportional to dose.
C. Half-life changes with increasing dose.
D. Clearance, volume of distribution, and half-life do not change with dose.

Q.11. Regarding the two-compartment model of classic toxicokinetics, which of the following is *true*?

A. There is rapid equilibration of chemical between central and peripheral compartments.
B. The logarithm of plasma concentration versus time data yields a linear relationship.
C. There is more than one dispositional phase.
D. It is assumed that the concentration of a chemical is the same throughout the body.
E. It is ineffective in determining effective doses in toxicity studies.

Q.12. When calculating the fraction of a dose remaining in the body over time, which of the following factors need not be taken into consideration?

A. Half-life
B. Initial concentration
C. Time
D. Present concentration
E. Elimination rate constant

Q.13. All of the following statements regarding apparent volume of distribution (V_d) are true *except* _____

A. V_d relates the total amount of chemical in the body to the concentration of chemical in the plasma.
B. V_d is the apparent space into which an amount of chemical is distributed in the body to result in a given plasma concentration.
C. A chemical that usually remains in the plasma has a low V_d.
D. V_d will be low for a chemical with high affinity for tissues.
E. V_d can be used to estimate the amount of chemical in the body if the plasma concentration is known.

Q.14. Chemical clearance _____

A. Is independent of V_d
B. Is unaffected by kidney failure
C. Is indirectly proportional to V_d
D. Is performed by multiple organs
E. Is not appreciable in the GI tract

Q.15. Which of the following chemical half-lives (T1/2) will remain in the body or the longest period of time when given equal dosage of each?

A. T1/2 = 30 min.
B. T1/2 = 1 day
C. T1/2 = 7 h
D. T1/2 = 120 s
E. T1/2 = 1 month

Q.16. With respect to first-order elimination, which of the following statements is *false*?

A. The rate of elimination is directly proportional to the amount of the chemical in the body.

B. A semilogarithmic plot of plasma concentration versus time shows a linear relationship.

C. Half-life (T1/2) differs depending on the dose.

D. Clearance is dosage-independent.

E. The plasma concentration and tissue concentration decrease similarly with respect to the elimination rate constant.

Q.17. The toxicity of a chemical is dependent on the amount of chemical reaching the systemic circulation. Which of the following does *not* greatly influence systemic availability?

A. Absorption after oral dosing
B. Intestinal motility
C. Hepatic first-pass effect
D. Intestinal first-pass effect
E. Incorporation into micelles

Q.18. Which of the following is *not* an advantage of a physiologically based toxicokinetic model?

A. Complex-dosing regimens are easily accommodated.

B. The time course of distribution of chemicals to any organ is obtainable.

C. The effects of changing physiologic parameters on tissue concentrations can be estimated.

D. The rate constants are obtained from gathered data.

E. The same model can predict toxicokinetics of chemicals across species.

Q.19. Which of the following will not help to increase the flux of a xenobiotic across a biological membrane?

A. Decreased size
B. Decreased oil: water partition coefficient
C. Increased concentration gradient
D. Increased surface area
E. Decreased membrane thickness

Q.20. Which of the following statements is true regarding diffusion-limited compartments?

A. Xenobiotic transport across the cell membrane is limited by the rate at which blood arrives at the tissue.

B. Diffusion-limited compartments are also referred to as flow-limited compartments.

C. Increased membrane thickness can cause diffusion-limited xenobiotic uptake.

D. Equilibrium between the extracellular and intracellular space is maintained by rapid exchange between the two compartments.

E. Diffusion of gases across the alveolar septa of a healthy lung is diffusion-limited.

Answers

1. B.   2. C.   3. A.   4. D.   5. A.   6. B.
7. C.   8. A.   9. C.   10. D.   11. C.   12. A.
13. D.   14. D.   15. E.   16. C.   17. B.
18. D.   19. B.   20. C.

Further Readings

Ehrnebo M (2010) Kinetic analysis of xenobiotics. In: Gupta PK (ed) Modern toxicology: basis of organ and reproduction toxicity, vol 1, 2nd reprint edn. PharmaMed Press, Hyderabad, pp 130–158

Gupta PK (2014) Essential concepts in toxicology. PharmaMed Press (A unit of BSP Books Pvt. Ltd), Hyderabad

Gupta PK (2016) Fundamentals of toxicology: essential concepts and applications, 1st edn. BSP/Elsevier, San Diego

Gupta PK (2018) Illustrative toxicology, 1st edn. Elsevier, San Diego

Gupta PK (2019) Concepts and applications in veterinary toxicology: an interactive guide. Springer-Nature, Switzerland

Gupta PK (2020) Brainstorming questions in toxicology. Francis and Taylor CRC Press, Boca Raton

van der Merwe D, Gehring R, Buur JL (2019) Toxicokinetics. In: Gupta RC (ed) Veterinary toxicology: basic and clinical principles, 3rd edn. Academic Press/Elsevier, San Diego, pp 133–144

Fruncillo RJ (2011) 2,000 Toxicology board review questions. Xlibris, Publishers, Bloomington

Shen Danny D (2015) Toxicokinetics. In: Klaassen CD, Watkins JB III (eds) Casarett & Doull's essentials of toxicology, 3rd edn. McGraw-Hill, New York, pp 109–120

Part III

Organ Toxicity

Target Organ Toxicity

7

Abstract

Several target organs such as liver, kidney, lungs, heart, ocular and visual apparatus, skin, reproductive organ, immune system, endocrine systems, etc. play an important role for various functions of the body. Damage to any system may lead to serious consequences. In addition to medicinal risks, liver and kidney damages accompany exposure to synthetic chemicals in the workplace or as environmental pollutants. Still other chemicals that harm the excretory organs are consumed as food contaminants. The vulnerability of the liver, kidney, and other organs to xenobiotic toxicity raises the question as to why such chemicals often display "organ selectivity" when inducing toxicity. This chapter briefly describes the overview, key points, and relevant text that are in the format of problem-solving study questions followed by multiple-choice questions (MCQs) along with their answers.

Keywords

Organ toxicity · Hepatotoxicity · Nephrotoxicity · Neurotoxicity · Cardiovascular toxicity · Hematotoxicity · Ocular toxicity · Visual system toxicity · Dermal toxicity · Reproductive system toxicity · Immune modulation · Endocrine system · MCQs · Question bank

1 Introduction

There is poor correlation of target organ toxicity across the species. The important target organs that are susceptible to exposure to xenobiotics include liver, kidney, heart, lungs, cardiovascular, hematopoietic, visual apparatus, skin, reproductive, and endocrine system exposed to different xenobiotics. Toxic responses may vary according to various situations, factors, or the previous or concomitant exposure to several foreign compounds. The chapter briefly describes the overview, key points, and relevant text that are in the format of problem-solving study questions followed by multiple-choice questions (MCQ's) along with their answers.

2 Overview

There is poor correlation of target organ toxicity across the species. For this reason, safety evaluation should not be based on the demonstration of target organ toxicity but on the absence of toxic signs. A step-by-step approach, based on the biological activity of the compound, would provide more meaningful data for safety evaluation than the standard toxicological studies in a rodent and non-rodent species. The standard animal studies in rats or mice that provide this information are 28-day, 90-day, or lifetime studies (up to 2 years)

P K Gupta, *Problem Solving Questions in Toxicology*, https://doi.org/10.1007/978-3-030-50409-0_7

that include hematological, clinic-chemical, and detailed macroscopic and microscopic examination to enable the toxic effects on target tissues/organs to be identified. Data from repeat-dose studies performed in other species may also be used. Other long-term exposure studies, e.g., for carcinogenicity, neurotoxicity, or reproductive toxicity, may also provide evidence of specific target organ/systemic toxicity. The information required to evaluate specific target organ/systemic toxicity comes either from repeated exposure in humans, e.g., exposure at home, in the workplace, or environment, or from studies conducted in experimental animals.

Key Points

- Several target organs such as liver, kidney, lungs, heart, ocular and visual apparatus, skin, reproductive organ, endocrine systems, etc. play an important role for various functions of the body. Damage to any system may lead to serious consequences.
- Damage to the liver could be enlargement and even cirrhosis. Prescription medications, herbal remedies, and natural chemicals or any toxicant/toxin can lead to hepatotoxicity.
- The liver contains most of the enzymes involved in xenobiotic biotransformation that have been identified in other tissues.
- The liver extracts ingested nutrients, vitamins, metals, drugs, environmental toxicants, and waste products of bacteria from the blood or catabolism, storage, and/or excretion into bile.
- Xenobiotics in the systemic circulation will be delivered to the kidney in relatively high amounts. Renal transport, accumulation, and biotransformation of xenobiotics contribute to the susceptibility of the kidney to toxic injury.
- The kidney contributes to total body homeostasis via its role in the excretion of metabolic wastes, the synthesis and release of renin and erythropoietin, and the regulation of extracellular fluid volume, electrolyte composition, and acid-base balance.
- Inhaled xenobiotics can affect lung tissues directly or distant organs after absorption. Particle size is usually the critical factor that determines the region of the respiratory tract in which a particle or an aerosol will deposit. Water solubility is a decisive factor in determining how deeply a given gas penetrates into the lung.
- Cardiac toxicity after a single or repeated exposure to a high dose of cardiotoxic chemicals may be manifested by cardiac hypertrophy and the transition to heart failure.
- Any xenobiotic that disrupts ion movement or homeostasis may induce a cardiotoxic reaction composed principally of disturbances in heart rhythm.
- Common mechanisms of vascular toxicity include (1) alterations in membrane structure and function, (2) redox stress, (3) vessel-specific bioactivation of protoxicants, and (4) preferential accumulation of the active toxin in vascular cells.
- Direct or indirect damage to blood cells and their precursors includes tissue hypoxia, hemorrhage, and infection.
- Xenobiotic-induced aplastic anemia is a life-threatening disorder characterized by peripheral blood pancytopenia, reticulocytopenia, and bone marrow hypoplasia.
- Idiosyncratic xenobiotic-induced agranulocytosis may involve a sudden depletion of circulating neutrophils concomitant with exposure that persists as long as the agent or its metabolites are in the circulation.

- Leukemias are proliferative disorders of hematopoietic tissue that originate from individual bone marrow cells.
- Xenobiotic-induced thrombocytopenia may result from increased platelet destruction or decreased platelet production, which lead to decreased platelet aggregation and bleeding disorders.
- Blood coagulation is a complex process involving a number of proteins whose synthesis and unction can be altered by many xenobiotics.
- The central nervous system (CNS) is protected from the adverse effects of many potential toxicants by an anatomical blood–brain barrier. Neurons are highly dependent on aerobic metabolism because this energy is needed to maintain proper ion gradients.
- Individual neurotoxic compounds typically target the neuron, the axon, the myelinating cell, or the neurotransmitter system.
- Neurotoxicants that cause axonopathies cause axonal degeneration and loss of the myelin surrounding that axon; however, the neuron cell body remains intact.
- Numerous naturally occurring toxins as well as synthetic chemicals may interrupt the transmission of impulses, block or accentuate transsynaptic communication, block reuptake of neurotransmitters, or interfere with second-messenger systems.
- Most electrophysiologic or neurophysiologic procedures for testing visual function after toxicant exposure involve stimulating the eyes with visual stimuli and electrically recording potentials generated by visually responsive neurons.
- Ophthalmologic procedures for evaluating the health of the eye include routine clinical screening evaluations using a slit-lamp biomicroscope and ophthal-moscope and an examination of the pupillary light reflex.
- The skin participates directly in thermal, electrolyte, hormonal, metabolic, and immune regulation. Percutaneous absorption depends on the xenobiotic's hydrophobicity, which affects its ability to partition into epidermal lipid, and rate of diffusion through this barrier.
- The cells of the epidermis and pilosebaceous units' express biotransformation enzymes.
- Irritant dermatitis is a nonimmune-related response caused by the direct action of an agent on the skin.
- Hypersensitivity reactions require prior exposure leading to sensitization in order to elicit a reaction on subsequent challenge. Xenobiotics that alter the immune system can upset the balance between immune recognition and destruction of foreign invaders and the proliferation of these microbes and/or cancer cells.
- The gonads possess a dual function: an endocrine function involving the secretion of sex hormones and a nonendocrine function relating to the production of germ cells (gametogenesis).
- Gametogenic and secretory functions of either the ovary or testes are dependent on the secretion for follicle-stimulating hormone (FSH) and luteinizing hormone (LH) from the pituitary.
- The blood–testis barrier between the lumen of an interstitial capillary and the lumen of a seminiferous tubule impedes or prevents the free exchange of chemicals/drugs between the blood and the fluid inside the seminiferous tubules.
- Xenobiotics can act directly on the hypothalamus and the adenohypophysis, leading to alterations in the secretion of hypothalamic-releasing hormones and/or gonadotropins.

- Steroid hormone biosynthesis can occur in several endocrine organs including the adrenal cortex, ovary, and the testes.
- Female reproductive processes of oogenesis, ovulation, the development of sexual receptivity, coitus, gamete and zygote transport, fertilization, and implantation of the conceptus may be sites of xenobiotic interference.
- May influence male reproductive organ structure, spermatogenesis, androgen hormone secretion, and accessory organ function.
- Each type of endocrine cell in the adenohypophysis is under the control of a specific releasing hormone from the hypothalamus.
- Toxicants can influence the synthesis, storage, and release of hypothalamic-releasing hormones, adenohypophyseal-releasing hormones, and the endocrine gland-specific hormones.

3   Terminology

Q. Define an organ
- An organ is a part of your body that has a particular purpose or function, for example, heart or lungs; muscles and internal organs; and the reproductive organs.

Q. Define organ toxicity
- Toxicity is the degree to which a substance can damage an organism. Toxicity can refer to the effect on a whole organism, such as an animal, bacterium, or plant, as well as the effect on a substructure of the organism, such as a cell (cytotoxicity), or an organ such as the liver (hepatotoxicity).

Q. What do you mean by target organ toxins?
- Target organ toxins are chemicals that can cause adverse effects or disease states manifested in specific organs of the body. Toxins do not affect all organs in the body to the same extent due to their different cell structures.

Q. Why are toxins often selective to tissues? Give suitable examples.
(a) Preferential accumulation: toxicant may accumulate in only certain tissues and cause toxicity to that particular tissue. For example, Cd in the kidney and paraquat in lung.
(b) Selective metabolic activation: enzymes needed to convert a compound to the active form may be present in highest quantities in a particular organ. For example, CCl_4 and nitrosamines in the liver.
(c) Characteristics of tissue repair: some tissues may be protected from toxicity by actively repairing toxic damage; some tissues may be susceptible because they lack sufficient repair capabilities, e.g., nitrosamines in the liver.
(d) Specific receptors and/or functions: toxicant may interact with receptors in a given tissue. For example, curare: a receptor-specific neuromuscular blocker.
(e) Physiological sensitivity: the nervous system is extremely sensitive to agents that block utilization of oxygen. For example, nitrite, oxidizes hemoglobin (methemoglobinemia); cyanide, inhibits cytochrome oxidase (cells not able to utilize oxygen); and barbiturates, interfere with sensors for oxygen and carbon dioxide content in the blood.

Q. What are the main target organs most frequently affected by toxicants?
(a) Central nervous system
(b) Circulatory system (blood, blood-forming system)
(c) Visceral organs (liver, kidneys, lung)
(d) Muscle and bone

Q. What are the pathways through which acetaminophen is metabolized?
- There are three pathways:
    (a) Sulfonation (about 52%)
    (b) Glucuronidation (about 42%)
    (c) P450 1A, 3A, and 2E1 (about 4%). (About 2% is excreted unchanged)

Q. What is the target where a toxicant produces its effect?

(a) Molecular

(b) Subcellular organelle

Q. What are the target organs on which toxic substance affect(s)?

(a) Localized

(b) Multiple organs

Q. In which tissues arsenic tends to accumulate and why?

- Arsenic accumulates in keratin-rich tissues such as hair and nails because arsenic has high affinity for sulfhydryl groups (-SH). Since hair and nails contain –SH-rich keratin, arsenic accumulates in them.

4 Hepatotoxicity

4.1 Problem-Solving Study Questions

Q. What is the function of the liver?

- In the liver three main functions occur: storage, metabolism, and biosynthesis. Glucose is converted to glycogen and stored; when needed for energy, it is converted back to glucose. Fat, fat-soluble vitamins, and other nutrients are also stored in the liver. Fatty acids are metabolized and converted to lipids, which are then conjugated with proteins synthesized in the liver and released into the bloodstream as lipoproteins. The liver also synthesizes numerous functional proteins, such as enzymes and blood-coagulating factors.

  In addition, the liver which contains numerous xenobiotic-metabolizing enzymes is the main site of xenobiotic metabolism.

Q. What is cholestasis?

- Cholestasis is the suppression or stoppage of bile flow and may have either intrahepatic or extrahepatic causes. Inflammation or blockage of the bile ducts results in retention of bile salts as well as bilirubin accumulation, an event that leads to jaundice. Other mechanisms causing cholestasis include changes in membranes permeability of either hepatocytes or biliary canaliculi.

Q. What is cirrhosis?

- Cirrhosis is a progressive disease that is characterized by the deposition of collagen throughout the liver. In most cases cirrhosis results from chronic chemical injury. The accumulation of fibrous material causes severe restriction in blood flow and in the liver's normal metabolic and detoxication processes. This situation can in turn cause further damage and eventually lead to liver failure. In humans, chronic use of ethanol is the single most important cause of cirrhosis.

Q. What is hepatitis?

- Hepatitis is an inflammation of the liver and is usually viral in origin; however, certain chemicals, usually drugs, can induce a hepatitis that closely resembles that produced by viral infections.

Q. Why liver is necessary for our survival?

- The liver is necessary for survival because it is essential for the coordination of metabolism in the body, including glucose homeostasis, xenobiotic metabolism, and detoxification. The liver is also a major site for steroid hormone synthesis and degradation and synthesis of plasma proteins. It continuously provides energy to the whole body by managing the systemic supply of nutrients. In addition, the liver is a mediator of systemic and local innate immunity and an important site of immune regulation.

Q. What is hepatotoxicity (liver)?

- Hepatotoxicity is damage produced to the liver such as liver enlargement and even cirrhosis. Prescription medications, herbal remedies, and natural chemicals or any toxicant/toxin can lead to hepatotoxicity. Approximately half of all cases of acute liver failure are related to hepatotoxicity. The type of liver damage caused by toxic substances/medications varies widely and depends upon the type of drug being taken, the dosage, and the overall health of the patient.

Q. What is the function of hepatocytes?
    • Hepatocytes have a rich supply of Phase I
      enzymes that often convert xenobiotics to
      reactive electrophilic metabolites and of
      Phase II enzymes that add a polar group to
      a molecule and thereby enhance its removal
      from the body. The balance between Phase
      I and Phase II reactions determines whether
      a reactive metabolite will initiate liver cell
      injury or be safely detoxified.
Q. Which reactive metabolite will initiate liver
    cell injury?
    • The pathogenesis of most chemical-
      induced liver injuries is initiated by the
      metabolic conversion of chemicals into
      reactive intermediate species, such as elec-
      trophilic compounds or free radicals, which
      can potentially alter the structure and func-
      tion of cellular macromolecules. Many
      reactive intermediate species can produce
      oxidative stress, which can be equally det-
      rimental to the cell.
Q. What is the mechanism of hepatotoxicity?
    • Chemically induced cell injury can be
      thought of as involving a series of events
      occurring in the affected animal and often
      in the target organ itself:
      (a) The chemical agent is activated to
           form the initiating toxic agent.
      (b) The initiating toxic agent is either
           detoxified or causes molecular changes
           in the cell.
      (c) The cell recovers or there are irrevers-
           ible changes.
      (d) Irreversible changes may culminate in
           cell death.
Q. What types of liver injury is induced by toxi-
    cants. Give examples.
    Hepatic response to insults by chemicals
    depends on the intensity of the insult, the popula-
    tion of cells affected, and whether the exposure
    is acute or chronic. Examples of types of hepato-
    biliary injury are summarized in Table 7.1.
Q. What is hepatitis?
    • Hepatitis is an inflammation of the liver
      and is usually viral in origin; however, cer-
      tain chemicals, usually drugs, can induce a

Table 7.1 Common toxins responsible for of hepatobili-
ary injury

Type of injury or damage	Representative toxins
Fatty liver	Amiodarone, CCl4, ethanol, fialuridine, tamoxifen, valproic acid
Hepatocyte death	Acetaminophen, allyl alcohol, Cu, dimethylformamide, ethanol
Immune-mediated response	Diclofenac, ethanol, halothane, tienilic acid
Canalicular cholestasis	Chlorpromazine, cyclosporin A,1,1-dichloroethylene, estrogens, Mn, phalloidin
Bile duct damage	Alpha-naphthyl isothiocyanate, amoxicillin, methylenedianiline, sporidesmin
Sinusoidal disorders	Anabolic steroids, cyclophosphamide, microcystin, pyrrolizidine alkaloids
Fibrosis and cirrhosis	CCl4, ethanol, thioacetamide, vitamin A, vinyl chloride
Tumors	Aflatoxin, androgens, arsenic, thorium dioxide, vinyl chloride

hepatitis that closely resembles that pro-
duced by viral infections.
Q. What is the function of bile?
    • Bile is essential for uptake of lipid nutri-
      ents from the small intestine, protection of
      the small intestine from oxidative insults,
      and excretion of endogenous and xenobi-
      otic compounds.
Q. Give four examples of hepatotoxicants.
    (a) Carbon tetrachloride
    (b) Ethanol
    (c) Bromobenzene
    (d) Acetaminophen
Q. Out of over-the-counter medications, which
    one is the most commonly associated with the
    development of liver damage?
    • The most common over-the-counter medi-
      cation associated with the development of
      liver damage is acetaminophen. Other
      types of drugs which have been linked to
      high rates of hepatotoxicity include che-
      motherapy drugs, carbon tetrachloride,
      alcohol, nitrosamines, chloroform, toluene,
      perchloroethylene, cresol, dimethyl sul-
      fate, etc.

Q. Name at least three industrial chemicals that have been identified as hepatotoxicants.

- There are several hundred industrial chemicals that have been identified as hepatotoxicants; examples include *N*-nitrosodimethylamine, hydrazine, and carbon disulfide.

4.2 Sample MCQ's

(Choose the correct statement, it may be one, two or more, or none.)

Q.1. Which of the following is thought to be important factor in the pathology of alcohol-induced liver disease?

- A. Inflammatory response
- B. Lipid peroxidation
- C. Oxidative stress
- D. All of the above

Q.2. Allyl alcohol is metabolized by ADH to ---

- A. Benzylaldehyde
- B. Acrolein
- C. Acetic anhydride
- D. Butyraldehyde

Q.3. All of the following statements are true *except* ---

- A. Xenobiotics can greatly slow down the proliferation of neutrophils and monocytes, increasing the risk of infection.
- B. Ethanol and cortisol decrease phagocytosis and microbe ingestion by the immune system.
- C. Agranulocytosis is predictable and can be caused by exposure to a number of environmental toxins.
- D. Heroin and methadone abusers have reduced ability to kill microorganisms due to drug-induced reduction in superoxide production.
- E. Toxic neutropenia may be mediated by the immune system.

Q.4. Ethyl alcohol is metabolized in humans by all of the following *except* --

- A. CYP3A4
- B. CYP2E1
- C. ADH
- D. Peroxisome catalase

Q.5. Idiosyncratic liver injury is characterized by all of the following *except* ----

- A. Can be immune or nonimmune-mediated
- B. Has a clear dose–response relationship
- C. Is relatively rare
- D. Has a probable genetic basis

Q.6. The liver cell process associated with cell swelling leakage of cell contents and an influx of inflammatory cells is -----

- A. Apoptosis
- B. Fibrosis
- C. Necrosis
- D. Steatosis

Q.7. All of the following are true regarding the hepatotoxicity of carbon tetrachloride *except* -----

- A. The reactive metabolite is formed by cytochrome P450 3A4
- B. The reactive metabolite is a free radical
- C. Chronic ethanol exposure can enhance the injury
- D. The injury involves lipid peroxidation

Q.8. All of the following are true regarding ethanol and the liver *except* ------

- A. Ethanol inhibits the transfer of triglycerides from the liver to adipose tissue.
- B. Alcohol dehydrogenase is the only inducible enzyme in chronic alcoholism.
- C. An inactive form of aldehydrogenase is formed in 50% of Asians.
- D. The catalase pathway is a minor route for ethanol metabolism.

Q.9. All of the following hepatic sites are matched with the appropriate preferential toxicant *except* ----

A. Zone 1 hepatocyte–iron
B. Bile duct cells–ethanol
C. Stellate cells–vitamin A
D. Zone 3 hepatocyte–carbon tetra-chloride

Q.10. All of the following cause nonimmune idiosyncratic live toxicity *except* -----

A. Tienilic acid
B. Isoniazid
C. Amiodarone
D. Ketoconazole

Answers
1. D.   2. B.   3. C.   4. A.   5. B.   6. C.
7. A.   8. B.   9. B.   10. A.

5   Nephrotoxicity

5.1   Problem-Solving Study Questions

Q. What is the function of the renal system?
The primary function of the renal system is the elimination of waste products, derived either from endogenous metabolism or from the metabolism of xenobiotics. The kidney also plays an important role in regulation of body homeostasis, regulating extracellular fluid volume and electrolyte balance.

Q. What is nephrotoxicity?
Nephrotoxicity is a toxic/poisonous effect of any substance on renal function. The nephrotoxic effect of most drugs is more profound in individuals already suffering from kidney failure.

Q. What is/are the most likely mechanism(s) by which glomerular nephrotoxicants such as antibiotics induce proteinuria?
The glomerulus is responsible for ultrafiltration of the plasma. Some toxicants reduce the anionic charge on the glomerular elements,

resulting in proteinuria. Since albumin is anionic, one often sees albuminuria if the charge-selective properties of the filtration barrier are decreased.
Explanation: The proximal tubule is often the site of toxicity; the tubule has a high rate of blood flow. The proximal tubule absorbs the bulk of the water and solute filtered at the glomerulus. The proximal tubule reabsorbs Na, K, Ca, Mg, Cl, PO_4, and HCO_3. Filtered sugar, amino acids, and some small organic acids are reabsorbed. The proximal tubule reabsorbs peptides and proteins which are filtered at the glomerulus. If the energy for sodium transport or other transport functions is decreased, the reabsorption rate in the proximal tubule can decline, producing glucosuria and proteinuria. The osmolality of urine is controlled in the collecting duct.

Q. How glomerulus is responsible for ultrafiltration of the plasma?
The glomerular basement membrane of the kidney contains anionic proteins which produce an electrostatic barrier that retards the passage of anionic macromolecules. Neutral molecules will pass through the glomerulus better than anionic molecules of the same size. The plasma protein concentration in the glomerular filtrate is low.
Some toxicants reduce the anionic charge on the glomerular elements, resulting in proteinuria. Since albumin is anionic, one often sees albuminuria if the charge-selective properties of the filtration barrier are decreased.

Q. Which area of the kidney is the site of toxicity?
The proximal tubule is often the site of toxicity.

Q. Why proximal tubule is often the site of toxicity
The proximal tubule has a high rate of blood flow. The proximal tubule absorbs the bulk of the water and solute filtered at the glomerulus. The proximal tubule reabsorbs Na, K, Ca, Mg, Cl, PO4, and HCO3. Filtered sugar, amino acids, and some small organic acids are reabsorbed. The proximal tubule reabsorbs peptides and proteins which are filtered

at the glomerulus. If the energy for sodium transport or other transport functions is decreased, the reabsorption rate in the proximal tubule can decline, producing glucosuria and proteinuria.

Q. What are nephrotoxin substances?
Nephrotoxins are substances displaying nephrotoxicity. Acute ethylene glycol poisoning is serious and with a fatal outcome in more than 88% of cases. Several other chemicals are known to cause edema, proteinuria, and other kidney problems. Some of these chemicals include halogenated hydrocarbons, uranium, chloroform, mercury, dimethyl sulfate, etc.

Q. Give some examples of nephrotoxins.
(a) Many heavy metals are potent nephrotoxicants. They interfere with enzymes of energy metabolism.
(b) Certain antibiotics, most notably the aminoglycosides, are known to be nephrotoxic in humans, especially in high doses or after prolonged therapy. The group of antibiotics includes streptomycin, neomycin, kanamycin, and gentamicin.
(c) Aristolochic acid, found in some plants and in some herbal supplements derived from those plants, has been shown to have nephrotoxic effects on humans.
(d) Rhubarb contains some nephrotoxins which can cause inflammation of the kidneys in some people.

Q. How do aminoglycosides cause nephrotoxicity?
Aminoglycosides preferentially affect the proximal tubular cells. They exert their main toxic effect within the tubular cell by altering phospholipid metabolism. In addition to their direct effect on cells, aminoglycosides cause renal vasoconstriction.

Q. How nephrotoxicants can lead to apoptosis or necrosis?
Numerous nephrotoxicants cause mitochondrial dysfunction via compromise respiration and ATP production, or some other cellular process, leading to either apoptosis or necrosis.

Q. What is acute kidney injury (AKI)?
One of the most common manifestations of nephrotoxic damage is acute renal failure (ARF) or acute kidney injury (AKI). AKI is characterized by an abrupt decline in GFR with resulting azotemia or a buildup of nitrogenous wastes in the blood. AKI describes the entire spectrum of the disease and is defined as a complex disorder that comprises multiple causative factors with clinical manifestations ranging from minimal elevation in serum creatinine to anuric renal failure.

Q. What are the causes of kidney injury?
Any decline in GFR is complex and may result from prerenal factors (renal vasoconstriction, intravascular volume depletion, an insufficient cardiac output), postrenal factors (ureteral or bladder obstruction), and intrarenal factors (glomerulonephritis, tubular cell injury, death, and loss resulting in back-leak; renal vasculature damage; interstitial nephritis).

5.2 Sample MCQ's

(Choose the correct statement, it may be one, two or more, or none.)

Q.1. Which of the following statements is *not* correct?

A. Many nephrotoxicants appear to have the primary site of action on (in) the proximal tubule.
B. The proximal convoluted tubule is the primary site of reabsorption of glucose and amino acids.
C. The pars recta (S3) has a greater capacity to absorb organic compounds than the distal tubule.
D. The loop of Henle is the site of damage produced by chronic administration of analgesic mixtures.
E. The collecting duct appears relatively insensitive to most nephrotoxicants.

Q.2. Which of the following does *not* contribute to filtrate formation in the nephron?

A. Capillary hydrostatic pressure
B. Positive charge of glomerular capillary wall
C. Hydraulic permeability of glomerular capillary wall
D. Colloid oncotic pressure
E. Size of filtration slits

Q.3. Which of the following is *not* a characteristic of the loop of Henle?

A. There is reabsorption of filtered Na+ and K+.
B. Tubular fluid in the thin descending limb is iso-osmotic to the renal interstitium.
C. Water is freely permeable in the thin ascending limb.
D. Na+ and Cl− are reabsorbed in the thin ascending limb.
E. The thick ascending limb is impermeable to water.

Q.4. Although the kidneys constitute 0.5% of total body mass, approximately how much of the resting cardiac output do they receive?

A. 0.5–1%
B. 5%
C. 10%
D. 20–25%
E. 50–60%

Q.5. Which of the following is most likely to occur after a toxic insult to the kidney?

A. GFR will decrease in the unaffected kidney.
B. Tight-junction integrity will increase in the nephron.
C. The unaffected cells will undergo atrophy and proliferation.
D. Clinical tests will likely show normal renal function.
E. Glomerulotubular balance is lost.

Q.6. Chronic renal failure *does not* typically result in------

A. Decrease in GFR of viable nephrons.
B. Glomerulosclerosis.
C. Tubular atrophy.
D. Increase glomerular pressures.
E. Altered capillary permeability.

Q.7. All of the following statements regarding toxicity to the kidney are true *except* ---

A. Concentration of toxins in tubular fluid increases the likelihood that the toxin will diffuse into tubular cells.
B. Drugs in the systemic circulation are delivered to the kidneys at relatively high amounts.
C. The distal convolute tubule is the most common site of toxicant-induced renal injury.
D. Immune complex deposition within the glomeruli can lead to glomerulonephritis.
E. Antibiotics and/or antifungal drugs affect the functioning of the nephron at multiple locations.

Q.8. Which of the following test results is *not* correctly paired with the underlying kidney problem?

A. Increase urine volume—effect in ADH synthesis
B. Glucosuria—effect in reabsorption in the proximal convoluted tubule
C. Proteinuria—glomerular damage
D. Proteinuria—proximal tubular injury
E. Brush-border enzymuria—glomerulonephritis

Q.9. Renal cell injury is *not* commonly mediated by which of the following mechanisms?

A. Loss of membrane integrity.
B. Impairment of mitochondrial function.
C. Increase cytosolic Ca2+ concentration.
D. Increase Na+, K+, and -ATPase activity.
E. Caspase activation.

Q.10. Which of the following statements is *false* with respect to nephrotoxicants?

    A. Mercury poisoning can lead to proximal tubular necrosis and acute renal failure.

    B. Cisplatin may cause nephrotoxicity because of its ability to inhibit DNA synthesis.

    C. Chronic consumption of NSAIDs results in nephrotoxicity that is reversible with time.

    D. Amphotericin B nephrotoxicity can result in ADH-resistant polyuria.

    E. Acetaminophen becomes nephrotoxic via activation by renal cytochrome P450.

Answers

1. C. 2. B. 3. C. 4. D. 5. D. 6. A.
7. C. 8. E. 9. D. 10. C.

---

6   Pulmonary Toxicity

6.1   Problem-Solving Study Questions

Q. What is pulmonary toxicity?
- Damage to the lungs is known as pulmonary toxicity. Lung damage often presents as inflammation, also called pneumonitis.

Q. What are the problems associated with pulmonary toxicity?
- Problems due to lung system include cough, tightness in chest, shortness of breath, etc. For example, in cystic fibrosis patients, mucus builds up impaired lung function by blocking airways. The mucus also traps pathogens that we inhale instead of clearing them out of the lungs, causing frequent lung infections.

Q. Name at least eight common chemicals responsible for lung toxicity?
- Substances known to damage lungs include paraquat herbicides, silica asbestos, nitrogen dioxide, ozone, hydrogen sulfide, chromium, nickel, alcohol, etc.

Q. What is acute lung toxicity?
- Damage to the lungs that resolves (returns to normal after time or after the cause has been removed) is called acute lung toxicity.

Q. What is chronic lung toxicity?
- Damage that is long-lasting or permanent is called chronic or late pulmonary toxicity. Lung damage often presents as inflammation, also called pneumonitis.

Q. What is amiodarone pulmonary toxicity?
- Interstitial pneumonitis usually presents after two or more months of therapy, especially in patients in whom the dose of amiodarone exceeds 400 mg per day. The incidence of pulmonary toxicity from amiodarone is not precisely known; it is estimated to be 1–5%, depending on the dose of amiodarone.

Q. How lungs get damaged?
- Allergies, infections, or pollution can trigger asthma's symptoms. Chronic obstructive pulmonary disease (COPD): Lung conditions defined by an inability to exhale normally, which causes difficulty breathing followed by emphysema. Lung damage allows air to be trapped in the lungs in this form of COPD.

Q. What is asthma?
Asthma is characterized by increased reactivity of the bronchial smooth muscle in response to exposure to irritants.

Q. What is emphysema?
- In emphysema, destruction of the gas-exchanging surface area results in a distended, hyperinflated lung that no longer effectively exchanges oxygen and carbon dioxide.

Q. What are inhalant toxicants?
- They include all types of inhalant toxicants, gases, vapors, fumes, aerosols, organic and inorganic particulates, and mixtures of any or all of these. Gasoline additives and exhaust particles, pesticides, plastics, solvents, deodorant and cosmetic sprays, and construction materials are all included.

Q. Which portion of the lungs is known as gas-exchange region?

The gas-exchange region consists of terminal bronchioles, respiratory bronchioles, alveolar ducts, alveoli, blood vessels, and lung interstitium. Gas exchange occurs in the alveoli, which comprise approximately 85% of the total parenchymal lung volume. Adult human lungs contain an estimated 300–500 million alveoli. Capillaries, blood plasma, and formed blood elements are separated from the airspace by a thin layer of tissue formed by epithelial, interstitial, and endothelial components.

Q. What is the mechanism of particle deposition in the respiratory tract?

In the respiratory tract, particles deposit by impaction, interception, sedimentation, diffusion, and electrostatic deposition (for positively charged particles only). Impaction occurs in the upper respiratory tract and large proximal airways where the airflow is faster than in the small distal airways because the cumulative diameter is smaller than in the proximal airways. In humans, most >10 μm particles are deposited in the nose or oral pharynx and cannot penetrate tissues distal to the larynx. For 2.5–10 μm particles, impaction continues to be the mechanism of deposition in the first generations of the tracheobronchial region.

Q. How biotransformation of xenobiotics takes place in the respiratory tract?

The CYP monooxygenase system responsible for metabolism is concentrated into a few lung cells: BSCs, alveolar type II cells, macrophages, and endothelial cells. Of these cell types, BSCs have the most CYP, followed by the type II cells. Phase II enzymes include glutathione S-transferases (GSTs) (alpha, mu, and pi), glucuronosyl transferases, and sulfotransferases (SULTs). GSTs (and glutathione) play a major role in the modulation of both acute and chronic chemical toxicity in the lung. The regulation of many of these enzymes is under coordinated control of the transcription factor, i.e., nuclear factor erythroid 2-related factor 2 (NRF2), also known as (nuclear factor erythroid-derived 2-like 2). Polymorphisms in glutathione transferase genes have been associated with a possible increase in risk of developing lung cancer, particularly in smokers.

Q. What is the role of particle size in determining the region of the respiratory tract in which a particle will be deposited?

Particle size is a critical factor in determining the region of the respiratory tract in which a particle will be deposited. In respiratory toxicology, aerosols (solid or liquid particles dispersed into air) include dusts, fumes, smoke, mists, fog, or smog (ranging from ≥ 1.0 μm or dusts to ≥ 0.01–50 μm or smog). Smaller aerosols include sub-micrometer particles, nanometer particles, or nanoparticles.

Q. What is pulmonary fibrosis?

Fibrotic lungs from humans with acute or chronic pulmonary fibrosis contain increased amounts of collagen. In lungs damaged by toxicants, the response resembles adult or infant respiratory distress syndrome. Excess lung collagen is usually observed not only in the alveolar interstitium but also throughout the alveolar ducts and respiratory bronchioles.

Q. What agents are known to produce lung injury in humans?

There are over several thousand unique chemicals that are commonly used in industry, many of which represent hazards to the respiratory tract. A few examples of such chemicals include isocyanates, iron oxides, manganese, nickel, nitrogen oxides, organic (sugar cane) dust (possibly contaminated with thermophilic actinomycete), perchloroethylene, phosgene, silica, tin, vanadium, etc.

6.2 Sample MCQ's

(Choose the correct statement, it may be one, two or more, or none.)

Q.1. Which of the following is *least* likely to increase occupational inhalation of a chemical?

    A. Increased airborne concentration
    B. Increased respiratory rate
    C. Increased tidal volume
    D. Increased particle size
    E. Increased length of exposure

Q.2. Which of the following lung diseases has the highest occupational death rate?

    A. Asbestosis
    B. Coal workers' pneumoconiosis
    C. Byssinosis
    D. Hypersensitivity pneumonitis
    E. Silicosis

Q.3. Which of the following will cause a right shift in the oxygen dissociation curve?

    A. Increased pH
    B. Decreased carbon dioxide concentration
    C. Decreased body temperature
    D. Increased 2,3-BPG concentration
    E. Fetal hemoglobin

Q.4. The free radicals that inflict oxidative damage on the lungs are generated by all of the following *except* ---

    A. Tobacco smoke
    B. Neutrophils
    C. Ozone
    D. Monocytes
    E. SO_2

Q.5. Which of the following gases would most likely pass all the way through the respiratory tract and be use into the pulmonary blood supply?

    A. O_3 (ozone)
    B. NO_2
    C. H_2O
    D. CO
    E. SO_2

Q.6. All of the following statements regarding particle deposition and clearance are true *except* -----

    A. One of the main modes of particle clearance is via mucociliary escalation.
    B. Diffusion is important in the deposition of particles in the bronchial regions.
    C. Larger volumes of inspired air increase particle deposition in the airways.
    D. Sedimentation results in deposition in the bronchioles.
    E. Swallowing is an important mechanism of particle clearance.

Q.7. Which of the following is not a common location to which particles are cleared?

    A. Stomach
    B. Lymph nodes
    C. Pulmonary vasculature
    D. Liver
    E. GI tract

Q.8. Pulmonary fibrosis is marked by which of the following?

    A. Increased type I collagen
    B. Decreased type III collagen
    C. Increased compliance
    D. Elastase activation
    E. Decreased overall collagen levels

Q.9. Activation of what enzyme(s) is responsible for emphysema?

    A. Antitrypsin
    B. Epoxide hydrolase
    C. Elastase
    D. Hyaluronidase
    E. Non-specific proteases

Q.10. Which of the following measurements would *not* be expected from a patient with restrictive lung disease?

    A. Decreased FRC
    B. Decreased RV
    C. Increased VC
    D. Decreased FEV1
    E. Impaired ventilation

Answers
1. D. 2. B. 3. D. 4. E. 5. D. 6. B.
7. D. 8. A. 9. C. 10. C.

7   Neurotoxicity

7.1   Problem-Solving Study Questions

Q. What is neurotoxicity?
Neurotoxicity refers to damage/or toxic effect to nervous system.

Q. What are neurotoxins?
Neurotoxins are an extensive class of exogenous chemical neurological insults that can adversely affect function in both developing and mature nervous tissue. These toxins may cause narcosis, behavioral changes, and decreased muscle coordination. The term can also be used to classify endogenous compounds, which, when abnormally contact, can prove neurologically toxic. Common examples of neurotoxins include lead, ethanol (drinking alcohol), manganese, glutamate, nitric oxide (NO), botulinum toxin (e.g., Botox), tetanus toxin, and tetrodotoxin, mercury, carbon disulfide, benzene, carbon tetrachloride, lead, mercury, and nitrobenzene.

Q. What are the functions of the nervous system?
Functions of the nervous system include motor, sensory, autonomic, and cognitive capabilities.

Q. What are common symptoms of neurotoxicity?
Neurotoxicity is a cause of brain damage. Common symptoms can include problems with memory, concentration, reaction time, sleep, thinking, language, as well as depression, confusion, personality changes, fatigue, and numbness of the hands and feet.

Q. How intercellular communication is achieved in the nervous system through the synapse.
Intercellular communication is achieved in the nervous system through the synapse. Neurotransmitters release from one neuron act as the first messenger. Binding of the transmitter to the postsynaptic receptor is followed by modulation of an ion channel for activation of a second-messenger system, leading to changes in the responding cell. Various therapeutic drugs and toxic compounds impact the process of neurotransmission.

Q. What are the factors relevant to neurodegenerative diseases?
Epidemiological studies indicate implication of exposure to several compounds such as pesticides, and metals act as risk factors for Parkinson's disease (PD). Environmental chemicals may cause heritable alterations in gene expression in the absence of changes in genome sequences.
Studies also suggest that miRNAs may be targeted by neurotoxicants, thus potentially affecting a broad spectrum of functions, encompassing cell differentiation and migration, neurogenesis, as well as synaptic function, to name a few.

Q. What are the basic components for the mechanisms of neurotoxicity?
Individual neurotoxic compounds typically have one of four targets: the neuron, the axon, the myelinating cell, or the neurotransmitter system.

Q. What are neuronopathies?
Certain toxicants are specific for neurons, resulting in their injury or death. Neuron loss is irreversible and includes degeneration of all of its cytoplasmic extensions, dendrites and axons, and the myelin ensheathing the axon.

Q. What are chemicals associated with neuronal injury (neuronopathies)?
A large number of compounds are known to result in toxic neuronopathies' all of these

toxicants share certain features. Each toxic condition is the result of a cellular toxicant that has a predilection for neurons. The initial injury to neurons is followed by apoptosis or necrosis, leading to permanent loss of the neuron. Important chemicals for neural injury include aluminum, arsenic, bismuth, carbon monoxide, carbon tetrachloride, chloramphenicol, cyanide, metals (lead, manganese, inorganic mercury, organic mercury–methylmercury), quinine, etc.

Q. What is axonopathy?

The neurotoxic disorders termed axonopathies are those in which the primary site of toxicity is the axon itself. The axon degenerates and with it the myelin surrounding that axon; however, the neuron cell body remains intact.

Q. What are chemicals associated with axonal injury (axonopathies)?

Several chemicals are known to be associated with axonal injury (axonopathies). The most significant exposures of humans to CS2 have occurred in the vulcan rubber and viscose rayon industries. High-level exposures of humans to CS2 cause a distal axonopathy that is identical pathologically to that cause by hexane. Other examples include acrylamide, carbon disulfide, clioquinol, colchicine, gold, nitrofurantoin, organophosphorus compounds (NTE inhibitors), vincristine (vinca alkaloids), etc.

Q. What is myelinopathy?

Myelin provides electrical insulation of neuronal processes, and its absence leads to a slowing of conduction and aberrant conduction of impulses between adjacent processes. Toxicants exist that result in the separation of the myelin lamellae, termed intramyelinic edema, and in the selective loss of myelin, termed demyelination. Intramyelinic edema may be caused by alterations in the transcript levels of myelin basic protein mRNA, and early its evolution is reversible. Demyelination may result from progressive intramyelinic edema or from direct toxicity to the myelinating cell.

Q. What is the neurotransmission-associated neurotoxicity?

A wide variety of naturally occurring toxins, as well as synthetic chemicals, alter specific mechanisms of intercellular communication. Although neurotransmitter-associated actions may be well understood for some agents, the specificity of the mechanisms should not be assumed. For example, nicotine, cocaine and amphetamines, excitatory amino acid s-glutamate and certain other acidic amino acids, manganese, etc. are known to cause neurotransmission-associated neurotoxicity.

7.2 Sample MCQ's

(Choose the correct statement, it may be one, two or more, or none.)

Q.1. Which of the following statements regarding the PNS and the CNS is *true*?

A. Nerve impulse transduction is much faster in the CNS than in the PNS.
B. PNS axons can regenerate, whereas CNS axons cannot.
C. Remyelination does not occur in the CNS.
D. Oligodendrocytes perform remyelination in the PNS.
E. In the CNS, oligodendrocyte scarring interferes with axonal regeneration.

Q.2. Platinum (cisplatin) results in which of the following neurologic problems?

A. Peripheral neuropathy
B. Trigeminal neuralgia
C. Spasticity
D. Gait ataxia
E. Tremor

Q.3. Which of the following is *NOT* character-istic of axonopathies?

A. There is degeneration of the axon.
B. The cell body of the neuron remains intact.
C. Axonopathies result from chemical transaction of the axon.
D. A majority of axonal toxicants caused motor deficits.
E. Sensory and motor deficits are first noticed in the hands and feet follow-ing axonal degeneration.

Q.4. All of the following statements regarding lead exposure are true *except* ---

A. Lead exposure results in peripheral neuropathy.
B. Lead slows peripheral nerve conduc-tion in humans.
C. Lead causes the transection of periph-eral axons.
D. Segmental demyelination is a com-mon result of lead ingestion.
E. Lead toxicity can result in anemia.

Q.5. Regarding excitatory amino acids, which of the following statements is *false*?

A. Glutamate is the most common excit-atory amino acid in the CNS.
B. Excitotoxicity has been linked to con-ditions such as epilepsy.
C. Overconsumption of monosodium glutamate (MSG) can result in a tin-gling or burning sensation in the face and neck.
D. An ionotropic glutamate receptor is couple to a G protein.
E. Glutamate is toxic to neurons.

Q.6. Which of the following statements regarding axons and/or axonal transport is *false*?

A. Single nerve cells can be over 1 m in length.

B. Fast axonal transport is responsible for movement of proteins from the cell body to the axon.
C. Anterograde transport is accomplished by the protein kinesin.
D. The motor proteins, kinesin and dynein, are associated with microtubules.
E. A majority of the ATP in nerve cells is used for axonal transport.

Q.7. Which of the following statements is not characteristic of Schwann cells in Wallerian degeneration?

A. Schwann cells provide physical guid-ance needed for the regrowth of the axon.
B. Schwann cells release trophic factors that stimulate growth.
C. Schwann cells act to clear the myelin fibers with the help of macrophages.
D. Schwann cells increase synthesis of myelin lipids in response to axonal damage.
E. Schwann cells are responsible for myelination of axons in the peripheral nervous system.

Q.8. Prenatal exposure to ethanol can result in mental retardation and hearing deficits in the newborn. What is the cellular basis of the neurotoxicity?

A. Neuronal loss in cerebellum
B. Acute cortical hemorrhage
C. Microcephaly
D. Loss of hippocampal neurons
E. Degeneration of the basal ganglia

Q.9. Which of the following characteristics is *least* likely to place a neuron at risk of toxic damage?

A. High metabolic rate
B. Ability to release neurotransmitters
C. Long neuronal processes supported by the soma
D. Excitable membranes
E. Large surface area

Q.10. The use of meperidine contaminate with MPTP will result in a Parkinson's disease like neurotoxicity. Where is the most likely site in the brain that MPTP exerts its toxic effects?

A. Cerebellum
B. Cerebral cortex
C. Brainstem
D. Substantia nigra
E. Hippocampus

Answers
1. B.   2. A.   3. D.   4. C.   5. D.   6. E.
7. D.   8. C.   9. B.   10. D.

---

8   Cardiovascular Toxicity

8.1   Problem-Solving Study Questions

Q. What is cardiovascular toxicity?
Cardiovascular toxicology is concerned with the adverse effects of extrinsic and intrinsic stresses on the heart and vascular system.

Q. What is extrinsic stress?
Extrinsic stress involves exposure to therapeutic drugs, natural products, and environmental toxicants. These toxic exposures result in alterations in biochemical pathways, defects in cellular structure and function, and pathogenesis of the affected cardiovascular system.

Q. What is intrinsic stress?
Intrinsic stress refers to exposure to toxic metabolites derived from nontoxic compounds such as those found in food additives and supplements. The intrinsic exposures also include secondary neurohormonal disturbance such as overproduction of inflammatory cytokines derived from pressure overload of the heart and counter-regulatory responses to hypertension. These toxic exposures result in alterations in biochemical pathways, defects in cellular structure and function, and pathogenesis of the affected cardiovascular system.

Q. What are the basic concepts in cardiac-induced toxic responses?
There is some interaction between environmental stresses and the heart and the balance between myocardial protection and deleterious dose and time effects (Fig. 7.1); chemicals can lead to heart failure without heart hypertrophy; a chemical can lead to activation of both protective and destructive responses in the myocardium; and long-term toxicologic responses often result in maladaptive hypertrophy, which primes the heart or malignant arrhythmia, leading to sudden cardiac death or transition to heart failure.

Q. What are myocardial degeneration and regeneration?
Myocardial degeneration is the ultimate response of the heart to toxic exposure, which can be measured by both morphologic and

Fig. 7.1 Triangle analytical model of cardiac responses to drugs and xenobiotics

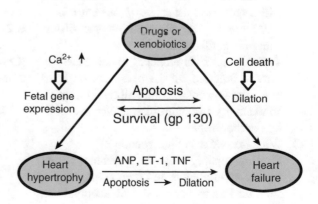

functional degenerative phenotypes. The heart was previously considered incapable of regenerating. However, evidence now indicates myocardial regeneration, and recovery from cardiomyopathy is possible in some instances.

Explanation: Drugs or xenobiotics can directly cause both heart failure and heart hypertrophy. Under severe acute toxic insults, myocardial cell death becomes the predominant response leading to cardiac dilation and heart failure. In most cases, myocardial survival mechanisms can be activated so that myocardial apoptosis is inhibited. The survived cardiomyocytes often become hypertrophy through activation of calcium-mediated fetal gene expression and other hypertrophic program. If toxic insult continues, the counter-regulatory mechanisms against heart hypertrophy such as activation of cytokine-medicated pathways eventually lead to myocardial cell death through apoptosis or necrosis, dilated cardiomyopathy, and heart failure.

Q. What is myocardial adaptation?

Myocardial adaptation refers to the general process by which the ventricular myocardium changes in structure and function. This process is often referred to as "remodeling." In response to pathologic stimuli, such as exposure to environmental toxicants, myocardial remodeling is adaptive in the short term, but is maladaptive in the long term, and often results in further myocardial dysfunction. The central feature of myocardial remodeling is an increase in myocardial mass associated with a change in the shape of the ventricle.

Q. What are typical chemical-induced disturbances in cardiac function?

Typical chemical-induced disturbances in cardiac function consist of effects on heart rate (chronotropic), contractility (inotropic), conductivity (dromotropic), and/or excitability (bathmotropic).

Q. What is typical cardiomyopathy?

Cardiomyopathy includes morphologic and functional alterations induced by toxic exposure, leading to decreased cardiac output and peripheral tissue hypoperfusion.

Q. What is concentric cardiac hypertrophy?

Concentric cardiac hypertrophy is an increased size of cardiac myocytes in which new contractile-protein units are assembled in parallel, resulting in a relative increase in the width of individual cardiac myocytes.

Q. What is heart failure?

Heart failure is the inability of the heart to maintain cardiac output sufficient to meet the metabolic and oxygen demands of peripheral tissues, including changes in systolic and diastolic function that reflect specific alterations in ventricular function and abnormalities in a variety of subcellular processes.

Q. What are cardiotoxic chemicals having primary concern?

Many substances can cause cardiac toxic responses directly or indirectly. However, only chemicals that primarily act on the heart or whose cardiac toxicity is established include:

(a) Alcohol and alcoholic cardiomyopathy, e.g., alcohol and ethanol

(b) Pharmaceutical chemicals, e.g., drugs used to treat cardiac disease such as digitalis, quinidine, and procainamide, and noncardiac such as anthracyclines and adriamycin

(c) Natural products such as catecholamines, hormones, and cytokines, as well as animal and plant toxins

(d) Environmental pollutants and industrial chemicals such as metals and metalloids, heavy metals, and cadmium

8.2   Sample MCQ's

(Choose the correct statement, it may be one, two or more, or none.)

Q.1. Which of the following is associated with pathological hypertrophy of the heart?

A. Hypertension
B. Exercise
C. Pregnancy
D. None of the above

Q.2. Myocardial accumulation of collagen is *not* associated with -------

    A. Ischemic cardiomyopathy
    B. Myocardial infarction
    C. Pathological hypertrophy
    D. Adaptive hypertrophy

Q.3. Counter-regulatory mechanism in response to compensatory mechanisms to cardiac hypertrophy lead to -----------

    A. Decrease in heart size
    B. Myocardial remodeling
    C. Decrease in cardiac fibrosis
    D. Decrease in salt/water retention

Q.4. Inflammatory lesions in the vascular system are termed -------------

    A. Vasculitis
    B. Embolitis
    C. Thrombitis
    D. Angio-inflammation

Q.5. The most prevalent vascular structural injury is --------------

    A. Capillary hyperplasia
    B. Varicose veins
    C. Angioma
    D. Atherosclerosis

Q.6. Cardiac glycosides like digoxin ------------

    A. Increase the sensitivity of myocytes to calcium.
    B. Inhibit sodium/potassium ATPase.
    C. Causes sinus tachycardia.
    D. Inhibit sympathetic outflow at high doses.

Q.7. Which of the following is the most sensitive clinical indicator of myocardial cell damage?

    A. Urine CPK
    B. Serum troponin

    C. Serum ALT
    D. Serum creatinine

Q.8. Which of the following is an indicator of fluid overload in congestive heart failure----?

    A. Urine pH
    B. Serum CPK
    C. Brain natriuretic peptide (BNP)
    D. First-degree AV block on ECG

Q.9. Moxifloxacin is associated with ----------

    A. Acute congestive heart failure
    B. Prolongation of the QT interval
    C. Coronary artery thrombotic events
    D. Toxic cardiomyopathy

Q.10. COX-2 inhibits presumably increase the risk for cardiovascular events by causing -----------

    A. Heart block
    B. Systolic dysfunction
    C. Toxic cardiomyopathy
    D. Coronary artery thrombotic events

Answers
1. A. 2. D. 3. B. 4. A. 5. D. 6. B.
7. B. 8. C. 9. B. 10. D.

9 Hematotoxicity

9.1 Problem-Solving Study Questions

Q. What is hematotoxicology?
Hematotoxicology is the study of adverse effects of exogenous chemicals on blood and blood-forming tissues.

Q. What type of direct or indirect damage to blood cells and their precursors is observed after exposure to various toxicants?
Direct or indirect damage to blood cells and their precursors includes tissue hypoxia, hemorrhage, and infection.

Q. What is aplastic anemia?

Aplastic anemia is a life-threatening disorder characterized by peripheral blood pancytopenia, reticulocytopenia, and bone marrow hypoplasia.

Q. What is agranulocytosis?

Agranulocytosis may involve a sudden depletion of circulating neutrophils concomitant with exposure that persists as long as the agent or its metabolites are in the circulation.

Q. What is leukemia?

Leukemia is proliferative disorder of hematopoietic tissue that originates from individual bone marrow cells.

Q. What is thrombocytopenia?

Thrombocytopenia may result from increased platelet destruction or decreased platelet production, which lead to decreased platelet aggregation and bleeding disorders.

Q. What is blood coagulation?

Blood coagulation is a complex process involving a number of proteins whose synthesis and function can be altered by many xenobiotics.

Q. How do abnormalities in hemoglobin synthesis take place?

Abnormalities that lead to decreased hemoglobin synthesis are relatively common (e.g., iron deficiency). An imbalance between α- and β-chain production is the basis of congenital thalassemia syndromes and results in decreased hemoglobin production and microcytosis. Xenobiotics can affect globin chain synthesis and alter the composition of hemoglobin within erythrocytes.

Q. What are xenobiotics associated with sideroblastic anemia?

Most common xenobiotics associated with sideroblastic anemia include chloramphenicol, isoniazid, copper chelation or deficiency, lead intoxication, cycloserine, pyrazinamide, ethanol, and zinc intoxication.

Q. What is hematopoiesis?

The *hematopoietic* system, which comprises all the cellular components of the blood, is one of the earliest organ systems to evolve during embryo development.

Q. Where does hematopoiesis occur?

Hematopoiesis is the production of all types of blood cells including formation, development, and differentiation of blood cells. Prenatally, hematopoiesis occurs in the yolk sack, then in the liver, and lastly in the bone marrow.

Q. How does hematopoiesis occur?

Hematopoiesis requires active DNA synthesis and frequent mitoses. Folate and vitamin B12 are necessary to maintain synthesis of thymidine or incorporation into DNA. Deficiency of folate and/or vitamin B12 results in megaloblastic anemia, a result of improper cell division.

Q. What are the mechanisms of toxic neutropenia?

In immune-mediated neutropenia, antigen–antibody reactions lead to destruction of peripheral neutrophils, granulocyte precursors, or both. As with RBCs, an immunogenic xenobiotic can act as a hapten, where the agent must be physically present to cause cell damage or, alternatively, may induce immunogenic cells to produce antineutrophil antibodies that do not require the drug to be present. Nonimmune-mediated toxic neutropenia often shows a genetic predisposition. Direct damage may cause inhibition of granulopoiesis or neutrophil function.

Q. What are human leukemias?

Leukemias are proliferative disorders of hematopoietic tissue that are monoclonal and originate from individual bone marrow cells. Historically they have been classified as myeloid or lymphoid, referring to the major lineages or erythrocytes, granulocytes, thrombocytes, or lymphocytes, respectively.

Q. What is acute lymphoblastic leukemia?

Poorly differentiated phenotypes have been designated as "acute," including acute lymphoblastic leukemia (ALL) and acute myelogenous leukemia (AML).

Q. What are chronic" leukemias?

Chronic" leukemias are well-differentiated which include chronic lymphocytic leukemia (CLL), chronic myelogenous leukemia

(CML), and the myelodysplastic syndromes (MDS).

Q. How do oral anticoagulants interfere with vitamin K metabolism?

Oral anticoagulants (e.g., warfarin) interfere with vitamin K metabolism by preventing the reduction of vitamin K epoxide, resulting in a functional deficiency of reduced vitamin K. These drugs are widely used for prophylaxis and therapy of venous and arterial thrombosis.

9.2 Sample MCQ's

(Choose the correct statement, it may be one, two or more, or none.)

Q.1. All of the following statements regarding oxidative hemolysis are true *except* -----

A. Reactive oxygen species are commonly generated by RBC metabolism.
B. Superoxide dismutase and catalase are enzymes that protect against oxidative damage.
C. Reduced glutathione (GSH) increases the likelihood of oxidative injuries to RBCs.
D. Glucose-6-phosphate dehydrogenase deficiency is commonly associated with oxidative hemolysis.
E. Xenobiotics can cause oxidative injury to RBCs by overcoming the protective mechanisms of the cell.

Q.2. Which of the following sets of leukocytes is properly characterized as granulocytes because of the appearance of cytoplasmic granules on a blood smear?

A. Neutrophils, basophils, and monocytes
B. Basophils, eosinophils, and lymphocytes
C. Eosinophils, neutrophils, and lymphocytes
D. Basophils, eosinophils, and neutrophils
E. Lymphocytes, neutrophils, and basophils

Q.3. All of the following statements are true *except*-----

A. Xenobiotics can greatly slow down the proliferation of neutrophils and monocytes, increasing the risk of infection.
B. Ethanol and cortisol decrease phagocytosis and microbe ingestion by the immune system.
C. Agranulocytosis is predictable and can be caused by exposure to a number of environmental toxins.
D. Heroin and methadone abusers have reduced ability to kill microorganisms due to drug-induced reduction in superoxide production.
E. *Toxic neutropenia may be mediated by the immune system.*

Q.4. Leukemias

A. Are often due to cytogenetic abnormalities, particularly damage to or loss of chromosomes 8 and 11.
B. Are rarely caused by agents used in cancer chemotherapy.
C. Originate in circulating blood cells.
D. Are characterized as "acute," and their effects are short-lived and severe.
E. Have long been associated with exposure to X-ray radiation.

Q.5. Regarding platelets and thrombocytopenia, which of the following statements is *false*?

A. Platelets can be removed from the circulation through a hapten-mediated pathway that is induced by drugs or chemicals.
B. Cortisol decreases platelet activity by inhibiting thromboxane prostaglandin synthesis.
C. *Toxins can induce a change in a platelet membrane glycoprotein, leading to recognition and removal of the platelet by phagocytes.*

D. Heparin administration can result in platelet aggregation and cause thrombocytopenia.

E. Thrombotic thrombocytopenic purpura is most commonly caused by infectious disease but can also be associated with administration of pharmacologic agents.

Q.6. Which of the following statements is *false* regarding true anemia?

A. Alterations of the mean corpuscular volume are characteristic of anemia.

B. Increased destruction of erythrocytes can lead to anemia.

C. Decreased production of erythrocytes is not a common cause of anemia because the bone marrow is continuously renewing the red blood cell pool.

D. Reticulocytes will live for a longer period of time in the peripheral blood when a person is anemic.

E. The main parameters in diagnosing anemia are RBC count, hemoglobin concentration, and hematocrit.

Q.7. Which of the following types of anemia is properly paired with its cause?

A. Iron deficiency anemia—blood loss

B. Sideroblastic anemia—vitamin B12 deficiency

C. Megaloblastic anemia—folate supplementation

D. Aplastic anemia—ethanol

E. Megaloblastic anemia—lead poisoning

Q.8. The inability to synthesize the porphyrin ring of hemoglobin will most likely result in which of the following?

A. Iron deficiency anemia

B. Improper RBC mitosis

C. Inability to synthesize thymidine

D. Accumulation of iron within erythroblasts

E. Bone marrow hypoplasia

Q.9. Which of the following will cause a right shift in the oxygen dissociation curve?

A. Increased pH

B. Decreased carbon dioxide concentration

C. Decreased body temperature

D. Increased 2,3-BPG concentration

E. Fetal hemoglobin

Q.10. All of the following statements regarding erythrocytes are true *except*-----

A. Aged erythrocytes are removed by the liver, where the iron is recycled.

B. Erythrocytes have a life span of approximately 120 days.

C. Red blood cells generally lose their nuclei before entering the circulation.

D. Reticulocytes are immature RBCs that still have a little RNA.

E. Persons with anemia have a higher than normal reticulocyte: erythrocyte ratio.

Answers

1. C.   2. D.   3. C.   4. E.   5. B.   6. C.
7. A.   8. D.   9. D.   10. A.

---

10   Ocular and Visual System Toxicity

10.1   Problem-Solving Study Questions

Q. Why the eye is highly vulnerable to local contacts of chemicals, toxins, pollutants, and occupational hazards and to toxic reactions of systemic agents?

The eye is highly vulnerable because it is exposed to the outside environment and perfused extensively by a rich blood supply.

Q. What part of the eye is most affected after exposure to chemicals?

Toxic chemicals and systemic drugs can affect all parts of the eye, including cornea, iris, ciliary body, lens retina, and optic nerve.

Q. What are common symptoms of ocular toxicity?

Ocular toxicity results from direct contact or after exposure to any toxicant that leads to conjunctivitis, corneal damage, etc.

Q. What are the factors that determine chemicals to reach a particular ocular site of action?

There are numerous barriers that restrict bioavailability, decrease therapeutic efficacy, and increase side effects. Development of nanoscale preparations or drug delivery is a new approach to drug delivery which can substantially enhance penetration from the cornea, deliver a wide variety of drugs and molecules, and increase the concentration and contact time of drugs with these tissues. Other common factors include:

(a) Physiochemical properties of the chemical
(b) Concentration and duration of exposure
(c) Movement across ocular compartments
(d) Barriers

The cornea, conjunctiva, and eyelids are often exposed directly to chemicals, gases, drugs, and particles.

Q. Describe briefly ocular drug metabolism?

Metabolism of xenobiotics occurs in all compartments of the eye by well-known Phase I and II xenobiotic-biotransforming enzymes. The activity of drug-metabolizing enzymes that are present in the tears, iris–ciliary body, choroid, and retina of many different species vary. The whole lens has low biotransformational activity.

Q. What arc important oxidizing agents that can cause damage to the eye?

The most important oxidizing agents are visible light and UV radiation, particularly UV A (320–400 nm) and UV-B (290–320 nm), and other forms of electromagnetic radiation. Light- and UV-induced photooxidation leads to generation of reactive oxygen species (ROS) and oxidative damage that can accumulate over time. Higher-energy UV-C (100–290 nm) is even more damaging. At sea level the atmosphere filters out virtually all UV-C and all but a small fraction of UV-B derived from solar radiance.

Q. Describe standard procedures for ocular irritancy and toxicity?

Draize test, with some additions and revisions, has formed the basis of standard procedures employed for evaluating ocular irritation and safety evaluations. Traditionally, albino rabbits are the subjects evaluated in the Draize test. This test has been criticized on several grounds, including high interlaboratory variability, the subjective nature of the scoring, poor predictive value for human irritants, and for causing undue pain and distress to the tested animals. These criticisms have spawned development of alternative methods or strategies to evaluate compounds or their potential to cause ocular irritation.

10.2 Sample MCQ's

(Choose the correct statement, it may be one, two or more, or none.)

Q.1. Which of the following statements regarding color vision deficits is *false*?

A. Inheritance of a blue–yellow color deficit is common.
B. Bilateral deficits in the visual cortex can lead to color blindness.
C. Disorders of the outer retina produce blue–yellow deficits.
D. Drug and chemical exposure most commonly results in blue–yellow color deficits.
E. Disorders of the optic nerve produce red–green deficits.

Q.2. A substance with which of the following pH values would be most damaging to the cornea?

A. 1.0
B. 3.0
C. 7.0
D. 10.0
E. 12.0

Q.3. Which of the following statements concerning the lens is *false*?

  A. UV radiation exposure is a common environmental risk factor for developing cataracts.
  B. Cataracts are opacities to the lens that can occur at any age.
  C. The lens continues to grow throughout one's life.
  D. Naphthalene and organic solvents both can cause cataracts.
  E. Topical treatment with corticosteroids can cause cataracts.

Q.4. Which of the following is *NOT* a reason why the retina is highly vulnerable to toxicant-induced damage?

  A. Presence of numerous neurotransmitter systems
  B. Presence of melanin in the RPE
  C. High choroidal blood flow rate
  D. High rate of oxidative mitochondrial metabolism
  E. Lack of gap junctions

Q.5. A deficiency in which of the following vitamins can result in degeneration of optic nerve fibers?

  A. Vitamin A
  B. Vitamin B3
  C. Vitamin C
  D. Vitamin B12
  E. Vitamin E

Q.6. In which of the following locations would one *not* find melanin?

  A. Iris
  B. Ciliary body
  C. Retinal pigment epithelium (RPE)
  D. Uveal tract
  E. Sclera

Q.7. Systemic exposure to drugs and chemicals is most likely to target which of the following retinal sites?

  A. RPE and ganglion cell layer
  B. Optic nerve and inner plexiform layer
  C. RPE and photoreceptors
  D. Photoreceptors and ganglion cell layer
  E. Inner plexiform layer and RPE

Q.8. Which of the following structures is *not* part of the ocular fundus?

  A. Retina
  B. Lens
  C. Choroid
  D. Sclera
  E. Optic nerve

Q.9. Drugs and chemicals in systemic blood have better access to which of the following sites because of the presence of loose endothelial junctions at that location?

  A. Retinal choroid
  B. Inner retina
  C. Optic nerve
  D. Iris
  E. Ciliary body

Q.10. All of the following statements regarding ocular irritancy and toxicity are true *except* ---

  A. The Draize test involves instillation of a potentially toxic liquid or solid into the eye.
  B. The effect of the irritant in the Draize test is scored on a weighted scale of the cornea, iris, and conjunctiva.
  C. The Draize test usually uses one eye for testing and the other as a control.
  D. The Draize test has strong predictive value in humans.
  E. The cornea is evaluated for opacity and area of involvement in the Draize test.

Answers
1. A.   2. E.   3. D.   4. E.   5. D.   6. E.
7. C.   8. B.   9. A.   10. D.

11 Dermal Toxicity

11.1 Problem-Solving Study Questions

Q. What is dermal toxicity?

Dermal toxicity is the ability of a substance to cause local reaction and/or systemic poisoning in people or animals by contact with the skin.

Q. Define the role of the skin in the body.

The skin protects the body against external insults in order to maintain internal homeostasis. It participates directly in thermal, electrolyte, hormonal, metabolic, and immune regulation. Skin acts as barrier by repelling noxious physical agents and may react to them with various defensive mechanisms that serve to prevent internal or widespread cutaneous damage.

Q. What are the three main factors that influence cutaneous responses?

Three main factors that influence cutaneous responses are:

(a) A variety of intrinsic and extrinsic factors including body site
(b) Duration of exposure
(c) Environmental conditions

Q. What are the main factors for absorption of toxic materials through the skin?

Absorption of substances through the skin depends on a number of factors, the most important of which are concentration, duration of contact, solubility of medication, and physical condition of the skin and part of the body exposed.

Q. Describe in brief the process of biotransformation in the skin.

The ability of the skin to metabolize agents that diffuse through the skin depends upon its barrier functions. This influences the potential biological activity of chemicals and topically applied drugs, leading to their degradation or their activation as skin sensitizers or carcinogens. The epidermis and pilosebaceous units are the major sites of such activity in the skin. Enzymes participating in

biotransformation that are expressed in the skin include multiple forms of cytochrome P450, epoxide hydrolase, UDP-glucuronosyltransferase, quinone reductase, and glutathione transferases. Other metabolic enzyme activities detected in human epidermal cells include sulfatases; β-corneum has catabolic activities (e.g., proteases, lipases, glycosidases, and phosphatase).

Q. What is contact dermatitis?

Contact dermatitis may be irritant or an allergic form. Both involve inflammatory processes and can have indistinguishable clinical characteristics of erythema (redness), induration (thickening and firmness), scaling (flaking), and vesiculation (blistering) on areas directly contacting the chemical agent.

Q. What are the symptoms of primary irritant dermatitis?

Primary irritant dermatitis is caused by chemical substances that directly irritate the skin (like caustic acids or bases). The symptoms may be similar to a *slight* burn (*redness*, *itching*, *pain*) or as severe as blisters, with peeling and open wounds (ulcerations). The absorption of toxic materials through the skin depends on various degrees, on their chemical composition, and solubility.

Q. What are chemical burns?

Extremely corrosive and reactive chemicals may produce immediate coagulative necrosis that results in substantial tissue damage, with ulceration and sloughing. In third-degree chemical burn, the damage does not have a primary inflammatory component and thus may not be classified as an irritant reaction because it leads to necrotic tissue. Necrotic tissue can act as a chemical reservoir resulting in either continued cutaneous damage for percutaneous absorption and systemic injury after exposure.

Q. Give examples of some selected chemicals causing skin burns.

Examples of selected chemicals causing skin burns include ammonia, calcium oxide (CaO), chlorine, ethylene oxide, hydrogen chloride (HCl), hydrogen fluoride (HF), hydrogen peroxide, methyl bromide, nitrogen oxides, phosphorus, phenol, sodium hydroxide, toluene diisocyanate, etc.

Q. What is allergic contact dermatitis?

Allergic contact dermatitis (ACD) is a form of contact dermatitis that is the manifestation of an allergic response caused by contact with a substance that irritates the skin or triggers an allergic reaction. The substance could be one of thousands of known allergens and irritants.

Q. What are granulomatous reactions?

A granulomatous reaction to a foreign body is one in which invading substances that cannot be readily removed are consequently isolated. These occur infrequently toward a variety of agents introduced into the skin through injection or after laceration or abrasion. Persistent lesions with abundant inflammatory cells can be produced, resembling chronic infectious conditions (e.g., tuberculosis, leprosy, leishmaniasis, and syphilis),

Q. What are adverse responses to electromagnetic/UV radiation exposure?

The most evident acute feature of UV radiation exposure is erythema (redness or sunburn). The smallest dose of UV light needed to induce an erythematous response varies greatly from person to person. Vasodilation responsible for the color change is accompanied by significant alterations in inflammatory mediators released from local inflammatory cells as well as from injured keratinocytes and may be responsible for several of the systemic symptoms associated with sunburn, such as fever, chills, and malaise. Environmental conditions that affect UV-induced injury include duration of exposure, season, altitude, body site, skin pigmentation, and previous exposure.

Q. What is photosensitivity?

Photosensitivity is an abnormal sensitivity to UV and visible light. It may result from endogenous or exogenous factors and various genetic diseases (such as xeroderma pigmentosum).

Q. What are hereditary or chemically induced porphyrias?

In hereditary or chemically induced porphyrias, enzyme abnormalities disrupt the biosynthetic pathways producing heme, leading to accumulation of porphyrin precursors or derivatives throughout the body.

Q. What is toxic epidermal necrolysis?

Toxic epidermal necrolysis (TEN) represents one of the most life-threatening dermatologic diseases that is caused by drugs and chemicals. At the most severe end of a spectrum, TEN involves detachment of $\geq 30\%$ of the epidermal surface from the dermis, commonly accompanied by severe erosions of mucous membranes, and has a fatality rate $\approx 30\%$. TEN commonly resembles an upper respiratory tract infection.

Q. Which substances are responsible for toxic epidermal necrolysis?

Nearly 200 drugs have been reported to cause this syndrome with major contributors being anticonvulsants, nonsteroidal anti-inflammatories, antibacterial sulfonamides, allopurinol, and nevirapine. Mechanisms leading to this idiosyncratic drug reaction are under scrutiny, and current hypotheses identify HLA genotype and ethnic background as contributing factors.

Q. What is the characteristic feature of toxic epidermal necrolysis syndrome?

A characteristic feature of the syndrome is the large-scale apoptosis of epidermal keratinocytes. Candidates for mediating apoptosis through cell surface death receptors include tumor necrosis factor and FAS ligand, which appear elevated; in addition, drug-sensitized natural killer and cytotoxic T lymphocytes, secreting granulysin, and other components of the innate immune response may participate in inducing keratinocyte death.

11.2 Sample MCQ's

(Choose the correct statement, it may be one, two or more, or none.)

Q.1. Acne is caused by all of the following *except*---

A. Clogged sebaceous glands
B. Hormones
C. Viruses
D. Genetics
E. Environmental factors

Q.2. Transdermal drug delivery does *not*----

A. Prevent drug exposure to low pH.
B. Avoid first-pass metabolism.
C. Provide steady infusion over an extended period of time.
D. Avoid large variation in drug plasma concentration.
E. Increase safety of drug delivery.

Q.3. Irritant and contact dermatitis are marked by all of the following characteristics *except*----

A. Softness
B. Erythema
C. Flaking
D. Induration
E. Blistering

Q.4. Nickel is a common cause of allergic contact dermatitis, which type of hypersensitivity reaction is this?

A. Type I
B. Type II
C. Type III
D. Type IV
E. Type V

Q.5. All of the following statements regarding phototoxicology are true *except*-----

A. Melanin is primarily responsible for the absorption of UV-B radiation.
B. UV-A is the most effective at causing sunburn in humans.
C. IL-1 release is responsible for systemic symptoms associated with sunburn.
D. Melanin darkening is a common response to UV exposure.
E. UV radiation exposure causes thickening of the stratum corneum.

Q.6. Photoallergies ----

A. Represent a form of type III hypersensitivity reaction.
B. Can occur without exposure to UV radiation.
C. Are hapten-mediated.
D. Cannot be tested or as contact dermatitis allergies can.
E. Often occur on first exposure.

Q.7. Diffusion through the epidermis would occur most slowly across the skin at which of the following locations?

A. Palm
B. Forehead
C. Scrotum
D. Foot sole
E. Abdomen

Q.8. Which of the following statements regarding photosensitivity is *false*?

A. Porphyrias cause light sensitivity because of the lack of heme synthesis.
B. Lupus patients are unable to repair damage caused by UV light.
C. Chronic phototoxic responses often result in hyperpigmentation.
D. Photoallergy represents a type IV hypersensitivity reaction.
E. UV radiation causes cycloadducts between pyrimidine bases.

Q.9. Which of the following statements is *false* regarding skin histology?

A. Blood supply to the epidermis originates in the epidermal–dermal junction.
B. Melanin is made and stored by melanocytes.

C. The stratum corneum is made up of nonviable cells.

D. It takes approximately 2 weeks for cells to be sloughed off from the stratum corneum.

E. Stem cells in the basal layer replenish the keratinocytes of the layers of epidermis.

Q.10. All of the following statements regarding urticaria are true *except* ----

A. Urticaria is a delayed-type hypersensitivity reaction.

B. Hives are mediated partly by histamine release from mast cells.

C. Latex is a common chemical cause of urticaria.

D. Select foods have been reported to elicit contact urticaria.

E. Urticaria is mediated by IgE antibodies.

Answers

1. C.   2. E.   3. A.   4. D.   5. B.   6. C.
7. D.   8. C.   9. B.   10. A.

12   Reproductive System Toxicity

12.1   Problem-Solving Study Questions

Q. What is reproduction toxicity?

Reproductive toxicity is a hazard associated with some chemical substances that interfere in some way with normal reproduction; such substances are called reprotoxic. It includes adverse effects on sexual function and fertility in adult males and females, as well as developmental toxicity in the offspring such as birth defects, sterility, etc.

Q. Draw a schematic diagram of processes of hormone regulation in the male and female reproductive through the hypothalamic-pituitary-gonadal (HPG) axis (Fig. 7.2).

Explanation: In females the hypothalamus, anterior pituitary gland, and gonads (ovaries) work together to regulate the menstrual cycle. Gonadotropin-releasing hormone (GnRH) from the hypothalamus stimulates luteinizing hormone (LH) and follicular-stimulating hormone (FSH) release from the anterior pituitary gland. LH and FSH are gonadotropins that act primarily on the ovaries in the female reproductive tract:

- FSH binds to granulosa cells to stimulate follicle growth, permit the conversion of androgens (from theca cells) to estrogens, and stimulate inhibin secretion.

- LH acts on theca cells to stimulate production and secretion of androgens.

- The menstrual cycle is controlled by feedback systems.

- Moderate estrogen levels: negative feedback on the HPG axis.

- High estrogen levels (in the absence of progesterone): positive feedback on the HPG axis.

- Estrogen in the presence of progesterone: negative feedback on the HPG axis.

- Inhibin: selectively inhibits FSH at the anterior pituitary.

Q. What are the functions of gonads?

The gonads possess a dual function: an endocrine function involving the secretion of sex hormones and a nonendocrine function relating to the production of germ cells (gametogenesis).

Q. Which hormones carry out gametogenic and secretory functions of the ovary or testes?

Gametogenic and secretory functions of either the ovary or testes are dependent on the secretion of follicle-stimulating hormone (FSH) and luteinizing hormone (LH) from the pituitary.

Q. Which barriers prevents the free exchange of chemicals/drugs between the blood and the fluid inside the seminiferous tubules?

The blood–testis barrier between the lumen of an interstitial capillary and the lumen of a seminiferous tubule impedes the free exchange of chemicals/drugs between the

Fig. 7.2 Processes of hormone regulation in the (**a**) male and (**b**) female reproductive systems. https://www.cliffsnotes.com/assets/277499.png

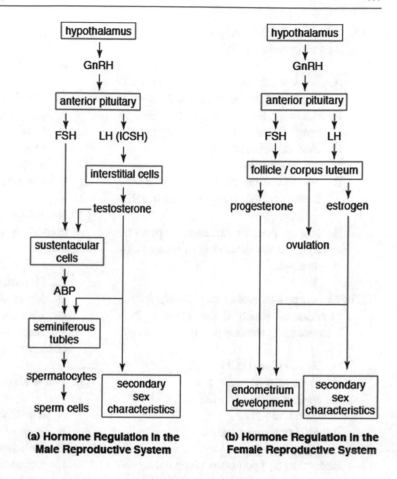

(a) Hormone Regulation in the Male Reproductive System

(b) Hormone Regulation in the Female Reproductive System

blood and the fluid inside the seminiferous tubules.

Q. In which gland or tissue biosynthesis of steroid hormone takes place?

Steroid hormone biosynthesis can occur in several endocrine organs including the adrenal cortex, ovary, and the testes.

Q. Which sites of female reproductive system do chemicals/xenobiotics interfere?

Usual sites with which xenobiotic interfere with the female reproductive system processes include oogenesis, ovulation, the development of sexual receptivity, coitus, gamete and zygote transport, fertilization, and implantation of the conceptus.

Q. Which sites of male reproductive system do chemicals/xenobiotics interfere?

Xenobiotics may influence male reproductive organ structure, spermatogenesis, androgen hormone secretion, and accessory organ function.

12.2   Sample MCQ's

(Choose the correct statement, it may be one, two or more, or none.)

Q.1. All of the following statements regarding the hypothalamo-pituitary-gonadal axis is true *except* ---

A. FSH increases testosterone production by the Leydig cells.
B. FSH and LH are synthesized in the anterior pituitary.
C. Estradiol provides negative feedback on the hypothalamus and the anterior pituitary.
D. GnRH from the hypothalamus increases FSH and LH release from the anterior pituitary.
E. The LH spike during the menstrual cycle is responsible for ovulation.

Q.2. Which of the following statements is *false* regarding gametal DNA repair?

  A. DNA repair in spermatogenic cells is dependent on the dose of chemical.
  B. Spermatogenic cells are less able to repair damage from alkylating agents.
  C. Female gametes have base excision repair capacity.
  D. Meiotic maturation of the oocyte decreases its ability to repair DNA damage.
  E. Mature oocytes and mature sperm no longer have the ability to repair DNA damage.

Q.3. The corpus luteum is responsible for the secretion of which of the following hormones during the first part of pregnancy?

  A. Estradiol and hCG
  B. Progesterone and estradiol
  C. Progesterone and hCG
  D. FSH and LH
  E. FSH and progesterone

Q.4. Reduction division takes place during the transition between which two cell types during spermatogenesis?

  A. Spermatogonium and primary spermatocyte
  B. Primary spermatocyte and secondary spermatocyte
  C. Secondary spermatocyte and spermatid
  D. Spermatid and spermatozoon
  E. Spermatozoon and mature sperm

Q.5. Which of the following cell types secretes anti-Müllerian hormone (AMH)?

  A. Spermatogonium
  B. Leydig cell
  C. Sertoli cell
  D. Primary spermatocyte
  E. Spermatid

Q.6. Which of the following cell types is properly paired with the substance that it secretes?

  A. Ovarian granulosa cells—progesterone
  B. Leydig cells—ABP
  C. Ovarian thecal cells—estrogens
  D. Sertoli cells—testosterone
  E. Gonadotrophin—LH

Q.7. Reduction of sperm production can be caused by all of the following diseases *except* ---

  A. Hypothyroidism
  B. Measles
  C. Crohn's disease
  D. Renal failure
  E. Mumps

Q.8. Penile erections are dependent on

  A. The CNS
  B. Sympathetic nerve stimulation
  C. Helicine (penile) artery constriction
  D. Corpora cavernosum smooth muscle relaxation
  E. A spinal reflex arc

Q.9. Of the following, which is *least* likely to be affected by estrogen?

  A. Nervous system
  B. Musculoskeletal system
  C. Digestive system
  D. Cardiovascular system
  E. Urinary system

Q.10. Which of the following statements regarding male reproductive capacity is *false*?

  A. Kline elder's syndrome males are sterile.
  B. FSH levels are often measured in order to determine male reproductive toxicity of a particular toxin.

C. Divalent metal ions, such as Hg and Cu, act as androgen receptor antagonists and affect male reproduction.

D. The number of sperms produced per day is approximately the same in all males.

E. ABP is an important biochemical marker for testicular injury.

Answers

1. A.   2. E.   3. B.   4. B.   5. C.   6. E.
7. B.   8. D.   9. C.   10. D.

---

13   Immune Modulation

13.1   Problem-Solving Study Questions

Q. Which is immunity?

Immunity is a condition of being able to resist a particular disease especially through preventing development of a pathogenic microorganism or by counteracting the effects of its products. It may be active immunity, natural immunity, or passive immunity.

Q. What are the main organs of the immune system?

The key primary lymphoid organs of the immune system include the thymus and bone marrow, as well as secondary lymphatic tissues including spleen, tonsils, lymph vessels, lymph nodes, adenoids, skin, and liver.

Q. What are the five parts of the immune system?

The main parts of the immune system are white blood cells, antibodies, the complement system, the lymphatic system, the spleen, the thymus, and the bone marrow.

Q. What are the four phases of the immune response?

The normal immune response can be broken down into four main components: pathogen recognition by cells of the innate immune system, with cytokine release, complement activation, and phagocytosis of antigens.

Q. What are accessory cells?

Accessory cells are nonlymphoid cells such as macrophages, dendritic cells, and Langerhans cells (epithelial dendritic cells) that function to present antigens to MHC-restricted T cells.

Q. What is acquired (adaptive) immunity?

If the primary defenses against infection (innate immunity) are breached, the acquired arm of the immune system is activated and produces a specific immune response to each infectious agent. This branch of immunity can protect the host from future infection by the same agent. Two key features that distinguish acquired immunity are specificity and memory.

Q. What are the types of acquired immunity?

Acquired immunity may be humoral and cell-mediated immunity (CMI). Humoral immunity is directly dependent on the production of antigen-specific antibody by B cells and involves the coordinated interaction of APCs, cells, and B cells. CMI is that part of the acquired immune system in which effector cells, such as phagocytic cells, helper T cells (T cells), T-regulatory cells (Tregs), APCs, CTLs, or memory T cells, play the critical role(s) without antibody involvement.

Q. What is hypersensitivity reaction?

Hypersensitivity reaction or intolerance refers to undesirable reactions produced by the normal immune system, including allergies and autoimmunity. There are four types of hypersensitivity reactions. One characteristic common to all four types of hypersensitivity reactions is the necessity of prior exposure leading to sensitization in order to elicit a reaction upon subsequent challenge. In the case of types I, II, and III, prior exposure to antigen leads to the production of allergen-specific antibodies (IgE, IgM, or IgG), and in the case of type IV, the generation of allergen-specific memory T cells.

Q. What is inflammation?

Inflammation refers to a complex reaction to injury, irritation, or foreign invaders characterized by pain, swelling, redness, and heat. Inflammation involves various stages, including release of chemotactic actors following the insult, increased blood flow, increased capillary permeability allowing for cellular infiltration, followed by either an acute resolution to tissue damage or persistence of the response that might contribute to fibrosis or subsequent organ failure.

Q. What are the possible adverse effects of xenobiotics on the immune system?

Many xenobiotics such as medical devices may have intimate and prolonged contact with the body. Possible immunologic consequences of this contact could lead to immunosuppression, immune stimulation, inflammation, and sensitization.

13.2   Sample MCQ's

(Choose the correct statement, it may be one, two or more, or none.)

Q.1. Which of the following types of hypersensitivity is *not* mediated by antibodies?

A. Type I
B. Type II
C. Type III
D. Type IV
E. Type V

Q.2. Which of the following is *not* a common mechanism of autoimmune disorders?

A. Subjection to positive selection in the thymus.
B. Anergic cells become activated.
C. Interference with normal immunoregulation by CD8+ suppressor cells.
D. Lack of subjection to negative selection in the thymus.
E. Decreased self-tolerance.

Q.3. Which of the following is *not* a step performed during an enzyme-linked immunosorbent assay (ELISA)?

A. A chromogen is added, and the color is detected.
B. The antigen of interest is fixed to a microtiter plate.

C. Radioactively labeled cells are added to the solution.
D. Enzyme-tagged secondary antibodies are added.
E. *Test* sera are added.

Q.4. The delayed hypersensitivity response (DHR) test does *not* -----

A. Evaluate memory cells' ability to recognize a foreign antigen.
B. Evaluate memory cells' ability to secrete cytokines.
C. Evaluate memory cells' ability to proliferate.
D. Evaluate memory cells' ability to lyse foreign target cells.
E. Evaluate memory cells' ability to migrate to the site of foreign antigen.

Q.5. The number of alveolar macrophages in smokers greatly increased relative to nonsmokers. What is a characteristic of the alveolar macrophages found in smokers?

A. They are in an inactive state.
B. They are far larger than normal.
C. They have increased phagocytic activity.
D. They are incapable of producing cytokines.
E. They have decreased bactericidal activity.

Q.6. Which of the following is *not* characteristic of a type I hypersensitivity reaction?

A. It is mediated by IgE.
B. It involves immune complex deposition in peripheral tissues.
C. It involves mast-cell degranulation.
D. Anaphylaxis is an acute, systemic, and very severe type I hypersensitivity reaction.
E. It is usually mediated by preformed histamine, prostaglandins, and leukotrienes.

Q.7. When an Rh− mother is exposed to the blood of an Rh+ baby during childbirth, the mother will make antibodies against the Rh factor, which can lead to the mother attacking the next Rh+ fetus. This is possible because of which antibody's ability to cross the placenta?

A. IgM
B. IgE
C. IgG
D. IgA
E. IgD

Q.8. Which of the following statements is *false* regarding important cytokine function in regulating the immune system?

A. IL-1 induces inflammation and ever.
B. IL-3 is the primary-cell growth actor.
C. IL-4 induces B-cell differentiation and isotype switching.
D. *T*ransforming growth factor-β (TGF-β) enhances monocyte/macrophage chemotaxis.
E. Interferon gamma (IFN-gamma) activates macrophages.

Q.9. Which of the following cells or substances is *not* part of the innate immune system?

A. Lysozyme
B. Monocytes
C. Complement
D. Antibodies
E. Neutrophils

Q.10. Myeloid precursor stem cells are responsible for the formation of all of the following *except*-----

A. Platelets
B. Lymphocytes
C. Basophils
D. Erythrocytes
E. Monocytes

Answers
1. D. 2. A. 3. C. 4. D. 5. E. 6. B.
7. C. 8. B. 9. D. 10. B.

14 Endocrine System

14.1 Problem-Solving Study Questions

Q. What is hormone?
A hormone is a chemical substance produced by a ductless endocrine gland that is secreted into the blood. The hormone-producing glands include the pituitary, the thyroid and parathyroids, the adrenals, the gonads, and the pancreas.

Q. What are chemical classes of hormones?
There are primarily three chemical classes of hormones: amino acid derivatives (catecholamines and thyroid hormones), peptide hormones (pancreatic), and steroids (derivatives of cholesterol). Endocrine glands are sensing and signaling devices that are capable of responding to changes in the internal and external environments and coordinating multiple activities that maintain homeostasis.

Q. What is endocrine system?
Endocrine glands are collections of specialized cells that synthesize, store, and release their secretions directly into the bloodstream.

Q. What does the endocrine system do?
The endocrine system is the collection of glands that produce hormones that regulate metabolism, growth and development, tissue function, sexual function, reproduction, sleep, and mood, among other things.

Q. What are the major endocrine glands in our body?
The major glands of the endocrine system are the hypothalamus, pituitary, thyroid, parathyroid, adrenals, pineal body, and the reproductive organs (ovaries and testes). The pancreas is also a part of this system; it has a role in hormone production as well as in digestion.

Q. How do endocrine systems function?

Endocrine systems function to maintain control over many of the other systems of the body via glands that release hormones that circulate in the bloodstream. Hormones act on target tissues and cells that respond to hormones via various signal transduction pathways, such as receptors. The endocrine system consists of many different glands that secrete hormones including the hypothalamus, pituitary, thyroid, adrenal, ovaries, and testes.

Q. How does endocrine toxicity occur?

Endocrine toxicity results when a chemical interferes with the synthesis, secretion, transport, metabolism, binding action, or elimination of hormones necessary for endocrine functions resulting in loss of normal tissue function, development, growth, or reproduction.

Q. What are endocrine disruptors?

Endocrine disruptors are chemicals that can interfere with endocrine (or hormone) systems at certain doses. These disruptions can cause cancerous tumors, birth defects, and other developmental disorders.

Q. What role toxicants can play on endocrine glands?

Toxicants can influence the synthesis, storage, and release of hypothalamic-releasing hormones, adenohypophyseal-releasing hormones, and the endocrine gland-specific hormones.

14.2   Sample MCQ's

(Choose the correct statement, it may be one, two or more, or none.)

Q.1. Chemical blockage of iodine transport in the thyroid gland ----

  A. Affects export of T3 and T4
  B. Prevents reduction to I2 by thyroid peroxidase
  C. Decreases RH release from the hypothalamus

  D. Interrupts   intracellular   thyroid biosynthesis
  E. Mimics goiter

Q.2. Which of the following statements regarding adrenal toxicity is *true*?

  A. The adrenal cortex and adrenal medulla are equally susceptible to fat-soluble toxins.
  B. Adrenal cortical cells lack the enzymes necessary to metabolize xenobiotic chemicals.
  C. Pheochromocytoma of the adrenal medulla can cause high blood pressure and clammy skin due to increased epinephrine release.
  D. Xenobiotics primarily affect the hydroxylase enzymes in the zona reticularis.
  E. Vitamin D is an important stimulus for adrenal cortex steroid secretion.

Q.3. 21-Hydroxylase deficiency causes masculinization of female genitals at birth by increasing androgen secretion from which region of the adrenal gland?

  A. Zona glomerulosa
  B. Zona reticularis
  C. Adrenal medulla
  D. Zona fasciculata
  E. Chromaffin cells

Q.4. Which of the following statements regarding pituitary hormones is *true*?

  A. The hypothalamic–hypophyseal portal system transports releasing hormones to the neurohypophysis.
  B. Dopamine enhances prolactin secretion from the anterior pituitary.
  C. Somatostatin inhibits the release of GH.
  D. The function of chromophobes in the anterior pituitary is unknown.
  E. Oxytocin and ADH are synthesized by hypothalamic nuclei.

Q.5. The inability to release hormones from the anterior pituitary would *not* affect the release of which of the following?

A. LH
B. PRL
C. ADH
D. SH
E. ACTH

Q.6. All of the following statements regarding glucose control are true *except* ---

A. Glucagon stimulates glycogenolysis, gluconeogenesis, and lipolysis.
B. Insulin stimulates glycogen synthesis, gluconeogenesis, and lipolysis.
C. Glucagon stimulates catabolic processes (mobilizes energy) to prevent hypoglycemia.
D. Insulin promotes storage of glucose, fatty acids, and amino acids by their conversion to glycogen, triglycerides, and protein, respectively.
E. Insulin and glucagon exert opposing effects on blood glucose concentrations.

Q.7. Which of the following vitamins increase calcium and phosphorus absorption in the gut?

A. Vitamin D
B. Niacin
C. Vitamin A
D. Vitamin B12
E. Thiamine

Q.8. Parathyroid adenomas resulting in increased pH levels would be expected to cause which of the following?

A. Hypocalcemia
B. Hyperphosphatemia
C. Increased bone formation
D. Osteoporosis
E. Rickets

Q.9. The parafollicular cells of the thyroid gland are responsible for secreting a hormone that

A. Increases blood glucose levels
B. Decreases plasma sodium levels
C. Increases calcium storage
D. Decreases metabolic rate
E. Increases bone resorption

Q.10. Chromaffin cells of the adrenal gland are responsible for secretion of which of the following?

A. Aldosterone
B. Epinephrine
C. Corticosterone
D. Testosterone
E. Estradiol

Answers
1. E.   2. C.   3. B.   4. D.   5. C.   6. B.
7. A.   8. D.   9. C.   10. B.

Further Reading

Fruncillo RJ (2011) 2,000 Toxicology board review questions. Xlibris, Publishers, USA

Gupta PK (ed) (2010) Modern toxicology, vol 3, 2nd reprint. PharmaMed Press, Hyderabad

Gupta PK (2014) Essential concepts in toxicology. BSP Pvt Ltd, Hyderabad

Gupta PK (2016) Fundamental in toxicology: essential concepts and applications in toxicology, 1st edn. Elsevier/BSP, San Diego

Gupta PK (2018) Illustrative toxicology, 1st edn. Elsevier, San Diego

Gupta RC (2018) Veterinary toxicology: basic and clinical principles, 3rd edn. Academic Press/Elsevier, San Diego

Gupta PK (2019) Concepts and applications in veterinary toxicology: an interactive guide. Springer-Nature, Switzerland

Gupta PK (2020) Brainstorming questions in toxicology. Francis and Taylor CRC Press, Boca Raton

Klaassen CD (ed) (2019) Casarett and Doull's toxicology: the basic science of poisons, 9th edn. McGraw-Hill, New York

Part IV

Non-Organ-Directed Toxicity

Chemical Carcinogenesis

8

Abstract

Carcinogenesis by *chemicals* is a multistage process. The first stage, initiation, occurs rapidly and appears to be irreversible. The available data indicate that initiation generally results from one or more mutations of cellular DNA. Studies on *mechanisms of chemical carcinogenesis* have led to the conclusion that cancer arises through three main mechanistic steps, namely initiation (the process of acquisition of genetic and epigenetic changes that sets the cell on path to cancer), promotion (a step during which the primed cells express). The use of the notion of three *risk factors* is adequate in approaching the complex process of carcinogenesis. The main carcinogenic factors can be grouped into: (a) primary determining factors; (b) secondary determining factors; and (c) favoring factors. There are cancers that are influenced by the hereditary factor. This chapter briefly describes the overview, key points, and relevant text that are in the format of problem-solving study questions followed by multiple-choice questions (MCQs) along with their answers.

Keywords

Cancer · Mutation · Chemical carcinogenesis · MCQs · Questions · Overview

1 Introduction

Cancer is a disease of cellular mutation, proliferation, and aberrant cell growth. It ranks as one of the leading causes of death in the world. Multiple causes of cancer have been either firmly established or suggested, including infectious agents, radiation, and chemicals. This chapter briefly describes the overview, key points, and relevant text that are in the format of problem-solving study questions followed by multiple-choice questions (MCQ's) along with their answers.

2 Overview

There is increasing evidence that carcinogens play a major role in causation of human cancer. The classes of carcinogens surveyed include polycyclic aromatic hydrocarbons, aromatic amines and amides, nitroarenes, heterocyclic amines formed in cooking, *N*-nitroso compounds, aflatoxins, natural oils such as safrole, and other natural products, such as the pyrrolizidine alkaloids. For each of these categories, a vast information is available on historical developments, environmental occurrence, the identities of the active metabolites, the pathways of enzymatic activation, and the structures of the adducts formed with DNA. Despite the chemical and structural diversity of the carcinogens, the evi-

P K Gupta, *Problem Solving Questions in Toxicology*, https://doi.org/10.1007/978-3-030-50409-0_8

dence indicates that their mechanisms of tumorigenesis are fundamentally similar. *The active metabolites of most carcinogens are electrophiles (or reactive oxygen species) that react with DNA to induce mutations and/or other genotoxic changes.*

those from biological sources), physical carcinogens, and oncogenic (cancer-causing) viruses.

Key Points

- The term cancer describes a subset of neoplastic lesions which has relatively autonomous growth of tissue with abnormal regulation of gene expression.
- The process of carcinogenesis may be divided into at least three stages: initiation, promotion, and progression.
- The first stage of carcinogenesis, initiation, results from an irreversible genetic alteration, most likely one or more simple mutations, transversions, transitions, and/or small deletions in DNA. Initiation requires one or more rounds of cell division for the "fixation" of the DNA damage.
- The second stage is promotion which results from the selective functional enhancement of the initiated cell and its progeny by the continuous exposure to the promoting agent.
- The third stage is progression which is the transition from early progeny of initiated cells to the biologically malignant cell population of the neoplasm.
- Stage 4 means the cancer has spread (metastasized) to another part of the body to form secondary cancers (metastases). As a general rule, cancers that have spread are difficult to treat and are unlikely to be cured in the long term, although treatment can help to shrink or control them.
- Carcinogen is any of a number of agents that can cause cancer in humans. They can be divided into three major categories: chemical carcinogens (including

3 Problem-Solving Study Questions

3.1 Terms Used for Chemical Carcinogenesis

Q. How do you define cancer?

The term cancer describes a subset of neoplastic lesions.

Q. How do you define neoplasm?

A neoplasm is defined as a heritably altered, relatively autonomous growth of tissue with abnormal regulation of gene expression.

Q. What is carcinogen?

A carcinogen is an agent whose administration to previously untreated animals leads to a statistically significant increased incidence of neoplasms of one or more histogenetic types as compared with the incidence in appropriate untreated animals.

Q. What is benign?

Lesions characterized by expansive growth, frequently exhibiting slow rates of proliferation that do not invade surrounding tissues

Q. What is malignant?

Lesions demonstrating invasive growth, capable of metastases to other tissues and organs

Q. What are metastases?

Metastases are secondary growths derived from a primary malignant neoplasm.

Q. What is tumor?

Tumor is a lesion characterized by swelling or increase in size and may or may not be neoplastic.

Q. What is genotoxic?

Genotoxic are carcinogens that interact with DNA resulting in mutation.

Q. What is nongenotoxic?

They are carcinogens that modify gene expression but do not damage DNA.

Q. How do you differentiate genotoxic and non-genotoxic carcinogens?

Common features of genotoxic and nongenotoxic carcinogens are summarized as under:

Genotoxic carcinogens	Nongenotoxic carcinogens
Mutagenic	Nonmutagenic
Can be complete carcinogens	Threshold, reversible
Tumorigenicity is dose responsive	Tumorigenicity is dose responsive
No theoretical threshold	May function at tumor promotion stage
	No direct DNA damage
	Species, strain, tissue specificity

Q. What is multistage carcinogenesis?

The carcinogenesis process involves a series of definable and reproducible stages. Operationally, these stages have been defined as initiation, promotion, and progression (Fig. 8.1).

Q. What is initiation?

Initiation is a process that is defined as a stable, heritable change. This stage is a rapid, irreversible process that results in a carcinogen-induced mutational event. Chemical and physical agents that interact with cellular components at this stage are referred to as initiators or initiating agents. Initiating agents lead to genetic changes including mutations and deletions. Chemical carcinogens that covalently bind to DNA and form adducts that result in mutations are initiating agents. Once initiated cells are formed, their fate has multiple potential outcomes:

(a) The initiated cell can remain in a static nondividing state.

(b) The initiated cell may possess mutations incompatible with viability or normal function and be deleted through apoptotic mechanisms.

(c) The cell may undergo cell division resulting in the proliferation of the initiated cell.

Q. What is promotion?

The second stage of the carcinogenesis process involves the selective clonal expansion of initiated cells to produce a preneoplastic lesion. This is referred to as the promotion stage of the carcinogenesis process. Both exogenous and endogenous agents that operate at this stage are referred to as tumor promoters. Tumor promoters are not mutagenic and generally are not able to induce tumors by themselves; rather they act through several mechanisms involving gene expression changes that result in sustained cell proliferation through increases in cell proliferation and/or the inhibition of apoptosis. Promotion is reversible upon removal of the promoting agent, and the focal cells may return to single initiated cell thresholds. Tumor promoters generally show organ-specific effects, e.g., a tumor promoter of the liver, such as phenobarbital, will not function as a tumor promoter in the skin or other tissues.

Q. What is progression?

Progression involves the conversion of benign preneoplastic lesions into neoplastic cancer. In this stage, due to an increase in DNA synthesis and cell proliferation in the preneoplastic lesions, additional genotoxic events may occur, resulting in further DNA damage including chromosomal aberrations and translocations. The progression stage is irreversible in that neoplasm formation, whether benign or malignant, occurs.

Fig. 8.1 Multistage model of carcinogenesis

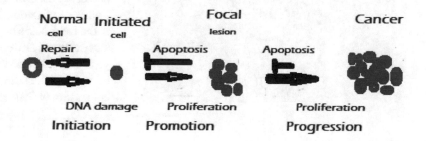

3.2   Mechanisms of Action

Q. What are the mechanisms of action of chemical carcinogens?

The formation of a neoplasm is a multistage, multistep process that involves the ultimate release of the neoplastic cells from normal growth control processes and creating a tumor microenvironment. Different properties/or mode of action of carcinogenesis is summarized in Table 8.1.

Q. Name different classes of genotoxic carcinogens

1. Polyaromatic hydrocarbons— Polyaromatic hydrocarbons such as benzo(a)pyrene are found at high levels in charcoal-broiled woods, cigarette smoke, and in diesel exhaust.

2. Alkylating agents—Some alkylating chemicals are direct-acting genotoxic agents; many require metabolic activation to produce electrophilic metabolites that can react with DNA. Alkylating agents readily react with DNA at more than 12 sites.

Table 8.1 Mode of action of different chemicals in causing carcinogenesis

Mode of action	Examples
Cytotoxicity	Chloroform, melamine
α2u-globulin binding	D-limonene, 1,4-dichlorobenzene
Receptor-mediated CAR	Phenobarbital
PPARα	Trichloroethylene, perchloroethylene, diethylhexylphthalate, fibrates (e.g., clofibrate)
AhR	TCDD, polychlorinated biphenyls (PCBs), polybrominated biphenyls (PBBs)
Hormonal	Biogenic amines, steroid and peptide hormones, DES, phytoestrogens (bisphenol-A), tamoxifen, phenobarbital
Altered methylation	Phenobarbital, choline deficiency, diethanolamine
Oxidative stress inducers	Ethanol, TCDD, lindane, dieldrin, acrylonitrile

3. Aromatic amines and amides—Aromatic amines and amides encompass a class of chemicals with varied structures. They can lead to liver and bladder carcinogenicity.

Q. What are inorganic carcinogens?

Several metals exhibit carcinogenicity in experimental animals and/or humans, including arsenic, beryllium, cadmium, chromium, nickel, and lead. The carcinogenic manifestations are varied as well and include increased risk for skin, lung, and liver tumors.

Q. Which are the most important targets for nongenotoxic (epigenetic) carcinogens?

The targets induced by nongenotoxic carcinogens are often in tissues where a significant incidence of background, spontaneous tumors is seen in the animal model. Prolonged exposure to relatively high levels of chemicals is usually necessary for the production of tumors.

Q. How do genotoxic/DNA-reactive carcinogens interact?

Genotoxic compounds directly interact with the nuclear DNA of a target cell. If this damage is unrepairable, DNA damage is inherited in subsequent daughter cells.

Q. How does mutagenesis occur?

Mutagenesis may result from misread DNA (through transitions or transversions), frameshifting, or broken DNA strands.

Q. How do alkylating electrophiles damage cells?

Some alkylating chemicals are strong reactive electrophiles that can readily form covalent adducts with nucleophilic targets. The stronger electrophiles display a greater range of nucleophilic targets, whereas weak electrophiles are only capable of alkylating strong nucleophiles. An important and abundant source of nucleophiles is contained not only in the DNA bases but also in the phosphodiester backbone. Different electrophilic carcinogens will often display different preferences or nucleophilic sites in DNA and, thus, different spectra of damage.

3.3 Modifying Factors

Q. What modifying factors affect chemical carcinogenesis?

Genetic and environmental factors have a significant impact on the way in which individuals and/or organisms respond to carcinogen exposure. Further, enzymes that metabolize carcinogens are expressed in a tissue-specific manner, and carcinogen-metabolizing enzymes are differentially expressed among species. These differences may represent an underlying factor explaining the differential responses to chemical carcinogens across species.

Q. What are factors associated with lifestyle that are responsible for cancer?

These factors include:
(a) Alcohol beverage, e.g., esophagus, liver, oropharynx, and larynx
(b) Aflatoxins, e.g., liver
(c) Betel chewing, e.g., mouth
(d) Dietary intake (protein, calories), e.g., breast, colon, endometrium, and gallbladder
(e) Tobacco smoking, e.g., mouth, pharynx, larynx, lung, esophagus, and bladder

3.4 Test Systems for Carcinogenicity Assessment

Q. What are test systems used for carcinogenicity?

Two test systems used for carcinogenicity:
(a) Chronic long-term tests: usually encompass 6 months to 2 years exposure to a chemical. Intermediate-term tests last from weeks up to a year.
(b) In vitro test systems: are typically for the duration of days to a few weeks.

Q. What is chronic testing for carcinogenicity?

Chronic (2-year) bioassay—Two-year studies over the life span of rodents remain the primary method by which chemicals or physical agents are identified as having the potential to be hazardous to humans. In the chronic bioassay, two- or three-dose levels (up to the maximum tolerated dose, MTD) of a test chemical and a vehicle control are administered to 50 males and 50 females (mice and rats), beginning at 8 weeks of age, continuing throughout their life span. During the study, food consumption and body weight gain are monitored, and the animals are observed clinically on a regular basis, and at necropsy the tumor number, location, and pathological diagnosis of each animal are thoroughly assessed.

Q. What are short-term tests or mutagenicity?

Short-term tests for mutagenicity were developed to identify potentially carcinogenic chemicals based on their ability to induce mutations in DNA either in vivo or in vitro. The majority of these tests measure the mutagenicity of chemicals as a surrogate for carcinogenicity.

Q. Name three in vitro gene mutation assays which can be used for mutagenicity.
(a) Ames assay
(b) Mouse lymphoma assay
(c) Mammalian cell mutation assay

4 Sample MCQ's

(Choose the statement, it may be one, two, more or none.)

Q.1. Which of the following is characteristic of a nongenotoxic carcinogen?

A. Has no influence on the promotional stage of carcinogenesis.
B. Would be expected to produce positive responses in in vitro assays for mutagenic potential.
C. Typically exerts other forms of toxicity and/or disrupts cellular homeostasis.
D. Generally shows little structural diversity.
E. Typically has little effect on cell turnover.

Q.2. All of the following are true of epoxide hydrolases *except*-----

A. They add oxygen to a double bond and form a three-member ring.
B. They are important in hydrolyzing electrophiles.
C. They play a role in converting benzo(a) pyrene to a carcinogen.
D. Some forms are inducible.

Q.3. Which of the following is *not* an initiating event in carcinogenesis?

A. DNA adduct formation
B. DNA strand breakage
C. Mutation of proto-oncogenes
D. Oxidative damage of DNA
E. Mitogenesis

Q.4. Which of the following is a nongenotoxic liver carcinogen in rats?

A. Aflatoxin
B. Vinyl chloride
C. Pyrrolizidine alkaloids
D. Clofibrate
E. Tamoxifen

Q.5. All of the following are true of apoptosis *except* --

A. Cell membrane remains intact.
B. Early in the process, caspases are activated.
C. Oxidative stress can initiate it.
D. It can lead to carcinogenesis.

Q.6. Asbestos exposure is unlikely to *cause* ----

A. Lung cancer
B. GI cancer
C. Emphysema
D. Pulmonary fibrosis
E. Mesothelioma

Q.7. All of the following are true of aromatic amine *except* ----

A. They are ultimate carcinogens.
B. Aniline dyes are example.
C. They are associated with bladder cancer.
D. They form reactive metabolites after phase 1 biotransformation.

Q.8. The most potent carcinogen derived from nicotine is ----

A. Naphthene
B. Styrene
C. Nicotine-derived nitrosamine ketone (NNK)
D. Meth tert-butyl ketone

Q.9. Xenobiotic toxicity that occurs after repair and adaptive processes are overwhelmed includes all of the following *except* -----

A. Fibrosis
B. Apoptosis
C. Necrosis
D. Carcinogenesis

Q.10. The carcinogenicity of nongenotoxic chemical that causes cytotoxicity is due to -----

A. Hormonal factors
B. Increase in spontaneous mutations from secondary hyperplasia
C. Acidosis
D. Active-phase reactants

Q.11. Which of the following statements is true?

A. Chemical carcinogens in animals are always carcinogens in animals.
B. A chemical that is carcinogenic in humans is usually carcinogenic in at least one animal species.
C. From a regulating perspective, carcinogens are considered to have a threshold dose-response curve.
D. Arsenic is an example of a chemical that is carcinogenic to humans and nearly all species treated.

Q.12. Which of the following is *not* associated with carcinogenesis?

A. Mutation
B. Normal p53 function
C. RAS activation
D. Inhibition of apoptosis
E. DNA repair failure

Q.13. Which of the following species develops cancer after exposure to a PPAR agonist?

A. Monkey
B. Human
C. Mouse
D. Guinea pig

Q.14. All of the following are PPAR agonist *except* ---

A. 3-methylcholanthrene
B. Clofibrate
C. Trichloroethylene
D. Diethylhexyl phthalate

Q.15. What do PPAR-alpha agonists, phenobarbital, and TCDD have in common?

A. They all cause human cancer.
B. They all bind to receptors that bind to response elements that modulate gene transcription.
C. They all bind to nuclear receptors that induce cytochrome 2D6.
D. They are all genotoxic in at least one species.

Q.16. All of the following are agonists at the estrogen receptor in humans *except* ---

A. DES
B. Bisphenol A
C. Nonylphenol
D. Tamoxifen

Q.17. Chemicals that increase reactive oxygen species can affect expression of gene regulating ---------

A. Proliferation
B. Differentiation
C. Apoptosis
D. All of the above

Q.18. Melamine causes nongenotoxic carcinogenicity by the mechanism of ------

A. Altered-DNA methylation
B. Induction of oxidative stress
C. Cytotoxicity
D. Stimulation of PPAR-alpha receptors

Answers
1. C.   2. A.   3. E.   4. D.   5. D.   6. C.
7. A.   8. C.   9. B.   10. B.   11. C.
12. B.   13. C.   14. A.   15. B.   16. D.
17. D.   18. C.

Further Reading

Choudhuri S, Chanderbhan R, Mattia A (2019) Carcinogenesis: mechanisms and models. In: Gupta RC (ed) Veterinary toxicology: basic and clinical principles, 3rd edn. Academic Press/Elsevier, San Diego, pp 339–356

Gupta PK (2010) Carcinogenicity and mutagenicity. In: Gupta PK (ed) Modern toxicology: basis of organ and reproduction toxicity, vol 1, 2nd reprint. PharmaMed Press, Hyderabad, pp 394–443

Gupta PK (2014) Essential concepts in toxicology. PharmaMed Press (A unit of BSP Books Pvt. Ltd), Hyderabad

Gupta PK (2016) Fundamentals of toxicology: essential concepts and applications, 1st edn. BSP/Elsevier, San Diego

Gupta PK (2018) Illustrative toxicology, 1st edn. Elsevier, San Diego

Gupta PK (2020) Brainstorming questions in toxicology. Francis and Taylor CRC Press, Boca Raton

Klaunig JE (2015) Chemical Carcinogenesis. In: Klaassen CD, Watkins JB III (eds) Casarett & Doull's essentials of toxicology, 3rd edn. McGraw-Hill, New York, pp 121–134

Genetic Toxicology

9

Abstract

Genetic toxicology is the study of the effects of chemical and physical agents on genetic material. It includes the study of DNA damage in living cells that leads to cancer, but it also examines changes in DNA that can be inherited from one generation to the next. Cellular changes induced by chemical and physical agents, the underlying molecular mechanisms for these changes, and how such information can be incorporated in risk assessments have been briefly discussed. This chapter provides the overview, key points, and relevant text that are in the format of problem-solving study questions followed by multiple-choice questions (MCQs) along with their answers.

Keywords

Genetic toxicology · DNA damage · Cellular changes · Risk assessments · Mutation · An overview · MCQs · Question and answer bank

1   Introduction

Genetic toxicology is the study of the effects of chemical and physical agents on genetic material. It includes the study of DNA damage in living cells

that leads to cancer, but it also examines changes in DNA that can be inherited from one generation to the next. Cellular changes induced by chemical and physical agents, the underlying molecular mechanisms for these changes, and how such information can be incorporated in risk assessments have been briefly discussed. This chapter also provides an overview, key points, and relevant text that are in the format of problem-solving study questions followed by multiple-choice questions (MCQ's) along with their answers.

2   Overview

Genotoxicity is a broader term. It includes mutagenicity, and it also includes DNA damage which may be mutagenic but may also be reversed by DNA repair or other cellular processes, and, thus, which may or may not result in permanent alterations in the structure or information content in a surviving cell or its progeny. Thus, genetic toxicology assesses the effects of chemical and physical agents on both DNA and on the genetic processes of living cells, the underlying molecular mechanisms for these changes, and how such information can be incorporated in risk assessments. A broad range of short-term assays or genetic toxicology serve to identify many mutagens and address the relationship between mutagens and cancer-causing agents.

P K Gupta, *Problem Solving Questions in Toxicology*, https://doi.org/10.1007/978-3-030-50409-0_9

Key Points

- The purpose of genotoxicity testing is to identify chemicals that can cause genetic alterations in somatic and/or germ cells.
- Genetic toxicology assesses the effects of chemical and physical agents on the hereditary material (DNA) and on the genetic processes of living cells.
- Mutagenicity is a subset of genotoxicity.
- Oncogenes are genes that stimulate the transformation of normal cells into cancer cells.
- Genetic toxicology assays serve to identify mutagens for purposes of hazard identification and to characterize dose–response relationships and mutagenic mechanisms.
- Two types of genetic toxicology studies are considered (in order of importance): (1) those measuring direct, irreversible damage to the DNA that is transmissible to the next cell generation, (i.e., mutagenicity) and (2) those measuring early, potentially reversible effects to DNA or the effect of mechanisms involved in the preservation of the integrity of the genome (genotoxicity).

3   Problem-Solving Study Questions

Q. What are somatic cells?

Somatic cells are any cell in the body that are not gametes (sperm or egg), germ cells (cells that go on to become gametes), or stem cells. Essentially, all cells that make up an organism's body and are not used to directly form a new organism during reproduction are somatic cells. Examples of somatic cells are cells of internal organs, skin, bones, blood, and connective tissues.

Q. What are germ cells?

A germ cell is any biological cell that gives rise to the gametes of an organism that reproduces sexually. In many animals, the germ cells originate in the primitive streak and migrate via the gut of an embryo to the developing gonads.

Q. What is germ cell mutation?

Germ cell mutations are mainly inherited from previous generations and are expressed when an individual inherits the mutant gene from both parents. New mutations make a larger contribution to the incidence of dominant diseases than to that of recessive diseases because only a single dominant mutation is required for expression mutations are mainly inherited from previous generations and are expressed when an individual inherits the mutant gene from both parents. New mutations make a larger contribution to the incidence of dominant diseases than to that of recessive diseases because only a single dominant mutation is required for expression.

Q. Where do germ cells originate?

Primordial germ cells, the earliest recognizable precursors of gametes, arise outside the gonads and migrate into the gonads during early embryonic development. Human primordial germ cells first become readily recognizable at 24 days after fertilization in the endodermal layer of the yolk sac.

Q. What are germ DNA mutations?

Germ DNA mutations are the cellular changes that turn a normal cell into a malignant cell that repeatedly and uncontrollably divides. This transformation occurs when there is genetic damage or an alteration in the structure of a cell's deoxyribonucleic acid (DNA), the coding machinery of life.

Q. What is cancer risk assessment?

Cancer risk assessment involves investigation of sensitivity of different species and subpopulations to tumor induction by a chemical and development of a dose–response curve of mutations to a chemical.

Q. What is genetic risk assessment?

To investigate genetic risk, the frequency of genetic alteration in human germ cells is estimated by extrapolation from data from rodent germ cells and somatic cells. For a complete estimate of genetic risk, it is necessary to obtain an estimate of the frequency of genetic alterations transmitted to the offspring.

Q. What are mutagens?

Chemicals that induce mutations in the DNA are called mutagens, and when these changes lead to cancer, the chemical is called a carcinogen. Not all mutagens are carcinogens, and not all carcinogens are mutagens.

Explanation: Heritable germ cell mutations and cancer are the major concerns when there is exposure to any genotoxic agent, and they provide the rationale for conducting assays to detect potential genotoxicity activity. In addition to being potential germ cell mutagens or carcinogens, there is evidence that the mutagenic events may play an important role in the cause and/or progression of human diseases other than cancer. It is now known that if a compound is genotoxic, then there is a reasonable probability that it will be a carcinogen. Types of genetic damage and methods for their detection are provided in Fig. 9.1.

3.1   Mechanisms of Induction of Genetic Alterations

The DNA is a double helix made of the compounds adenine (A), guanine (G), thymine (T), and cytosine (C). These chemicals are bound in long stretches as AT and CG pairs and wrapped in sugar molecules that hold them together (Fig. 9.2). Long stretches of these AT and CG combinations form genes which when "read" produce the proteins that drive our cells. Ideally the DNA sequence would not change except in the recombining that occurs during reproduction. However, DNA damage occurs regularly as part of the cell process and from interaction with both normal cellular chemicals and with toxic chemicals. A very robust repair mechanism rapidly and very accurately repairs the DNA damage, but if for some reason the DNA is repaired incorrectly, a mutation occurs. The mutation is a subtle or not-so-subtle change in the A, G, C, or T that make up the DNA. Many of the mutations have no effects, some have minor effects, and a small number have life-threatening effects. If a mutation occurs in the wrong place, a cell can start to divide uncontrollably, becoming a malignant cell

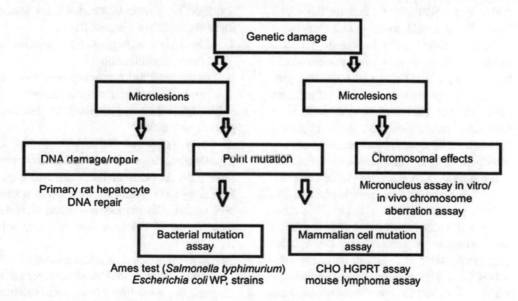

Fig. 9.1 Types of genetic damage and methods for their detection

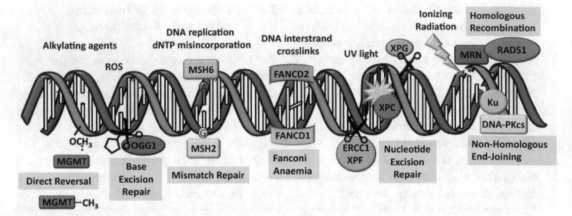

Fig. 9.2 Damage and repair of DNA after different agents. https://media.springernature.com/lw785/sringerstatic/image/
art%3A10.1007%2Fs00018-018-2833-9/MediaObjects/18_2018_2833_Fig2_HTML.gif

and causing a cancer. If a mutation occurs in our germ line cells, the mutation can be passed on to our offspring.

Q. What are the types of DNA damages? Give suitable examples.

The different types of damages include the types of DNA damage produced by radiations, and chemicals are many and varied, including single- and double-strand breaks in the DNA backbone, cross-links between DNA bases or between DNA bases and proteins, and chemical addition to the DNA bases. For example, ionizing radiations such as X-rays, gamma rays, and alpha particles produce DNA single- and double-strand breaks and a broad range of base damages. Chemicals can produce DNA alterations either directly (DNA-reactive) as adducts or indirectly by intercalation of a chemical between the base pairs (e.g., 9-aminoacridine). Endogenous agents are responsible for several hundred DNA damages per cell per day (e.g., 8-oxoguanine and thymine glycol). The cellular processes that can lead to DNA damage are oxygen consumption that results in the formation of reactive oxygen species (e.g., superoxide $O_2(-)$, hydroxyl free radicals •OH, and hydrogen peroxide) and deamination of cytosines and 5-methylcytosines leading to uracils and thymines, respectively.

Spectrum of DNA damage induced by physical and chemical agents and repair has been summarized in Fig. 9.2.

3.2 Assays for Detecting Genetic Alterations

Q. What are the purposes of assays used for detecting genetic alterations?

There are two main purposes of assays used for detecting genetic alterations in the toxicologic evaluation of chemicals:

1. Identifying mutagens for purposes of hazard identification
2. Characterizing dose–response relationships and mutagenic mechanisms

Q. What types of assays are used for detecting genetic alterations?

A broad range of short-term assays or genetic toxicology are used to identify many mutagens. At present, there are more than 200 assays for mutagens that are available, and useful information has been obtained from many of them. A few of these tests include:

(a) In silico *assays:* in silico assays include computational and structural programs and the modeling of quantitative structure–activity relationships.

(b) *DNA damage and repair assays:* A rapid method of measuring DNA damage is the comet assay. In this assay, cells are incorporated into agarose on slides, lysed so as to liberate their DNA, and subjected to electrophoresis.

(c) *Gene mutations in prokaryotes:* In this assay microorganisms are used that have a specific nutritional requirement.

(d) *Genetic alterations in nonmammalian eukaryotes:* In this the fruit fly, *Drosophila* is used, and the test sex-linked recessive lethal (SLRL) yields information about mutagenesis in germ cells, which is lacking in microbial and cell culture systems.

(e) *Mammalian cytogenetic assays:* These tests are in vivo assays for chromosome aberrations that involve treating intact animals, and later cells are collected for cytogenetic analysis.

(f) *Mammalian germ cell assays:* Mammalian assays permit the measurement of mutagenesis at different germ cell stages.

4   Sample MCQ's

(Choose the statement, it may be one, two or more, or none.)

Q.1. Which of the following tumor suppressor gene-neoplasm pairs is incorrect?

    A. p16–melanoma
    B. Rb1–small cell lung carcinoma
    C. BRCA1–osteosarcoma
    D. WT-1–lung cancer

Q.2. All of the following are true of the p53 gene *except* ----

    A. It is essential for checkpoint control during cell division.
    B. The active form is a hexamer of six identical units.
    C. Enhanced MDM2 in tumor cell decreases functional p53.

    D. Mutations are associated with lung, colon, and breast cancer.

Q.3. All of the following are true of carcinogen that inhibit at lower doses and demonstrate protection against carcinogenesis *except*---

    A. Induction of P450 enzyme as a possible mechanism.
    B. Exhibit a J-shaped dose–response curve.
    C. Stimulation of adaptive response that dominate at low doses.
    D. A mechanism that is only exhibited by tumor promoters.

Q.4. Which of the following chemoprotective agent-mechanism pairs is *incorrect*?

    A. Vitamin D—inhibition of cytochrome P450
    B. Vitamin C—antioxidant
    C. Vanillin—increase DNA repair
    D. Folic acid—correct DNA methylation imbalances

Q.5. Big Blue and Muta Mouse are examples of ----

    A. In vitro gene mutation assays
    B. Assays that test for tumor promoters and non-initiator
    C. Transgenic models
    D. None of the above

Q.6. All the following statements are true regarding gap-junctional, intracellular communication *except* -------

    A. Small molecule less than 1Ka can be exchanged through neighboring cells.
    B. It is inhibited by tumor promoters.
    C. Carcinogens that interfere with it are not tissue and species specific.
    D. It is achieved by connexin hexamers that form a pore between adjacent cells.

Q.7. All of the following statements are true regarding GSTM1 *except* ---

   A. It demonstrates high reactivity toward epoxides.
   B. Humans possessing the null isoform have a higher risk for bladder and gastric cancer.
   C. It is primarily a detoxication enzyme.
   D. The null isoform is protective in breast cancer.

Q.8. All of the following are true regarding proto-oncogenes *except* ----

   A. There are no known oncogenic virus analogues.
   B. They are dominant.
   C. Somatic mutations can be activated during all stages of carcinogenesis.
   D. Germ line inheritance of these genes is rarely involved in cancer development.

Q.9. All of the following are true regarding oncogenes *except* --------

   A. No known oncogenic virus analogue.
   B. They are recessive.
   C. Broad tissue specificity for cancer development.
   D. Somatic mutations activated during all stages of carcinogenesis.

Q.10. All of the following are true regarding tumor suppressor genes *except* -----

   A. BCRA1 is an example.
   B. They are recessive.
   C. No oncogenic virus analogues.
   D. Germ line inheritance is never involved in cancer development.

Q.11. All of the following statements regarding nondisjunction during meiosis are true *except* ----

   A. Nondisjunction events can happen during meiosis I or meiosis II.

   B. All gametes from nondisjunction events have an abnormal chromosome number.
   C. Trisomy 21 (Down syndrome) is a common example of nondisjunction.
   D. In a nondisjunction event in meiosis I, homologous chromosomes fail to separate.
   E. The incorrect formation of spindle fibers is a common cause of nondisjunction during meiosis.

Q.12. Which of the following diseases does *not* have a recessive inheritance pattern?

   A. Phenylketonuria
   B. Cystic fibrosis
   C. Tay–Sachs disease
   D. Sickle cell anemia
   E. Huntington's disease

Q.13. What is the purpose of the Ames assay?

   A. To determine the threshold of UV light that bacteria can receive before having mutations in their DNA
   B. To measure the frequency of aneuploidy in bacterial colonies treated with various chemicals
   C. To determine the frequency of a reversion mutation that allows bacterial colonies to grow in the absence of vital nutrients
   D. To measure rate of induced recombination in mutagen-treated fungi
   E. To measure induction of phenotypic changes in *Drosophila*

Q.14. In mammalian cytogenetic assays, chromosomal aberrations are measured after treatment of the cells at which sensitive phase of the cell cycle?

   A. Interphase
   B. M-phase
   C. S-phase
   D. G1
   E. G2

Q.15. Which of the following molecules is used to gauge the amount of a specific gene being transcribed to mRNA?

    A. Protein
    B. mRNA
    C. DNA
    D. cDNA
    E. CGH

Answers

1. C.   2. B.   3. D.   4. A.   5. C.   6. C.
7. D.   8. A.   9. B.   10. D.   11. B.   12.
E.   13. C.   14 C.   15. D.

Further Reading

Gupta PK (2010) Carcinogenicity and mutagenicity. In: Gupta PK (ed) Modern toxicology: basis of organ and reproduction toxicity, vol 1, 2nd reprint. PharmaMed Press, Hyderabad, pp 394–443

Gupta PK (2016) Fundamentals of toxicology: essential concepts and applications, 1st edn. BSP/Elsevier, San Diego

Gupta PK (2018) Illustrative toxicology, 1st edn. Elsevier, San Diego

Gupta PK (2020) Brainstorming questions in toxicology. Francis and Taylor CRC Press, Boca Raton

Julian PR, Hofmann GR (2015) Genetic toxicology. In: Klaassen CD, Watkins JB III (eds) Casarett & Doull's essentials of toxicology, 3rd edn. McGraw-Hill, New York, pp 135–148

Developmental Toxicology

10

Abstract

Developmental toxicology is the study of pharmacokinetics, mechanisms, pathogenesis, and outcomes following exposure to agents or conditions leading to abnormal development. Developmental toxicology includes teratology, or the study of structural birth defects. In 1960, a large increase in newborns with rare limb malformations of amelia (absence of the limbs) or various degrees of phocomelia (reduction of the long bones of the limbs) was recorded in West Germany. Congenital heart disease; ocular, intestinal, and renal anomalies; and malformations of the external and inner ears were also involved. This chapter briefly describes the overview, key points, and relevant text that are in the format of problem-solving study questions followed by multiple-choice questions (MCQs) along with their answers.

Keywords

Developmental toxicology · Teratology · Reproduction · Test procedures · Endocrine disruption · Overview · questions and answers · MCQ's

1 Introduction

Developmental toxicology is the study of pharmacokinetics, mechanisms, pathogenesis, and outcomes following exposure to agents or conditions leading to abnormal development. Developmental toxicology includes teratology or the study of structural birth defects. This chapter briefly describes an overview and relevant text that is in the format of problem solving study questions followed by multiple choice questions (MCQ's) along with their answers.

2 Overview

Developmental and reproductive toxicology (DART) is the discipline that deals with adverse effects on male and female resulting from exposures to harmful chemical and physical agents. The developmental stage during which treatment occurred is the critical factor in determining which organ was affected. The concept of developmental phase specificity and other core principles of experimental developmental toxicology grew out of that early work. Mass media coverage of the thalidomide tragedy brought the field of developmental toxicology to the attention of the public. For the first time, it was tragically demonstrated that a chemical agent had the potential to profoundly affect human develop-

P K Gupta, *Problem Solving Questions in Toxicology*, https://doi.org/10.1007/978-3-030-50409-0_10

ment. An understanding of how exposure to a toxicant can result in an adverse developmental outcome is needed to develop intervention and preventive public health practices. Risk assessors seek to obtain mechanism-based toxicity results from animal tests in order to make justifiable extrapolations to humans. The process by which a toxicant can produce dysmorphogenesis, growth retardation, lethality, and functional alterations commonly is referred to as the "mechanism" by which developmental toxicity is produced. In general, it has been difficult to analyze mechanisms in sufficient detail and depth for risk assessment purposes due to several reasons including the toxicant that might interact with an important molecular component and cause developmental toxicity.

> **Key Points**
>
> - The term developmental toxicity has widely replaced the early term for the study of primarily structural congenital abnormalities, teratology, to enable inclusion of a more diverse spectrum of congenital disorders.
> - Developmental toxicity is any structural or functional alteration, reversible or irreversible, which interferes with homeostasis, normal growth, differentiation, development or behavior and which is caused by environmental insult (including drugs, lifestyle factors such as alcohol, diet, and environmental toxic chemicals or physical factors).
> - The first-trimester exposure is considered the most potential for developmental toxicity.
> - Typical factors and xenobiotics causing developmental toxicity are radiation, infections (e.g., rubella), maternal metabolic imbalances (e.g., alcoholism, diabetes, folic acid deficiency), drugs (e.g., anticancer drugs, tetracyclines, many hormones, thalidomide), and environ-

> mental chemicals (e.g., mercury, lead, dioxins, PBDEs, tobacco smoke).
> - Testing for developmental toxicant is done in different stages such as fertilization to implantation, implantation to gastrulation, organogenesis, and morphogenesis, and postnatal to puberty and environmental toxicant exposures.

3   Problem-Solving Study Questions

Q. What is developmental toxicology?
Developmental toxicology encompasses the study of pharmacokinetics, mechanisms, pathogenesis, and outcomes following exposure to agents or conditions leading to abnormal development. It includes teratology or the study of structural birth defects.

Q. What is teratology?
Teratology is the study of abnormalities of physiological development. It is often thought of as the study of human congenital abnormalities, but it is broader than that, taking into account other non-birth developmental stages, including puberty, and other organisms, including plants.

Q. What are teratogens?
Teratogens are environmental factors that result in permanent structural or functional malformations or death of the embryo or fetus. Many congenital malformations are of unknown origin, but known teratogens include drugs, maternal illnesses and infections, metal toxicity, and physical agents (e.g., radiation).

Q. Which one is the most dangerous and common teratogens?
The tranquilizer thalidomide is one of the most famous and notorious teratogens. The common malformations include craniofacial dysmorphisms, cleft palate, thymic aplasia, and neural tube defects.

Q. At which stage are teratogens most harmful in human beings?
Only between days 28 and 50 of pregnancy.

Q. What factors influence the effects of teratogens?

The adverse effects of a teratogen depend on several factors, such as the dose or level of exposure, heredity, age, and any other negative influences.

Q. What is gametogenesis?

Gametogenesis is the process of forming the haploid germ cells: the egg and the sperm. These gametes are use in the process of fertilization to form the diploid zygote or one-celled embryo.

3.1   Principles of Developmental Toxicology

Q. What are the general principles of teratology?

These principles include:

(a) Susceptibility to teratogenesis depends on the genotype of the conceptus and the manner in which this interacts with adverse environmental actors.

(b) Susceptibility to teratogenesis varies with the developmental stage at the time of exposure to an adverse influence.

(c) Teratogenic agents act in specific ways (mechanisms) on developing cells and tissues to initiate sequences of abnormal developmental events (pathogenesis).

(d) The access of adverse influences to developing tissues depends on the nature of the influence (agent).

(e) The four manifestations of deviant development are death, malformation, growth retardation, and functional deficit.

(f) Manifestations of deviant development increase in frequency and degree as dosage increases from the no effect to the totally lethal level.

3.2   Pathogenesis of Developmental Toxicity

Q. What are the mechanisms of abnormal development?

The term mechanism refers to cellular-level events that initiate the process leading to abnormal development.

Q. What is pathogenesis?

Pathogenesis comprises the cell-, tissue-, and organ-level sequelae that ultimately manifest in abnormality.

Q. What are mechanisms of teratogenesis?

Mechanisms of teratogenesis include mutations, chromosomal breaks, altered mitosis, altered nucleic acid integrity or function, diminished supplies of precursors for substrates, decreased energy supplies, altered membrane characteristics, osmolar imbalance, and enzyme inhibition. Although these cellular insults are not unique to development, they may trigger unique pathogenetic responses in the embryo, such as reduced cell proliferation, cell death, altered cell–cell interactions, reduced biosynthesis, inhibition of morphogenetic movements, or mechanical disruption of developing structures.

Explanation: Cell death plays a critical role in normal morphogenesis. The term programmed cell death refers specifically to apoptosis, which is under genetic control in the embryo. Apoptosis is necessary for sculpting the digits from the hand plate and for assuring appropriate functional connectivity between the central nervous system and distal structures. Cell proliferation rates change both spatially and temporally during ontogenesis. There is a delicate balance between cell proliferation, cell differentiation, and apoptosis in the embryo. DNA damage might lead to cell cycle perturbations and cell death.

Q. What are end point effects of prenatal exposure to toxicants?

The major effects of prenatal exposure, observed at the time of birth in developmental toxicity studies, are embryo lethality, malformations, and growth retardation. For some agents, these end points may represent a continuum of increasing toxicity, with low dosages producing growth retardation and increasing dosages producing malformations and then lethality.

3.3   Maternal Factors Affecting Development

Q. What are the factors that affect development toxicity?
(a) Genetics—the genetic makeup of the pregnant female has been well-documented. For example, the incidence of cleft lip and/or palate [CL(P)] occurs more frequently in whites than in Blacks.
(b) Disease—certain infections in the mother (i.e., *Cytomegalovirus* and *Toxoplasma gondii*) are leading causes of several types of defects in the fetus.
(c) Chronic hypertension—chronic hypertension in the mother and uncontrolled maternal diabetes mellitus.
(d) Hyperthermia—exposure to hyperthermia (such as febrile illness in the mother) is also implicated in neural defects in the fetus.
(e) Nutrition—nutrition is a wide spectrum of dietary insufficiencies.
(f) Stress—stress may cause, diverse forms of maternal toxicity.
(g) Placental toxicity—the placenta is the interface between the mother and the conceptus, providing attachment, nutrition, gas exchange, and waste removal.
(h) Maternal toxicity—adverse developmental outcomes include increased intrauterine death, decreased fetal weight, supernumerary ribs, and enlarged renal pelvises.
(i) Drug toxicity—developmentally toxic dosages resulted in severe maternal toxemia and several other abnormalities including teratogenicity.
(j) Endocrine-disrupting chemicals—estrogenic or antiestrogenic developmental toxicants include antiandrogens, DES, estradiol, antiestrogenic drugs such as tamoxifen and clomiphene citrate, and some pesticides and industrial chemicals.

3.4   Safety Assessment (Test Systems)

Q. What are the end points in safety assessment in development toxicity studies?
The various end points that may be examined include:
1. Maternal toxicity
2. Embryo – fetal toxicity
3. External malformations
4. Soft tissue and skeletal malformations

Q. What are the key elements of various safety assessment tests used in development toxicity?
The aim of developmental and reproductive testing is to examine the potential for a compound to interfere with the ability of an organism to reproduce. This includes testing to assess reproductive risk in mature adults as well as in developing individuals at various stages of life, from conception to sexual maturity. Therefore, the goal of these studies is to identify the NOAEL, which is the highest dosage level that does not produce a significant increase in adverse effects in the offspring of juvenile animals.

Guidelines by the US FDA
Q. What are formal testing guidelines for reproduction studies for safety evaluation established by the US FDA?
These guidelines include:
Segment (I): During a premating period, the adults are treated, and continuation is optional for the female through implantation or lactation (one rodent species).
Segment (II): This is known as teratogenicity studies. Treatment of pregnant animals during the major period of organogenesis (one rodent species).
Segment (III): Treatment of pregnant/lactating animals from the completion of organogenesis through lactation (perinatal and postnatal study).

In adults, these include development of mature egg and sperm, fertilization, implantation, delivery of offspring (parturition), and lactation. In the developing organism, these include early embryonic development, major organ formation, fetal development and growth, and postnatal growth including behavioral assessments and attainment of full reproductive function. These evaluations are usually best performed in several separate studies.

Guidelines by the International Council for Harmonization (ICH)

Q. What are ICH guidelines of fertility protocol?

As per ICH guidelines for fertility protocol, the males are treated 4 weeks prior to mating and females 2 weeks prior to mating (shorter treatment duration than segment I). Males are examined for reproductive organ weights and histology, sperm counts, and motility. The females are examined viability of conceptuses at midpregnancy or later. The aim is to assess male reproductive system end points.

Q. What are ICH guidelines for studying effects on prenatal and postnatal development including maternal function?

As per ICH guidelines, implantation or mating is done through end of lactation. End points include relative toxicity to pregnant versus nonpregnant females, postnatal viability, growth, development, and functional deficits (including behavior, maturation, and reproduction).

Q. What are ICH guidelines for studying effects on embryo – fetal development?

As per ICH guidelines (similar to segment II study, usually conducted in two species, rodent and nonrodent), implantation or mating is done through end of organogenesis. End points include viability and morphology (external, visceral, and skeletal) of fetuses just prior to birth.

OECD Guidelines

Q. What are OECD guidelines for studying prenatal developmental?

Segment II study is usually conducted in two species (rodent and nonrodent). Implantation (or mating) through the day prior to cesarean section. End points include viability and morphology (external, visceral, and skeletal) of fetuses just prior to birth.

Alternative Testing Strategies

Q. What are alternative testing strategies for parental toxicity?

Various alternative test systems have been proposed to refine, reduce, or replace the standard regulatory mammalian tests or assess prenatal toxicity. These tests can be grouped into assays based on:

(a) Cell cultures,
(b) Cultures of embryos in vitro (including sub-mammalian species)
(c) Short-term in vivo tests

It was initially hoped that the alternative approaches would become generally applicable to all chemicals and help prioritize full-scale testing; this has not yet been accomplished.

Indeed, given the complexity of embryogenesis and the multiple mechanisms and target site of potential teratogens, it is perhaps unrealistic to have expected a single test, or even a small battery, to accurately prescreen the activity of chemicals in general.

---

4   Sample MCQ's

(Choose the statement, it may be one, two, more, or none.)

Q.1. The FDA protocol that primarily examines fertility and preimplantation and postimplantation viability is ___

A. Segment I
B. Segment II
C. Segment III
D. Segment IV

Q.2. The FDA protocol that primarily examines postnatal, survival, growth, and external morphology is___

A. Segment I
B. Segment II
C. Segment III
D. Segment IV

Q.3. All of the following maternal diseases have been assumed with adverse pregnancy outcomes *except* ___

A. Allergic rhinitis
B. Febrile illness during the first trimester
C. Hypertension
D. Diabetes mellitus

Q.4. All of the following are true of the development toxicity of cadmium *except* ___

A. It appears to involve placental toxicity.
B. It appears to involve inhibition of nutrient transport across the placenta.
C. Zinc can affect the developmental toxicity of cadmium.
D. Cadmium induces transferrin, which binds zinc in the placenta.

Q.5. All of the following are necessary for a normally developing embryo *except* ___

A. Apoptosis
B. Cell proliferations
C. Cell differentiation
D. Necrosis

Q.6. The fetal period is characterized by all of the following *except* ___

A. Beginning organ development
B. Tissue differentiation
C. Growth
D. Physiological maturation

Q.7. Toxic exposure during the fetal period is likely to cause effects on ___

A. Organogenesis
B. Implantation
C. Growth and maturation
D. All of the above

Q.8. Approximately what percentage of marked drugs belong to FDA pregnancy category?

A. 1%
B. 10%
C. 20%
D. 30%

Q.9. Diethylstilbestrol (DES)

A. Was used to treat morning sickness from the 1940s to the 1970s.
B. Was found to affect only female of spring in exposed pregnancies.
C. Greatly affects the development of the fetal brain.
D. Exposure increases the risk of clear cell adenocarcinoma of the vagina.
E. Is now used to treat leprosy patients.

Q.10. Early (prenatal) exposure to which of the following teratogens is most often characterized by craniofacial dysmorphism?

A. Thalidomide
B. Retinol
C. Ethanol
D. Tobacco smoke
E. Diethylstilbestrol (DES)

Q.11. The nervous system is derived from which of the following germ layers?

A. Ectoderm
B. Mesoderm
C. Epidermal placodes
D. Paraxial mesoderm
E. Endoderm

Q.12. Toxin exposure during which of the following periods is likely to have the *least* toxic effect on the developing fetus?

  A. Gastrulation
  B. Organogenesis
  C. Preimplantation
  D. Third trimester
  E. First trimester

Q.13. Regarding prenatal teratogen exposure, which of the following statements is *false*? Major effects include growth retardation and malformations.

  A. Exposure to teratogens during critical developmental periods will have more severe effects on the fetus.
  B. There is considered to be a toxin level threshold below which the fetus is capable of repairing itself.
  C. The immune system of the fetus is primitive, so the fetus has little to no ability to fight off chemicals and repair itself.
  D. Embryo lethality becomes more likely as the toxic dose is increased.

Q.14. Which of the following stages of the cell cycle are important in monitoring DNA damage and inhibiting?

  A. Progression of the cell cycle
  B. G1–S, anaphase, and M–G1

  C. G1–S, S, G2–M
  D. S, prophase, and G1
  E. G2–M, prophase
  F. M–G1, anaphase

Q.15. Which of the following molecules is *not* important in determining the ultimate outcome of embryonal DNA damage?

  A. p53
  B. Bax
  C. Bcl-2
  D. c-Myc
  E. NF-κB

Answers

1. A.   2. C.   3. A.   4. D.   5. D.   6. A.
7. C.   8. A.   9. D.   10. C.   11. A.   12. C.
13. D.   14. B.   15. E.

Further Reading

Gupta PK (2018) Illustrative toxicology, 1st edn. Elsevier, San Diego
Gupta PK (2020) Brainstorming questions in toxicology. Francis and Taylor CRC Press, Boca Raton
Rogers JM (2015) Developmental toxicology. In: Klaassen CD, Watkins JB III (eds) Casarett & Doull's essentials of toxicology, 3rd edn. McGraw-Hill, New York, pp 149–162
Vettorazzi G (2010) Reproduction toxicity and teratogenicity. In: Gupta PK (ed) Modern toxicology: basis of organ and reproduction toxicity, vol 1, 2nd reprint edn. PharmaMed Press, Hyderabad, pp 340–393

Part V
Toxic Agents

Pesticides

11

Abstract

This chapters deals with the toxic effects of different pesticides such as organochlorine insecticides, organophosphorus insecticides, carbamate insecticides, pyrethroids, formamidines, nicotinamides, botanical insecticides, fumigants, fungicides, herbicides, and various rodenticides by the farmers. Pesticides chemicals are among the most widely used group of chemicals in modern world and have provided immense benefits to mankind by controlling pests, significantly enhancing food production and improving health. However, their massive and indiscriminate use in crop protection, food preservation, and insect pests control has led to acute or chronic poisoning incidents in human, domestic animals, and wildlife and resulted in widespread ecological adverse effects. This chapter briefly describes the overview, key points, and relevant text that are in the format of problem-solving questions (MCQs) along with their answers.

Keywords

Pesticides · Agrochemicals · Organochlorine (OC) insecticides · Organophosphorus (OP) insecticides · Carbamate (CM) insecticides · Pyrethroids · Formamidines · Nicotinamides · Botanical insecticides · Question and answer bank · MCQ's

1 Introduction

Toxic effects of different pesticides such as organochlorine insecticides, organophosphorus insecticides, carbamate insecticides, pyrethroids, formamidines, nicotinamides, botanical insecticides, fumigants, fungicides, herbicides, rodenticides, and insect repellents in human beings and animals have been well-documented. This chapter briefly describes an overview, key points, and relevant text that are in the format of problem-solving study questions followed by multiple-choice questions (MCQ's) along with their answers.

2 Overview

Pesticides can be defined as any substance or mixture of substances intended for preventing, destroying, repelling, or mitigating pests (such as insects, rodents, weeds, and a host of other unwanted organisms). Ideally, their injurious action would be highly specific for undesirable targets; in reality, however, many pesticides are not highly selective and are often toxic to many nontarget species, including humans. Until the

P K Gupta, *Problem Solving Questions in Toxicology*, https://doi.org/10.1007/978-3-030-50409-0_11

1930s, pesticides were mainly of natural origins or inorganic compounds. Arsenicals have played a major role in pest control, first as insecticides and then as herbicides. Sulfur has been widely used as a fumigant since the early 1800s and remains one of the most widely used fungicides as of today. Nicotine has been widely used as an insecticide all over the world. In 1939 Paul Mueller found that DDT (dichlorodiphenyltrichloroethane), which had been first synthesized in 1874, acted as a poison on flies, mosquitoes, and other insects. DDT was commercialized in 1942 and was used extensively and successfully for the control of typhus epidemics and particularly of malaria. Indeed, at the time, the public health benefits of DDT were viewed so great that its discoverer, Paul Mueller, was awarded the Nobel Prize in Medicine in 1948. Subsequently, several compounds were synthesized as potential insecticides and chemical warfare agents.

ysis of muscles of respiration, bronchoconstriction, and airway obstruction from profuse respiratory tract secretions.
- OP compounds such as triaryl phosphates (e.g., triorthocresyl phosphate) are weak cholinesterase inhibitors but do inhibit "neurotoxic esterase" (NTE) present in the brain and spinal cord.
- In OP and CM poisoning, antidotal treatment such as the combined use of atropine sulfate and pyridine-2-aldoxime methochloride is used.
- Organochlorine (OC) insecticide toxicosis has no specific treatment. Acute poisoning treatment should mainly be directed toward symptomatic and control of convulsions

Key Points

- The chlorinated hydrocarbons are neurotoxicants and cause acute effects by interfering with the transmission of nerve impulses.
- Cholinesterase inhibitors fall into two classes, organophosphorus compounds and carbamates. The former one has higher toxicity, longer duration of action, and more commonly cause CNS toxicity.
- Organophosphorus (OP) and carbamate (CM) insecticides share a common mode of toxicological action associated with their ability to inhibit the ChE enzyme within the nervous tissue and at the neuromuscular junction (NMJs).
- Poisoning cases of OP or CM are usually diagnosed based on clinical signs and quantified levels of AChE inhibition in the blood.
- Fatalities due to OP compounds occur mainly due to effects on respiration due to depression of respiratory drive, paral-

3 Problem-Solving Study Questions

3.1 Pesticide Regulation

Q. Define in brief regulatory mandate of pesticides in the United States.

For safe use and the protection of the population, the primary authority for pesticide regulation resides with the Environmental Protection Agency (EPA) under the Federal Insecticide, Fungicide and Rodenticide Act (FIFRA), and the Federal Food, Drug and Cosmetic ACT (FFDCA).

Explanation: Under FIFRA, the EPA registers pesticides for use, while under FFDCA, the EPA establishes maximum allowable levels of pesticide residues (tolerances) in foods and animal feeds, which are enforced by other federal agencies. The first legislation passed in the United States was the Federal Insecticide Act of 1910 which only prohibited the manufacture of any insecticide or fungicide that was adulterated or misbranded. In 1970, the primary federal authority for the regulation of pesticides was transferred from

USDA and FDA to the newly formed EPA. Between 1970 and 1990, FIFRA was amended several other times to address various issues related to pesticide safety and registration processes.

Q. What is Delaney clause?

Delaney clause stated that "...no additive shall be deemed safe if it is found to induce cancer when ingested by man or animal or if it is found, after tests which are appropriate for the evaluation of the safety of food additives, to induce cancer in man or animal...." Pesticides were included in this "additive" legislation. However, pesticide residues are excluded from the definition of food additive, and the Delaney clause no longer applies to residues in food.

3.2   Insecticides

Q. What is the difference between pesticides and insecticides?

Pesticides are chemicals that may be used to kill fungus, bacteria, insects, plant diseases, snails, slugs, or weeds among others. Insecticides are a type of pesticide that is used to specifically target and kill insects. They include ovicides and larvicides used against insect eggs and larvae, respectively. Insecticides are used in agriculture, medicine, industry, and by consumers.

Q. What are organochlorine (OC) insecticides? Give examples?

An organochloride, organochlorine compound, chlorocarbon, or chlorinated hydrocarbon is an organic compound containing at least one covalently bonded atom of chlorine that has an effect on the chemical behavior of the molecule. For example, aldrin, chlordecone, DDT, dieldrin, endosulfan, endrin, heptachlor, hexachlorobenzene, lindane (gamma-hexachlorocyclohexane), dicofol, mirex, kepone, and pentachlorophenol.

Q. What makes OC insecticides toxic?

OC insecticides are persistent organic pollutants (POPs) because they are:
(a) Highly lipophilic (soluble in oils and fats)
(b) Stable

(c) Mobile
(d) Resistant to break down in the environment.

Insecticides such as the DDT are persistent organic pollutants and accumulate in food chains and cause reproductive problems (e.g., eggshell thinning) in certain bird species. Due to their cumulative effects, the use of some of them has been banned. Some organochlorine compounds, such as sulfur mustards, nitrogen mustards, and Lewisite, are even used as chemical weapons due to their toxicity.

Q. What is the mechanism of action of DDT?

In insects, DDT opens sodium ion channels in neurons, causing them to fire spontaneously, which leads to spasms and eventual death. Insects with certain mutations in their sodium channel gene are resistant to DDT and similar insecticides.

Q. What are organophosphate (OP) insecticides? Give examples.

An organophosphate (sometimes abbreviated OP) or phosphate ester is the general name for esters of phosphoric acid. They are used as insecticides, acaricides, soil nematicides, fungicides, herbicides, defoliants, rodenticides, insecticides synergists, insect repellents, chemosterilants, and warfare agents. Examples of OP compounds include acephate, chlorpyrifos, chlorpyriphos-methyl, diazinon, malathion, parathion, etc. They are known to inhibit esterases (ChE).

Q. Define carbamate (CM) insecticides? Give examples.

Carbamates are often used as insecticides. Unlike OPs, CM compounds are not structurally complex and are not considered to be persistent, because these are readily hydrolyzed. For example, carbaryl and benthiocarb.

Q. Why OP and CMs are preferred over OC insecticides?

As compared to OC, OP and CMs are:
(a) Much less environmentally persistent.
(b) Much more biodegradable.
(c) Less subject to biomagnification
(d) Usually unstable in presence of sunlight.
(e) Much more acutely toxic to nontarget species.

Q. Out of OC, OP, and CM insecticides, which of them have more acute toxic effects?

Both OP and CM insecticides are often involved in serious fatal human, animal, and wildlife poisoning incidences. Victims are usually children, farmers, and unskilled labor and are considered most dangerous orally or through the skin.

Q. Describe in brief OP nerve agents/gases.

OP nerve agents include tabun (GA), sarin (GB), soman (GD), cyclosarin (GF), venom toxin (VX), and Russian VX (VR). These compounds are highly toxic and pose continuous threats for the lives of humans as well as animals, because they can be used as chemical weapons of mass destruction (WMD). So far these agents have been used by dictators and terrorists. In some incidents, animals have been victims of military operations. These compounds produce toxicity by directly inhibiting AChE, and much more potent than OP insecticides, as they cause lethality to animals in the micrograms range.

Q. Which pesticides are commonly used for malicious poisoning in animals?

The most common pesticides used for malicious poisoning in animals are:

(a) Organophosphorus insecticides

(b) Carbamates

(c) Rodenticides

(d) Fumigants such as aluminum phosphide and zinc phosphide

(e) Pyrethroid insecticides

Q. How animals are exposed to pesticides?

(a) Accidental

(b) Suicidal poisonings

(c) Occupational exposure,

(d) By exposure to off-target drift

(e) Through environmental contamination, e.g., aerial spray

Q. What is acetylcholine?

Acetylcholine is a chemical neurotransmitter found widely in the body. It triggers the stimulation of postsynaptic nerves, muscles, and exocrine glands.

Q. What is acetylcholinesterase?

Acetylcholinesterase (generally referred to as cholinesterase) is an enzyme that rapidly breaks down the neurotransmitter, acetylcholine, so that it does not overstimulate postsynaptic nerves, muscles, and exocrine glands.

Q. What is acetylcholinesterase inhibitor?

Acetylcholinesterase inhibitor (generally referred to as cholinesterase inhibitor) is a chemical that binds to the enzyme, cholinesterase, and prevents it from breaking down the neurotransmitter, acetylcholine. With toxic doses, the result is that excessive levels of the acetylcholine build up in the synapses and neuromuscular junctions and glands.

Q. Why fever is observed in atropine poisoning?

Atropine poisoning causes decreased secretions in the body, and, occasionally, therapeutic doses dilate cutaneous blood vessels, particularly in the "blush" area (atropine flush), and may cause atropine "fever" due to suppression of sweat gland activity especially in infants and small children.

Q. What is OP-induced delayed neuropathy (OPIDP)?

Some OP compounds such as tri-o-cresyl phosphate (TOCP) was known to produce delayed neurotoxic effects in man and chicken, characterized by ataxia and weakness of the limbs, developing 10 to 14 days after exposure. This syndrome was called OP-induced delayed neuropathy (OPIDN). TOCP and certain other compounds have minimal or no anti-AChE property; however, they cause phosphorylation and aging (dealkylation) of a protein in neurons called neuropathy target esterase (NTE) and subsequently lead to OPIDP. Today, many compounds, such as mipafox, tetraethyl pyrophosphate (TEPP), parathion, o-cresyl saligenin phosphate, and haloxon, are known to produce this syndrome. Some OPs as well as non-OP inhibitors (such as carbamates and sulfonyl fluorides) also covalently react with NTE but cannot undergo the aging reaction. As a result, these inhibitors do not cause OPIDP.

Q. What is the treatment for OP poisoning?

In OP insecticide poisoning, atropine sulfate can be used as an antidote in conjunction with pralidoxime (2-PAM) or other pyridinium oximes (such as trimedoxime or obidoxime); atropine sulfate acts a muscarinic antagonist and thus blocks the action of acetylcholine peripherally. Pralidoxime or other pyridinium oximes act as anticholinergic drugs and counteract the effects of excess acetylcholine and reactivate AChE. The use of morphine, aminophylline, phenothiazine, reserpine etc. is to be avoided.

Q. What is the treatment for CM poisoning?
CM insecticides have similar cholinesterase inhibiting toxicity as OP insecticides and nerve agents. However, the carbamate-cholinesterase bond spontaneously hydrolyzes, therefore, in the past, 2-PAM was contraindicated in CM poisoning. However, its use in carbamate toxicity can reduce the clinical severity.

Q. Why OC insecticides are being discouraged/banned?
OC insecticides are not degradable and are persistent in the environment. And due to high lipid solubility, they accumulate in the food chain and enter human and animal bodies. Hence, OC compounds are being discouraged.

Q. Why OP compounds are preferred as insecticides for the crops?
OP compounds are biodegradable and hence are not persistent in environment. Further, they are easily destroyed by sunlight, water, microbes, alkalis, metals, etc. Hence, within 2–4 weeks of application, OP compounds are destroyed. However, they have considerable toxicity for mammals if consumed directly.

Q. How the binding of carbamates and OP compounds to AChE differs?
(a) Carbamates bind with both anionic and esteratic sites, whereas OP compounds bind only with esteratic site.
(b) Carbamates cause carbamylation, whereas OP compounds cause phosphorylation.
(c) Binding of carbamates is reversible, whereas that of OP compounds is irreversible (aging).

Q. Name two two main types of cholinergic receptors. Why they are so named?
Main cholinergic receptors are:
(a) Nicotinic
(b) Muscarinic
They are so named because their effects are similar to those of nicotine and muscarine.

Q. What is the location and function of nicotinic and muscarinic receptors?
(a) Are present in different anatomical locations
(b) Have different functions
(c) Have different mechanisms by which they trigger signal transmission

Q. What is the key function of nicotinic receptors?
A key function of nicotinic receptors is to *trigger rapid* neural and neuromuscular transmission.

Q. Where nicotinic receptors are found in the body?
(a) The somatic nervous system (neuromuscular junctions in skeletal muscles)
(b) The sympathetic and parasympathetic nervous system (autonomic ganglia)

Q. What are the key response differences between muscarinic and nicotinic receptors?
The response of muscarinic receptors
(a) Is slower.
(b) May be excitatory or inhibitory.
(c) Does not affect skeletal muscles, but does influence the activity of smooth muscle, exocrine glands, and the cardiac conduction system. In contrast to skeletal muscle and neurons, smooth muscle and the cardiac conduction system normally exhibit intrinsic electrical and mechanical rhythmic activity. This activity is modulated, rather than initiated, by the muscarinic receptors.

Q. Where muscarinic receptors are located?
Muscarinic receptors are located in the
(a) Parasympathetic nervous system
(b) Cardiac conduction system
(c) Exocrine glands
(d) Smooth muscles
(e) Sympathetic nervous system

(f) Sweat glands

(g) Central nervous system

Q. Why the binding of carbamates with AChE is reversible?

Carbamates causes carbamylation of AChE, which is weaker than phosphorylation caused by OP compounds. Hence, the binding is reversible.

Q. Why carbamates cannot cause delayed neuropathy?

Carbamates cannot bind with neurotoxic esterase. Hence delayed neuropathy is not caused.

Q. What are the metabolic active forms of malathion and parathion?

Maloxon and paroxon

Q. Why carbamates are the most preferred insecticides in veterinary use?

Carbamates have broad spectrum of activity, low in mammalian toxicity, and undergo rapid degradation in environment. Hence, carbamates are preferred for veterinary use (e.g., carbaryl, propoxur, etc.)

Q. Draw a schematic diagram representing mechanism of action of OP and CM insecticides.

Both these groups of insecticides inhibit the acetylcholinesterase enzyme from breaking down acetylcholine, thereby increasing both the level and duration of action of the neurotransmitter acetylcholine. Schematic diagram representing mechanism of action is given in Fig. 11.1.

In brief OP and CMs bind ChE and inhibit its functions. This result in excess of ACh in synapses and neuromuscular junction leading to muscarinic and nicotinic symptoms and signs.

Q. How normally acetylcholine is broken down by cholinesterase enzyme?

The positively charged nitrogen in the acetylcholine molecule is attracted to the ionic site on acetylcholinesterase, and hydrolysis is catalyzed at the esteratic site to form choline and acetic. The breakdown of acetylcholine by cholinesterase is shown in Fig. 11.2.

Q. How do cholinesterase inhibitors attach with acetylcholinesterase?

Figure 11.3 shows how a cholinesterase inhibitor (in this case, a nerve agent) attaches to the serine hydroxyl group on acetylcholinesterase. This prevents acetylcholine from

Fig. 11.1 Schematic representation of mechanism of action of OP and CM insecticides

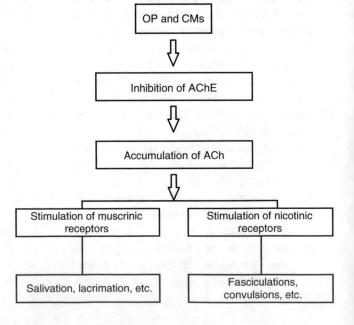

Fig. 11.2 Breakdown of acetylcholine. https://www.atsdr.cdc.gov/csem/cholinesterase/images/acetylcholinesterase.png

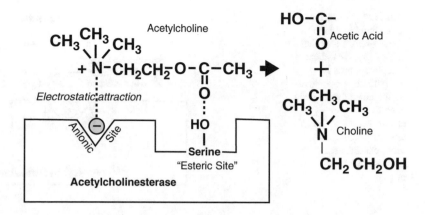

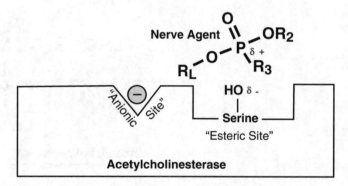

Fig. 11.3 Partially electropositive phosphorus is attracted to partially electronegative serine. δ+ indicates that phosphorus is partially electropositive. δ– indicates that oxygen is partially electronegative. https://www.atsdr.cdc.gov/csem/cholinesterase/images/agent_binding.png

interacting with the cholinesterase enzyme and being broken down.

Q. How do cholinesterase inhibitors work?

Figure 11.4 shows transition state indicating which bonds break and which one's form, and Fig. 11.5 shows cholinesterase inhibitor attached to acetylcholinesterase preventing the attachment of acetylcholine.

Q What are the adverse effects of blocked acetylcholine breakdown?

The adverse effects of blocked acetylcholine break down leads to the buildup of excessive levels of the neurotransmitter, acetylcholine, at the skeletal neuromuscular junction and those synapses where acetylcholine receptors are located. Thus, the primary manifestations of acute cholinesterase inhibitor toxicity are those of cholinergic (neurotransmitter) hyperactivity.

Q. What is aging due to cholinesterase inhibitors?

After some time, some inhibitors can develop a permanent bond with cholinesterase, known as aging, where "-doximes" such as pralidoxime cannot reverse the bond. Pralidoxime is often used with atropine (a muscarinic antagonist) to help reduce the parasympathetic effects of organophosphate poisoning.

Q. How do cholinesterase inhibitors can lead to aging?

Phosphorylated cholinesterases may undergo a dealkylation reaction of the organophosphorus moiety leading to "aged" enzyme, i.e., conversion of the inhibited enzyme into a

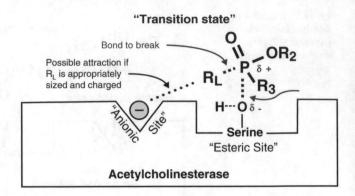

Fig. 11.4 Transition state showing which bonds break and which one's form. δ+ indicates that phosphorus is partially electropositive. δ− Indicates that oxygen is partially electronegative. https://www.atsdr.cdc.gov/csem/cholinesterase/images/transition_state.png

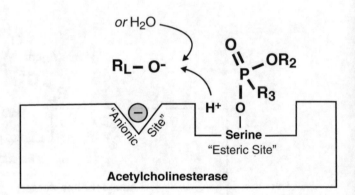

Fig. 11.5 Cholinesterase inhibitor attached to acetylcholinesterase preventing the attachment of acetylcholine. https://www.atsdr.cdc.gov/csem/cholinesterase/images/esteric_binding.png

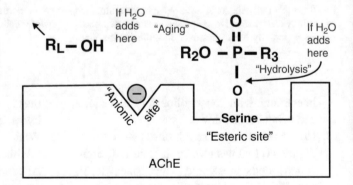

Fig. 11.6 Cholinesterase is blocked, but it can hydrolyze to original state (slow); regenerate with an oxime (fast); and "age" (cannot regenerate). http://www.atsdr.cdc.gov/csem/cholinesterase/images/cholinesterase_aging.png

non-reactivable form. Aging occurs rapidly when the inhibitor is soman, a powerful nerve agent (Figs. 11.6 and 11.7).

Q. Which are two important classes of cholinesterase inhibitors? How they differ from each other?

Cholinesterase inhibitors fall into two classes, organophosphorus compounds, and carbamates. The former has generally higher toxic-

ity, longer duration of action, and usually causes CNS toxicity.

Q. What are toxic symptoms of OP and CM insecticides?

Signs and symptoms of cholinesterase inhibitor poisoning include central nervous system effects that are due to the presence of both nicotinic and muscarinic receptors, and death is usually due to respiratory failure caused by

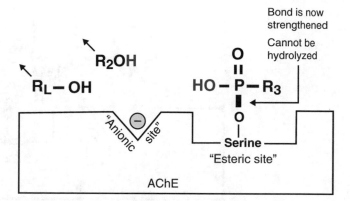

Fig. 11.7 The "aged" bond (after addition of H2O to the P-R3 bond. Prior to aging, R2 was pulling the electrons away from "P." Upon it being removed during the aging process, these electrons are shared with "O"-serine, strengthening its bond, so that it can no longer be hydrolyzed).   http://www.atsdr.cdc.gov/csem/cholinesterase/images/cholinesterase_aging2.png

Fig. 11.8 2-PAM and phosphorylated enzyme. http://www.atsdr.cdc.gov/csem/cholinesterase/images/2pam_action1.png

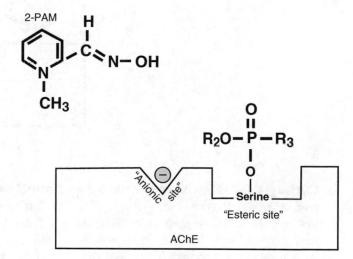

bronchoconstriction, bronchorrhea, central respiratory depression, weakness, and paralysis of respiratory muscles.

Q. Describe the mechanism of action of 2-PAM
In organophosphate poisoning, an organophosphate bind to just one end of the acetylcholinesterase enzyme (the esteratic site), blocking its activity (Fig. 11.8). Pralidoxime is able to attach to the other half (the unblocked, anionic site) of the acetylcholinesterase enzyme (Fig. 11.9). It then binds to the organophosphate; the organophosphate changes conformation and loses its binding to the acetylcholinesterase enzyme. The conjoined poison/antidote then unbinds from the site and thus regenerates the enzyme, which is now able to function again (Fig. 11.10).

Q. How does 2-PAM reactivate the enzyme ChE?
2-PAM attaches to ChE inhibitors that have blocked ChE and removes them from the enzyme, thereby reactivating it.

Q. How does aging takes place?
Some ChE inhibitors after a time will form a permanent bond with ChE in a process called aging, after which 2-PAM is no longer effective.

Fig. 11.9 Partially electropositive nitrogen on 2-PAM is attracted to electronegative anionic site on cholinesterase. http://www.atsdr.cdc. gov/csem/cholinesterase/ images/2pam_action2. png

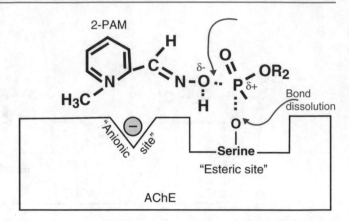

Fig. 11.10 Regeneration of cholinesterase. http://www.atsdr.cdc. gov/csem/cholinesterase/ images/2pam_action3. png

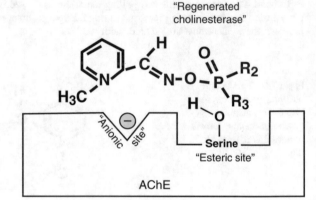

Q. Can we give 2-PAM in conjunction with atropine in OP poisoning?

Yes. 2-PAM should be given in conjunction with atropine, with which it has a notable synergistic effect. Although it has been suggested that 2-PAM was absolutely contraindicated in carbamate poisoning, data are lacking to support this recommendation.

Q. When does 2-PAM treatment failure occurs?

(a) With an inadequate dose

(b) When aging has already occurred

(c) When active cholinesterase inhibitor absorption or redistribution (e.g., from fat tissue) is continuing to occur

Q. Does aging takes place in carbamate poisoning?

No. The carbamate-cholinesterase bond does not age.

Natural and Synthetic Insecticides

Q. Define natural insecticides. Give examples.

Natural insecticides, such as rotenone, nicotine, pyrethrum, and neem extracts, made by plants as defenses against insects. Natural insecticides are usually nontoxic to humans and pets and safe for the environment.

Q. Name at least three plants having insecticidal properties.

(a) Nicotine

(b) *Chrysanthemum*

(c) Derris

Q. Name the plant from which pyrethrin is obtained.

Chrysanthemum

Q. What are pyrethrins and pyrethroids insecticides? Give examples.

A pyrethroid is an organic compound similar to the natural pyrethrins produced by the flowers of pyrethrums (*Chrysanthemum cinerariaefolium* and *C. coccineum*) Pyrethroids now constitute the majority of commercial household insecticides. For example, allethrin, bifenthrin, cyfluthrin, cypermethrin, etc.

Q. Describe the important properties of pyrethrins and pyrethroids insecticides.

These compounds are:

(a) More persistent,

(b) Have greater insecticidal activity,

(c) Photostable,

(d) Low doses are effective,

(e) Have low mammalian toxicities.

Q. Classify pyrethroids?

There are two broad classes of pyrethroids. Type I pyrethroids resemble natural pyrethrins in their structure and activity (e.g., allethrin, pyrethrin, and permethrin) and type II pyrethroids contain a --CYANO group in their structure and are more active and toxic (e.g., deltamethrin, cypermenthrin, and fenvalarate).

Q. Describe mechanism of action of pyrethrins and pyrethroids.

Pyrethroids (types I and II) activate nerve membranes by modifying the sodium channels, resulting in depolarization of the membranes.

1. The length of tail current is characteristic for each pyrethroid.

2. Both classes have little effect on the activation of channels and current flow but prolong the inactivation, creating tail currents. Type I pyrethroids produce relatively short tail currents, whereas type II is substantially the longer ones.

Formulations of these insecticides frequently contain the insecticide synergist piperonyl butoxide [5-{2-(2-butoxyethoxy) ethoxymethyl}-6-propyl-1,3-benzodioxole], which acts to increase the efficacy of the insecticide by inhibiting the cytochrome P450 enzymes responsible for the breakdown of the insecticide.

Q. Describe symptoms of pyrethroid poisoning.

The usual signs of poisoning include restlessness, incoordination, hyperactivity sensory to external stimuli, fine tremors progressing to other parts of body, and hyperthermia.

Formamidine and Neonicotinoid Insecticides

Q. Do formamidine and neonicotinoid insecticides are very toxic to human beings?

No. Both formamidine and neonicotinoid are new class of insecticides that are applied at low dosages and are extremely effective but are relatively nontoxic to humans.

Q. Define neonicotinoids. Give examples.

Neonicotinoids (sometimes shortened to neonics/ˈniːoʊnɪks) are a class of neuroactive insecticides chemically similar to nicotine. The neonicotinoid family includes acetamiprid, clothianidin, imidacloprid, nitenpyram, nithiazine, thiacloprid, and thiamethoxam. Imidacloprid is the most widely used insecticide in the world.

Q. Define formamidine inscticides. Give examples.

Formamidine insecticides are a relatively new group of acaricides which are particularly useful for the control of Lepidoptera, Hemiptera, phytophagous mites, and cattle ticks. Because of the widespread use for control of cotton insects and cattle ticks, their toxicity is extremely important. This group includes amitraz, chlordimeform, formetanate, formparanate, medimeform, and semiamitraz.

3.3 Herbicides

Q. What are herbicides?

Herbicides control weeds and are the most widely used class of pesticides. This class of pesticide can be applied to crops using many strategies to eliminate or reduce weed populations, for example, imidazolinones, chlorophenoxy herbicides such as 2,4-D (2,4-dichlorophenoxy acetic acid) and 2,4,5-T (2,4,5-trichlorophenoxy-acetic acid), triazines, bipyridylium family such as paraquat (1,1-dimethyl-4,4-bipyridinium ion as the chloride salt), diquat, and so on.

Q. Classify herbicides
  (a) Inorganic (arsenicals, chlorates)
  (b) Organic (chlorophenoxy and its deriva-
      tives, dinitrophenols, bipyridyls, ureas,
      and other herbicides)
Q. What are the main signs and symptoms of
   herbicide toxicity?
  (a) Ingestion: burning pain in the mouth,
      throat, chest, and upper abdomen; pul-
      monary edema; pancreatitis; and renal
      and CNS effects such as nervousness,
      irritability, combativeness, disorienta-
      tion, and diminished reflexes.
  (b) Dermal: dry and fissured hands, horizon-
      tal ridging or loss of fingernails, ulcer-
      ation, and abrasion. Direct spilling may
      lead to severe skin injury.
Q. Describe mode of action of paraquat
   herbicide.
   Paraquat is one of bipyridinium compounds.
   It is caustic and irritant agent which causes
   ulceration and necrosis of the skin and
   mucous membranes. Paraquat is actively
   taken up by the alveolar cells via a diamine or
   polyamine transport system where it undergoes NADPH-dependent reduction. These are
   easily reduced to the radical ions, which generates superoxide radical that reacts with
   unsaturated membrane lipids. The excess of
   superoxide anion radical O_2- and H_2O_2
   cause damage to the cellular membrane in
   lungs, which reduces the functional integrity
   of lung cells, affects efficient gas transport
   and exchange, and results in respiratory
   impairment including pulmonary fibrosis.
Q. Despite being highly toxic, bipyridyl herbicides don't produce toxicity after being
   sprayed on plants, why?
  (i). Bipyridyl herbicides are used in very low
       doses, which are not toxic
  (ii). They are inactivated immediately upon
        contact with soil.
Q. Why lung tissue is primarily affected by
   paraquat?
  (a) Paraquat accumulates up to 10 times in
      lungs.

  (b) Lung tissue is deficient in superoxide
      dismutase (SOD) enzyme, which
      destroys superoxide radical. Hence,
      lungs are primarily affected.
Q. Despite being highly toxic, why bipyridyl herbicides don't produce toxicity after being
   sprayed on plants?
  (a) Bipyridyl herbicides are used in very low
      doses, which are not toxic.
  (b) They are inactivated immediately upon
      contact with soil.
Q. 81 How do paraquat and diquat differ in their
   toxicity?
   During paraquat exposure, toxicity results
   from lung injury resulting from both the preferential uptake of paraquat by the lungs and
   the redox cycling mechanism. Pulmonary
   fibrosis is the usual cause of death in paraquat
   poisoning. During diquat poisoning, renal
   damage result from both the preferential
   uptake of diquat by the kidney and the redox
   cycling mechanism. No progressive pulmonary fibrosis has been noted in diquat poisoning. However, diquat has severe toxic effects
   on the central nervous system that are not
   typical of paraquat poisoning.
Q. Does use of oxygen is beneficial in paraquat
   poisoning?
   Use of supplemental oxygen is contraindicated until the patient develops severe hypox-
   emia. High concentrations of oxygen in the
   lung increase the injury induced by paraquat
   and possibly by diquat as well.
Q. Describe mode of action of diquat herbicide.
   Diquat is a very reactive compound and
   exerts its action in a similar manner to paraquat but affects liver and kidney but does not
   cause pulmonary edema or alter lung functions. Signs of CNS excitement and renal
   impairment occur in severely affected
   patients
Q. Can we use phenothiazine derivatives as
   treatment in pyrethroid insecticide
   poisoning?
   No. Use of phenothiazine derivatives is
   contraindicated.

3.4 Rodenticides

Q. What are rodenticides? Give examples?
Rodenticides are used to control rodents. The list of rodenticides included anticoagulants (warfarin, coumatetralyl, chlorophacinone, flocoumafen, difenacoum, bromadiolone, brodifacoum), hypercalcemia (Calciferol), metal phosphides, aluminum phosphide (fumigant only), calcium phosphide (fumigant only), magnesium phosphide (fumigant only), zinc phosphide (bait only), ANTU (α-naphthylthiourea; specific against brown rat, *Rattus norvegicus*), arsenic trioxide, barium carbonate, chloralose (a narcotic prodrug), and so on.

Q. What is the chemical nature of rodenticides?
The compounds used as rodenticides comprise a diverse range of chemical structures having a variety of mechanisms of action.

Q. What are "second-generation" anticoagulant rodenticides?
A few of the "second-generation" anticoagulant rodenticides are coumarins, such as the "superwarfarins" brodifacoum, or difenacoum, while others are indan-1,3-dione derivatives (diphacinone, chlorophacinone). These compounds essentially act like warfarin, have prolonged half-lives (e.g., brodifacoum 16–34 days vs. warfarin 15–37 hours), and cause very long-lasting inhibition of coagulation; in addition, they are mostly "single-dose" rodenticides.

Q. Describe one nonanticoagulant rodenticides.
Bromcthalin is a "single-dose" nonanticoagulant rodenticide. Toxic metabolite of bromethalin is desmethylbromethalin. The targets of toxicity for desmethylbromethalin are the mitochondria, where this metabolite, and to a lesser extent the parent compound, uncouples oxidative phosphorylation resulting in decreased ATP synthesis. In the CNS this leads to retention of water causing edema of the myelin sheath.

Q. What is secondary poisoning?
The poisoning that is seen in dogs and cats as a result of consumption of rodenticide poisoned rodents

Q. Why the use of fluoroacetate is restricted?
Fluoroacetate is highly toxic and nonspecific affecting other species.

Q. What is bait shyness?
A rodent surviving the exposure to a particular rodenticide will avoid the same rodenticide in the future. This phenomenon is called bait shyness.

Q. Why sodium fluoroacetate does not produce bait shyness?
Sodium fluoroacetate needs lag period for developing toxicity. Hence, the rodents do not remember the exposure.

Q. Why zinc phosphide preparations contain antimony potassium tartrate?
Antimony potassium tartrate is an emetic, which can prevent accidental zinc phosphide toxicity in nontarget species through vomiting.

Q. Why zinc phosphide is more toxic on full stomach than empty?
On full stomach, the acid production in stomach is increased. As zinc phosphide releases phosphine gas in acidic medium, full stomach increases the toxicity.

Q. What are signs and symptoms aluminum phosphide?
Aluminum phosphide has a metallic taste. Symptoms include garlicky odor, nausea, pain in gullet, stomach, abdomen, vomiting, diarrhea, cough dyspnea, respiratory failure, headache, anxiety, hypotension tachycardia/bradycardia, myocarditis, hepatosplenomegaly, renal failure, coma, etc.

Q. What is the mode of action of warfarin?
Warfarin interferes with normal function of vitamin K and causes coagulation defects characterized by decreased blood concentrations of coagulation protein factors. The decreased coagulation factors lead to massive internal hemorrhages, and the affected individuals died due to tissue hypoxia.

Q. Despite being very specific to rats, why ANTU is banned?
Due to carcinogenic potential of alpha naphthylamine impurities

Q. What is the difference between pulmonary toxicity caused by ANTU (rodenticide) and paraquat (herbicide)?
ANTU causes pulmonary edema and is fatal, whereas paraquat causes pulmonary fibrosis which is not fatal.

Q. Describe in brief aluminum phosphide.
Aluminum phosphide is a solid fumigant pesticide, widely used as a grain preservative. It is used as suicidal and homicidal poisoning. On exposure to air or moisture, it liberates phosphine and can produce multi-organ damage.

Q. Why zinc phosphide preparations contain antimony potassium tartrate?
Antimony potassium tartrate is an emetic, which can prevent accidental zinc phosphide toxicity in nontarget species through vomiting.

Q. What are signs and symptoms aluminum phosphide?
Aluminum phosphide has a metallic taste. Symptoms include garlicky odor, nausea, pain in gullet, stomach, abdomen, vomiting, diarrhea, cough dyspnea, respiratory failure, headache, anxiety, hypotension tachy/bradycardia, myocarditis, hepato-spleenomegaly, renal failure, coma, etc.

Q. What is the mode of action of warfarin?
Warfarin interferes with normal function of vitamin K and causes coagulation defects characterized by decreased blood concentrations of coagulation protein factors. The decreased coagulation factors lead to massive internal hemorrhages, and the affected individuals died due to tissue hypoxia.

Q. John is a 60-year-old business agent with a past history of rheumatic fever and a mechanical mitral valve replacement. He takes warfarin to prevent clots forming from the valve replacement. While showering one day, he notices extensive bruising on his abdomen and thighs. He visits his general practitioner, who determines the warfarin dose is too high. What drug could be administered to rectify this problem?
- Vitamin K is the antidote for warfarin overdose.

3.5 Fungicides

Q. What are fungicides?
A chemical that destroys fungus

Q. What are the examples of fungicides?
Examples of broad-spectrum fungicides include captan, sulfur, and mancozeb. Some fungicides have a very narrow spectrum of activity; for example, mefenoxam is effective only against oomycetes like *Phytophthora*. Alternatively, a fungicide may affect a broad range of fungi but by only a specific mode of action.

Q. How are fungicides classified?
Fungicides can be classified based on:
(a) Mobility in the plant: Contact vs. mobile (types of systemics).
(b) Preventive vs. curative: Preventive fungicides work by preventing the fungus from getting into the plant.
(c) Mode of action: This refers to how the fungicide affects the fungus.

Q. What are fungicides? Give examples
Fungicides are chemicals that destroy fungus. Important fungicides include chlorothalonil (tetrachloroisophthalonitrile), captan, captafol, folpet, dithiocarbamates, sulfur derivatives of dithiocarbamic acid, metallic dimethyldithiocarbamates, mancozeb, maneb, zineb (zinc ethylenebisdithiocarbamate), and ethylthiourea (ETU) compounds.

3.6 Fumigants

Q. What are fumigants?
Fumigants are extremely toxic gases used to protect stored products, especially grains, and to kill soil nematodes.

Q. Classify fumigants
   (a) Inorganic (aluminum phosphide, hydrogen cyanide, carbon disulfide, sulfur dioxide),
   (b) Organic (methyl bromide, ethylene dibromide, dibromochloropropane)

3.7   Insect Repellents

Q. Name a few best insect repellents used in the world?
   The best known and most widely used insect repellent is DEET, and a newer compound picaridin is encountering increasing success. Botanical insect repellents based on citronella or oil of eucalyptus and a biopesticide structurally similar to the amino acid alanine are also commercialized in Europe and the United States.
Q. What is the repellent mechanism of DEET?
   The exact repellent mechanism of DEET is still unknown, but it may be related to disturbances of the mosquito antennae that allow the insect to locate humans.

4   Sample MCQ's

(Choose the correct statement, it may be one, two, more, or none.)

Q.1. Inhibition of acetylcholinesterase (AChE) is the mechanism of action of which pesticide?

   A. Organochlorines
   B. Pyrethrins
   C. Organophosphates
   D. Rotenone
   E. Fipronil

Q.2. Which of the following is considered treatment for organophosphate but cannot be used for carbamate poisoning?

   A. Atropine sulfate (muscarinic antagonism).
   B. 2-PAM.

C. Gastric lavage.
D. Activated charcoal.
E. All can be used to treat both organophosphates and carbamate poisoning.

Q.3. What is the specific antidote for organochlorine exposure?

   A. Atropine sulfate
   B. 2-PAM
   C. Methylene blue
   D. Physostigmine
   E. None

Q.4. Which of the following statements regarding organochlorines is *false*?

   A. Toxicity is neurological.
   B. Organochlorines are highly persistent and bioaccumulate.
   C. Chronic organochlorine exposure can lead to eggshell thinning and reduced fertility in birds.
   D. Mechanism of action is either by inhibition of Na+ influx and K + efflux or inhibiting GABA receptors.
   E. Organochlorines are highly volatile, and exposure is most likely via inhalation.

Q.5. . Which of the following statements is *true* regarding pyrethrins and pyrethroids?

   A. Pyrethrins and pyrethroids are rapidly hydrolyzed and metabolized with majority eliminated 12–24 hours.
   B. Inhalation exposure of pyrethrins and pyrethroids is low
   C. Pyrethrins and pyrethroids are hydrophilic in nature and do not distribute in fat or nervous tissue
   D. Mammalian Na+ channels are 1000x more sensitive than the insect counterpart
   E. Cats do not have adverse reactions to pyrethrins and pyrethroids because they are a more intelligent species and know not to lick this product of a dog.

Q.6. What is the mechanism of action of fipronil (frontline)?

A. Fipronil inhibits the oxidation of
NADH to NAD+ which leads to an
energy deficiency in cells.
B. Fipronil binds to the membrane lipid
phase near the Na+ channel.
C. Fipronil inhibits Na+ influx and K
efflux.
D. Fipronil noncompetitively binds
GABA receptors and blocks Cl- influx
E. Fipronil is an AChE inhibitor

Q.7. Which of the following pesticides is toxic
to herding breeds with a mutation in the
ABCB1 transporter?

A. Ivermectin
B. Imidacloprid
C. Rotenone
D. Fipronil
E. Pyrethrins

Q.8. Amitraz is an alpha-2 agonist of the CNS
which results in sedation. Which drug
would be used to treat amitraz poisoning?

A. Atropine sulfate
B. Yohimbine
C. 2-PAM
D. Atipamezole
E. Both yohimbine and atipamezole

Q.9. Paraquat is a highly toxic herbicide that
causes damage through generation of
reactive oxygen species. Which organ
does paraquat accumulate in?

A. Heart
B. Brain
C. Lung
D. Spleen
E. Small intestine

Q.10. Which of the following statements is *false*
regarding bromethalin?

A. Uncouples oxidative phosphorylation
in mitochondria, thus depleting ATP
B. Highly lipophilic with the brain and fat
having high concentrations
C. Causes a buildup of vitamin D3 metabolites which causes an increase in
plasma Ca+ and P+
D. Developed for use against warfarin-
resistant rodents
E. Secondary poisoning can occur in
dogs and cats that eat rodents killed by
bromethalin

Q.11. Organochlorine insecticides protect
against the acute toxicity of several
organophosphorus insecticides by ____

A. Stimulating enzymatic detoxification
of organophosphates
B. Increasing noncatalytic-binding sites
of organophosphates
C. Stimulating enzymatic detoxification
as well as increasing noncatalytic-
binding sites of organophosphates

Q.12. Ethylene dibromide in high concentrations
produces ____

A. Lung edema
B. Nephritis
C. Hepatitis

Q.13. Carbamate insecticides interact with ____

A. Esteratic site of acetylcholine enzyme
(AChE)
B. Anionic site of AChE
C. Esteratic as well as anionic site of
AChE

Q.14. Red squill is obtained from the plant ____

A. *Urginea maritima*
B. *Strophanthus* sp.
C. *Croton tiglium*
D. *Cassia fistula*

Q.15. Cypermethrin-induced toxicity in laboratory animals is also known as _____

A. Turner's syndrome
B. T syndrome
C. X disease
D. CS syndrome

Q.16. The diagnostic symptom of chronic pyrethroid toxicity is _____

A. Muscular twitching
B. Grinding of teeth
C. Hypothermia
D. Irritation

Q.17. The avian toxicant 4-aminopyridine is toxic to dogs and causes clinical effects similar to those of _____

A. Arsenic
B. Ethylene glycol
C. Lead
D. Organophosphates
E. Strychnine

Q.18. All of the following are characteristic of DDT poisoning *except* _____

A. Paresthesia
B. Hypertrophy of hepatocytes
C. Increased potassium transport across the membrane
D. Slow closing of sodium ion channels
E. Dizziness

Q.19. Which of the following is used as rodenticide?

A. Warfarin
B. Sulfur
C. Nicotine
D. Pyrethrum

Q.20. Which of the following does *not* contribute to the environmental presence of organochlorine insecticides?

A. High water solubility
B. Low volatility
C. Chemical stability
D. Low cost
E. Slow rate of degradation

Answers
1. C.   2. B.   3. E.   4. E.   5. A.   6. D.
7. A.   8. E.   9. C.   10. C.   11. C.   12. D.
13. A.   14. A   15. D.   16. A.   17. E.
18. C.   19. A.   20. A.

Further Reading

Gupta PK (1986) Pesticides in the Indian environment. Interprint, New Delhi

Gupta PK (2010a) Epidemiology of anticholinesterase pesticides: India. In: Satoh T, Gupta RC (eds) Anticholinesterase pesticides: metabolism, neurotoxicity, and epidemiology. Wiley, Hoboken, pp 417–431

Gupta PK (2010b) Pesticides. In: Gupta PK (ed) Modern toxicology: the adverse effects of xenobiotics, vol 2, 2nd reprint edn. PharmaMed Press, Hyderabad, pp 1–60

Gupta PK (2014) Essential concepts in toxicology. PharmaMed Press (A unit of BSP Books Pvt. Ltd), Hyderabad

Gupta PK (2016a) Fundamentals of toxicology: essential concepts and applications, 1st edn. BSP/Elsevier, San Diego

Gupta PK (2016b) Herbicide poisoning. In: The Merck veterinary manual, 11th edn. Merck & Co. Inc, Whitehouse Station, pp 2969–2999

Gupta PK (2017) Herbicides and fungicides. In: Gupta RC (ed) Reproductive and developmental toxicology, 2nd edn. Academic Press/Elsevier, San Diego, pp 657–680

Gupta PK (2018a) Illustrative toxicology, 1st edn. Elsevier, San Diego

Gupta PK (2018b) Toxicity of herbicides. In: Gupta RC (ed) Veterinary toxicology: basic and clinical principles, 3nd edn. Academic Press/Elsevier, San Diego, pp 553–568

Gupta PK (2018c) Toxicity of fungicides. In: Gupta RC (ed) Veterinary toxicology: basic and clinical principles, 3rd edn. Academic Press/Elsevier, San Diego, pp 569–582

Gupta PK (2019a) Herbicides and fungicides. In: Gupta RC (ed) Biomarkers in toxicology, 3rd edn. Elsevier, USA, pp 409–432

Gupta PK (2019b) Concepts and applications in veterinary toxicology: an interactive guide. Springer-Nature, Switzerland

Gupta PK (2020) Brainstorming questions in toxicology. Francis and Taylor CRC Press, Boca Raton

Gupta Ramesh C (2018) Veterinary toxicology: basic and clinical principles, 3rd edn. Academic Press/Elsevier, San Diego

Klaassen CD (ed) (2019) Casarett & Doull's toxicology: the basic science of poisons, 9th edn. McGraw-Hill, New York

Metals and Micronutrients

12

Abstract

This chapters deals with the adverse effects of a wide range of metals and micronutrients such as arsenic, lead, mercury, copper, fluoride, iron, molybdenum, selenium, zinc, salt poisoning, etc. that have important role in animal practice. These metals have also been used to make utensils, machinery, and so on. These activities increased environmental levels of metals. More recently metals have found a number of uses in industry, agriculture, and medicine. These activities have increased exposure not only to metal-related occupational workers but also to animals through environmental contamination or through other sources. Despite the wide range of metals and their toxic properties, there are a number of toxicological features that are common to many metals. This chapter briefly describes the overview, key points, and relevant text that are in the format of problem-solving study questions followed by multiple-choice questions (MCQs) along with their answers.

Keywords

Metals · Micronutrients · Lead · Mercury · Arsenic · Cadmium · Aluminum · Micronutrients · Copper · Iron · Chromium · Nickel · Molybdenum · Zinc deficiency ·
Questions and answers · MCQs · Toxicity · Metalloids · Interactions

1 Introduction

Metals are elements that form cations when compounds of it are in solution, and oxides of the elements form hydroxides rather than acids in water. Micronutrient is a chemical element or substance required in trace amounts for the normal growth and development of living organisms. Despite the wide range of metal toxicity and toxic properties, there are a number of toxicological features that are common to many metals. The chapter briefly describes an overview, key points, and relevant text that are in the format of problem-solving study questions followed by multiple-choice questions (MCQ's) along with their answers.

2 Overview

Metals are element in the solid state having high reflectivity (luster), high electrical conductivity, high thermal conductivity, and mechanical ductility and strength. Metals are unique among pollutant toxicants in that they are all naturally occurring and are already ubiquitous to some level within the human environment. Regardless of how safely metals are used in industrial processes or consumer products, some level of human exposure is inevitable. Human use of metals has influenced environmental levels of metals in air, water, soil, and food. Metals are redistributed naturally in the environment by both geological and biological cycles. Biological cycles moving metals include biomagnification by plants and animals resulting in incorporation into food cycles. Reports of metal intoxication are common in plants, aquatic organisms, invertebrates, fish, sea mammals, birds, and domestic animals. For example, chronic arsenic poisoning from high levels of naturally occurring inorganic arsenic in drinking water is a major health issue in many parts of the world. Endemic intoxication from excess fluoride, selenium, or thallium can all occur from natural high environmental levels. A toxicologically important characteristic of metals is that they may react in biological systems by losing one or more electrons to form cations.

Key Points

- Metals are elements that form cations when compounds of it are in solution, and oxides of the elements form hydroxides rather than acids in water.
- Micronutrient is a chemical element or substance required in trace amounts for the normal growth and development of living organisms.
- Young children or elderly people are more susceptible to toxicity from exposure to a particular level of metal or micronutrient than most adults.
- Metals that provoke immune reactions include mercury, gold, platinum, beryllium, chromium, and nickel.
- Complexation is the formation of a metal-ion complex in which the metal ion is associated with a charged or uncharged electron donor, referred to as a ligand. Chelation occurs when bidentate ligands form ring structures that

include the metal ion and the two ligand atoms attached to the metal.
- Metal–protein interactions include binding to numerous enzymes, the metallothioneins, nonspecific binding to proteins such as serum albumin or hemoglobin, and specific metal carrier proteins involved in the membrane transport of metals.
- Arsenic, certain chromium compounds, and nickel are known human carcinogens; beryllium, cadmium, and cisplatin are probable human carcinogens.
- Metals lose electrons easily, and they often corrode easily. The oxides of metals tend to be basic, but the oxides of non-metals tend to be acidic.
- Non-metals show more variability in their properties than do metals. Non-metals if solid generally have a submetallic or dull appearance and are brittle, as opposed to metals, which are lustrous, ductile, or malleable.
- Exposure to non-metals act as irritant poisons and produce inflammation on the site of contact, especially in the GI tract, respiratory tract, and the skin.
- Selenium (Se), a non-metal, is sometimes classified instead as a metalloid.

---

3   Problem-Solving Study Questions

Q. Describe in brief general mechanism of enzyme inhibition/activation by metals
   Chemically, metals in their ionic form can be very reactive and can interact with biological systems in a large variety of ways. In this regard, a cell presents numerous potential metal-binding ligands. A major site of toxic action for metals is interaction with enzymes, resulting in either enzyme inhibition or activation. Two mechanisms are of particular importance: inhibition may occur as a result

of interaction between the metal and sulfhydryl (SH) groups on the enzyme, or the metal may displace an essential metal cofactor of the enzyme. Another key chemical reaction in metal toxicology is metal-mediated oxidative damage. Many metals can directly act as catalytic centers for redox reactions with molecular oxygen or other endogenous oxidants, producing oxidative modification of biomolecules such as proteins or DNA. This may be a key step in the carcinogenicity of certain metals. Besides oxygen-based radicals, carbon- and sulfur-based radicals may also occur.

Q. Give one example of metal-binding protein.

The metallothioneins are the best known example of metal-binding proteins. These thiol ligands provide the basis for high affinity binding of several essential and toxic metals including zinc, cadmium, copper, and mercury.

Q.1. List some common metals used in industrial processes which can give rise to toxicity. Indicate what element forms are involved and what kind of toxicity is produced.

(a) *Lead (II) ions*: These ions possibly reduce fertility; possible effects on baby in the womb; anemia; brain and kidney damage; and death.

(b) *Mercury–elemental mercury*: The vapors are well absorbed from the lungs; may be absorbed through the skin; and inhibit nerve and kidney functions.

(c) *Mercuric ions*: These ions are poorly absorbed; inhibit enzymes dependent on SH groups; and affect nervous system and kidneys.

(d) *Alkoxymercury*: It is broken down to inorganic mercuric ions (see mercuric ions).

(e) *Alkylmercury*: It is readily absorbed through skin, gut, or lungs; accumulates in fatty tissue and the nervous system; and causes paralysis and death; developing baby in the womb is especially sensitive and may die though mother is unaffected.

Q. Name one general metal detoxicant protein?

Ferritin is primarily a storage protein for iron. It may serve as a general metal detoxicant protein, because it binds a variety of toxic metals including cadmium, zinc, beryllium, and aluminum.

Q. What are the factors that affect metal toxicity?

(a) Exposure-related factors include dose, route of exposure, duration, and frequency of exposure.

(b) Host-based actors that can impact metal toxicity include age at exposure, gender, and capacity for biotransformation. For example, younger subjects are often more sensitive to metal intoxication. Elderly persons are also believed to be generally more susceptible to metal toxicity than younger adults.

(c) Lifestyle factors such as smoking or the composition of dict (i.e., alcohol ingestion).

(d) Adaptive mechanisms: Adaptation can be at the level of uptake, excretion, or long-term storage in a toxicologically inert form.

Q. Which metal (s) have kidney as the target organ?

• The following metals can cause nephrotoxicity:

(a) Cadmium

(b) Inorganic mercury compounds, which are more water soluble

(c) Organic lead compounds

Q. Which metal (s) have nervous system as the target organ?

• The nervous system is the target organ for organic metal compounds such as methylmercury because it is lipid soluble, readily crosses the blood–brain barrier, and enters the nervous system.

Q. Name two metals which are known to have endocrine and reproductive effects.

(a) Cadmium is known to produce testicular injury after acute exposure.

(b) Lead accumulation in the testes is associated with testicular degeneration, inhibition of spermatogenesis, and Leydig-cell atrophy.

3.1 Lead

Q. What is Burtonian line?

- The Burton line or Burtonian line is a clinical sign found in patients with chronic lead poisoning. It is a stippled blue line seen at the junction of the gums usually nearer to tooth caries, especially in the upper jaw. This is due to the deposition of lead sulfide formed by the action of lead with hydrogen sulfide due to decomposed food debris in the caries tooth.

Q. Define the effect of lead on the blood.

- Lead causes hypochromic, microcytic anemia with reticulocytosis, and punctate basophilia (Fig. 12.1). Lead can combine with sulfhydryl enzymes and can decrease synthesis of heme leading to anemia and can bring about hemolysis as well as release immature RBCs into circulation (reticulocytosis and basophilic stippling of RBCs). Platelet count decreases. Anemia is probably due to decreased survival time of RBCs and inhibition of heme synthesis by interference with the incorporation of iron into protoporphyrin.

Q. What is the effect of lead on the bone?

- Lead can accumulate in bones.

Q. Why milk from lead-affected animals is dangerous for young ones?

- Considerable amount of lead is excreted in milk (about 5% of blood concentration). Since young animals have greater capacity to absorb lead than adults, milk from lead-affected animals is dangerous to young ones.

Q. Why lead poisoning is more common in veterinary cases?

- Lead is ubiquitous in nature. Most of the animals live at a closer level to soil and hence get more exposure. Further, habits like frequent digging of soil seen in dogs and cats increase exposure. Ultimately, increasing vehicular and industrial pollution is the major reason for lead toxicosis.

Q. Why acute lead toxicosis is not common?

- Because >90% of ingested lead is eliminated from GIT without absorption. Even after absorption, only <1% of lead is in free form. Therefore, acute lead toxicosis is not common.

Q. Is it true that lead directly enters the bone and gets deposited?

- NO. Initially, lead is distributed to various soft tissues and later gets redistributed to the bone from these soft tissues.

Q. Why only whole blood is recommended for estimation of lead?

- Majority of lead (90%) is bound to hemoglobin in RBC. Hence, plasma or serum samples are not appropriate.

Q. Animals with depraved appetite (pica) are more commonly affected with lead poisoning. Why?

- In pica, animals tend to lick walls, chew on dry peelings of paint, eat wall posters, etc. Since paints are lead based, the animals are affected with lead poisoning. Even children chewing on toys painted with cheap lead paints are also reported to be affected with lead toxicosis.

Fig. 12.1 Basophilia (arrows) of RBCs in humans after drinking repeatedly from glasses decorated with lead paint. https://upload. wikimedia.org/ wikipedia/ commons/3/3b/ Lead_poisoning_-_ blood_film.jpg

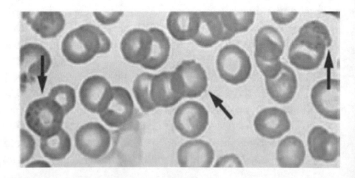

3.2   Mercury

Q. What is Minamata disease?

Minamata disease was identified in Japan. This disease is caused due to the consumption of fish contaminated with methylmercury. Analysis of fish led to the detection of organic Hg as the root of the problem.

Q. What was the outcome of studies done in 1974 on methylmercury poisoning?

- The studies indicated that women who gave birth to congenitally poisoned children had exhibited none of the early symptoms of methylmercury poisoning. This was because the methylmercury easily crosses the placenta and concentrates in the developing fetus. Concentrations in fetal brains were up to 4 times those in the mother, and fetal blood levels were 28% greater than the mothers.

Q. What are major target organs of three forms of mercury?

(a) Elemental mercury: the vapors target the respiratory system.

(b) Inorganic mercury: mainly affects kidneys and GI tract.

(c) Organic mercury: mainly affects the central nervous system.

Q. Give reasons as to why mercury (Hg) poisoning is not common in animals?

- Hg compounds are completely replaced by better alternatives in medicinal, agricultural, and industrial use. Hence, Hg poisoning is not common in animals. (Predatory animals at the end of food chain are more likely to accumulate Hg, which causes poisoning).

Q. Why young animals are more susceptible for mercury poisoning?

- Developing nervous system is more susceptible to mercury. Hence young ones are more susceptible.

Q. What were the symptoms of methylmercury poisoning outbreak?

Symptoms of methylmercury poisoning outbreak include primitive oral and grasping reflexes, poor coordination, character disorders (unfriendly, nervous, shy, and restless), seizures and epilepsy, deformed limbs, and slow growth.

Q. Draw a schematic diagram of environmental cycling of mercury.

The less toxic inorganic mercury gets converted through biomethylation to more toxic form of mercury. The schematic representation of mercury's environmental cycling, biomethylation, and food chain transfer is shown in Fig. 12.2.

Q. Where does mercury in fish come from?

Anthropogenic sources, such as coal burning and mining of iron, can contaminate water sources with methylmercury. Methylmercury is absorbed in the bodies of fish through the process of biomagnification; mercury levels in each successive predatory stage increase (Fig. 12.3).

Q. Describe in brief toxic potential of different forms of mercury.

Both inorganic and organic forms of mercury are associated with genotoxicity, teratogenicity,

Fig. 12.2 Environmental cycling and conversion of inorganic mercury to methylmercury

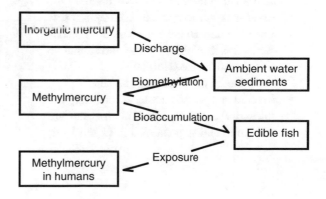

Fig. 12.3 Through the process of biomagnification, mercury levels in each successive predatory stage increase in fish. https://upload. wikimedia.org/ wikipedia/commons/ thumb/0/07/ MercuryFoodChain. svg/1200px- MercuryFoodChain.svg. png

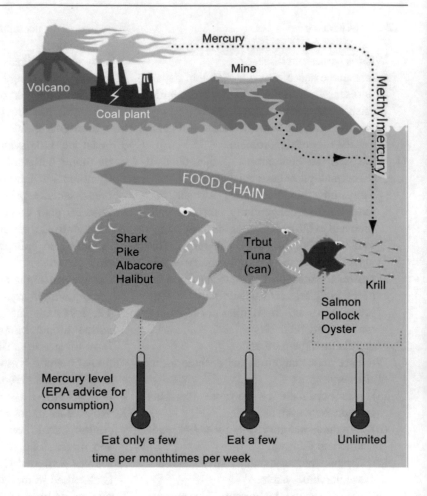

and embryotoxicity. Major organs affected along with their manifestation in mercury poisoning are summarized in Table 12.1.

3.3 Arsenic

Q. Which form of arsenic is nonpoisonous?
- Arsenic is a heavy metallic inorganic irritant poison. Metallic arsenic is not poisonous as it is insoluble in water and cannot be absorbed from the GI tract.

Q. What is the mode of action of arsenic?
- Arsenic compounds act by inactivating the sulfhydryl enzymes, which in turn interfere with the cellular metabolism, in the liver,

Table 12.1 Major organs affected along with their manifestation in mercury poisoning

Organ or system affected	Manifestations
Brain	Memory loss, attention deficit, ataxia, impairment of hearing and vision, sensory disturbances, fatigue, autism in children
Motor system	Disruption of motor function, decreased muscular strength, late walking in children
Kidney	Increased plasma creatinine level
Heart	Alteration of normal cardiovascular homeostasis
Immune	System decreased immunity, multiple sclerosis, autoimmune thyroiditis
Reproductive system	Decreased fertility rate, abnormal offspring

lungs, intestinal wall, and spleen. Arsenic can replace phosphorus in the bones where it may remain for years. It also gets deposited in the hairs.

Q. What is raindrop pigmentation in arsenic poisoning?
- Raindrop pigmentation is known to produce milk and roses complexion followed by patchy brown pigmentation of the skin (especially face), which resembles the raindrops. It might also show hyperkeratosis of the skin of the palm and soles, which is prone to change into basal cell carcinoma at a later stage. The scalp may also show alopecia (baldness).

Q. What are Meese's lines?
- Meese's lines are *lines* of discoloration across the nails of the fingers and toes (whitish lines 1–2 mm breadth) across the mail of the finger and toes. These symptoms represent chronic arsenic poisoning as a result of high sulfhydryl content of the keratin.

Q. In arsenic poisoning, why milk is considered unfit, whereas meat is passed for human consumption?
- Arsenic gets methylated and gets rapidly excreted through urine, milk, sweat, etc. Hence, milk is considered unfit for consumption. As arsenic tends to accumulate only in visceral organs and not in muscles, flesh of surviving animal is considered fit for human consumption.

Q. Is arsenic cumulative in animals?
- No, arsenic is rapidly detoxified and is completely eliminated in few days.

Q. In which species of animals organic arsenicals cause nervous symptoms?
- Swine are mostly affected. Nervous symptoms include ataxia, incoordination, etc.

Q. Which form of arsenic is more toxic?
- Arsenite (As3+ or trivalent) is 5–10 times more toxic than arsenate (As5+ or pentavalent) due to higher solubility.

Q. Malicious poisoning is very common with which arsenic compound?
- Arsenic trioxide

Q. Why arsenic can cause abortions but not nervous symptoms?
- Arsenic can cross placental barrier and hence can cause abortions, but in most of species, it cannot cross blood–brain barrier (BBB), and, hence, is unable to cause nervous symptoms.

Q. How is arsenic differentiated from lead poisoning?
- In arsenic poisoning, severe gastroenteritis and absence of nervous symptoms are observed, whereas in lead poisoning, the symptoms are just the reverse.

Q. Why arsenic tends to accumulate in keratin-rich tissues such as hair and nails?
- Arsenic has high affinity for sulfhydryl groups (–SH). Since hair and nails contain –SH-rich keratin, arsenic accumulates in them.

Q. What are the prominent postmortem findings in arsenic poisoning?
- Severe gastroenteritis

Q. What is arsenical neuritis?
- The victim presents with polyneuritis, optic neuritis, anesthesias, paresthesias, atrophy of extensors resulting in wrist drop, etc.

Q. Which form of arsenic is poisonous?
- Arsenious oxide or arsenic trioxide (sankhyal or somalker) is poisonous. They are found in shellfish, codfish, and haddock. Sources of poisoning include soil, well water, shellfish, and arsenic compounds. Inorganic arsenicals, a by-product of smelting of ore containing copper, lead, and zinc, are more toxic than the organic.

3.4 Cadmium

Q. Which is metal-binding protein for cadmium?
- Metal-binding protein for cadmium is cysteine-rich and readily binds to and induces the production of metallothionein; binding to metallothionein does not have a major effect on the uptake of cadmium but

is, in part, responsible for retention of cadmium within cells. Metallothionein does this by decreasing cadmium elimination, especially in bile.

Q. What is itai-itai disease?

• Itai-itai disease was the name given to the mass cadmium poisoning of Toyama Prefecture, Japan, starting around 1912. The term "itai-itai disease" was coined by locals for the severe pains felt in the spine and joints of victims. The disease resulted from consumption of cadmium-contaminated rice.

Q. What is the mechanism of toxicity of cadmium?

• Cadmium is present in the circulatory system bound primarily to the metal binding protein, metallothionein (CdMT), produced in the liver. Following glomerular filtration in the kidney, CdMT is reabsorbed efficiently by the proximal tubule cells, where it accumulates within the lysosomes. Subsequent degradation of the CdMT complex releases $Cd+2$, which inhibits lysosomal function, resulting in cell injury. The mechanism of chromium ($Cr+6$) carcinogenicity in the lung is believed to be its reduction to $Cr+3$ and generation of reactive intermediates, leading to bronchogenic carcinoma.

Q. What is half-life of cadmium?

• Half-life of cadmium is about 30 years.

3.5   Nickel

Q. What are the sources of nickel poisoning?
Nickel is used in various metal alloys, including stainless steels, and in electroplating. Occupational exposure to nickel occurs by inhalation of nickel-containing aerosols, dusts, or fumes, or dermal contact in workers engaged in nickel production (mining, milling, refinery, etc.) and nickel-using operations (melting, electroplating, welding, nickel–cadmium batteries, etc.). Nickel is ubiquitous in nature, and the general population is exposed to low levels of nickel in air, cigarette smoke, water, and food.

3.6   Copper

Q. What are the major sources of exposure to copper in the general population?
Food, beverages, and drinking water are major sources of exposure in the general population. Copper exposure in industry is primarily from inhaled particulates in mining or metal fumes in smelting operations, welding, or related activities.

Q. What are the commonly adverse health effects of excess oral copper intake?
The most commonly reported adverse health effects of excess oral copper intake are gastrointestinal distress. Nausea, vomiting, and abdominal pain have been reported shortly after drinking solutions of copper sulfate or beverages stored in containers that readily release copper. Ingestion of large amounts of copper salts, most frequently copper sulfate, may produce hepatic necrosis and death.

Q. Which salts of copper are poisonous?

• Copper, an inorganic metallic irritant, is not poisonous in metallic state, but some of its salts are poisonous, e.g., copper sulfate (blue vitriol) and copper subacetate (verdigris). *Copper toxicity*, also called copperiedus, refers to the consequences of an excess of overuse of copper sulfate as an algicide has been speculated to have *caused a copper poisoning* epidemic on Great Palm Island in 1979.

Q. Define hereditary disease of copper metabolism?
The disease is known as Menkes disease. The Menkes disease can be linked to deficiencies in copper-containing proteins. The gene responsible for Menkes disease, ATP7A, belongs to the family of ATPases and is a copper transporter. This is a rare sex-linked genetic defect in copper metabolism resulting in copper deficiency in male infants. It is characterized by severe mental retardation,

neurological impairment, connective tissue dysfunction, and death usually by 3–5 years of age. Bones are osteoporotic with altered metaphases of the long bones and bones of the skull. There is extensive degeneration of the cerebral cortex and of white matter.

Q. What is Wilson's disease?

Wilson's disease is an autosomal recessive genetic disorder of copper metabolism characterized by the excessive accumulation of copper in the liver, brain, kidneys, and cornea. Clinical abnormalities of the nervous system, liver, kidneys, and cornea are related to copper accumulation. Patients with Wilson's disease have impaired biliary excretion of copper.

Q. Which breed of animal is more susceptible to copper toxicosis?

Some animals show genetic variations. For example, Bedlington terrier (breed of dog) is highly susceptible to copper toxicosis due to genetic predisposition. This breed has autosomal recessive gene that causes retention of copper due to failure of excretion.

Q. What are signs and symptoms of copper deficiency?

- Copper deficiency is likely to occur in winter on free draining or peaty soils, especially when there has been lots of rain. Young stock is more prone to copper deficiency and shows poor growth and loss of coordination of the hind limbs, and adult cattle gets diarrhea (scours), dehydration, jaundice, and blood in the urine.

3.7   Cobalt

Q. Why animals need cobalt?

- All ruminants (including sheep, cattle, and goats) require cobalt in their diet for the synthesis of vitamin B12. Vitamin B12 is essential for energy metabolism and the production of red blood cells. Normally microorganisms in the rumen are able to synthesize vitamin B12 needs of ruminants if the diet is adequate in cobalt. Cobalt defi-

ciency in soils can cause vitamin B12 deficiency in livestock.

Q. What are the symptoms of cobalt deficiency?

- Cobalt deficiency causes lack of appetite, lack of thrift, severe emaciation, weakness, anemia, decreased fertility, decreased milk and wool production, and weeping eyes, leading to a matting of wool on the face. Sheep are more susceptible to cobalt deficiency than cattle. Cobalt deficiency also impairs the immune function of sheep which may increase their vulnerability to infection with worms.

3.8   Chromium

Q. In which form chromium is available?

- Chromium occurs in a number of oxidation states from Cr+2 to Cr+6, but only the trivalent (Cr+3) and hexavalent (Cr+6) forms are of biological significance.

Q. Which form of chromium is toxic?

- The trivalent compound is the most common form found in nature. The hexavalent form is of greater industrial importance. In addition, hexavalent chromium, which is not water soluble, is more readily absorbed across cell membranes than is trivalent chromium. In vivo the hexavalent form is reduced to the trivalent form, which can complex with intracellular macromolecules, resulting in toxicity. Chromium is a known human carcinogen and induces lung cancers among exposed workers.

3.9   Iron

Q. What are the sources of iron toxicity?

Iron is an inorganic metallic irritant. Most exposures involve children less than 6 years of age who have ingested pediatric multivitamin preparations. Concentrated iron supplement overdoses more often result in serious poisoning.

Q. Why iron is considered an essential metal?

Iron is an essential metal for erythropoiesis and a key component of hemoglobin, myoglobin, heme enzymes, metalloflavoprotein enzymes, and mitochondrial enzymes. In biological systems, iron mainly exists as the ferrous (+2) and ferric (+3) forms.

Q. What are the complications of iron overload in human beings?

Iron overload and complications of iron toxicity are summarized in Table 12.2.

Q. Numerate various steps involved in the catabolism of heme.

Various steps involved in the catabolism of heme include:

- Generation of bilirubin
- Transport to the liver
- Conjugation in the liver
- Excretion of bilirubin in the intestine
- Fate of conjugated bilirubin in the intestine
- Enterohepatic circulation
- Final excretion

Q. What are common problems associated with chronic iron toxicity?

Chronic iron toxicity from iron overload in adults is a relatively common problem. There are three basic ways in which excessive amounts of iron can accumulate in the body:

(a) Hereditary hemochromatosis due to abnormal absorption of iron from the intestinal tract

(b) Excess intake via the diet or from oral iron preparations

(c) Repeated blood transfusions for some form of refractory anemia (transfusional siderosis).

Table 12.2 Iron toxicity and overload

Iron is essential for cellular metabolism, but too much can be toxic
Upper limit has been set at 45 mg/day from all sources
Iron poisoning can be life-threatening. It can damage the intestine lining and cause abnormalities in body pH, shock, and liver failure
Iron overload can happen over time and accumulates in tissues such as the heart and the liver
The most common form of iron overload is hemochromatosis

Increased body iron may play a role in the development of cardiovascular disease. It is suspected that iron may act as a catalyst to produce free radical damage resulting in atherosclerosis and ischemic heart disease. Some neurodegenerative disorders associated with aberrant iron metabolism in the brain include neuroferritinopathy, aceruloplasminemia, and manganism.

Q. Name the specific antidote of iron toxicity?

Deferoxamine (desferrioxamine) is the specific antidote.

3.10 Zinc

Q. What is the source of exposure to zinc?

Zinc is present in most food stuffs, water, and air. Occupational exposure to dusts and fumes of metallic zinc occurs in zinc mining and smelting. The zinc content of substances in contact with galvanized copper or plastic pipes may be high.

Q. What is zinc deficiency?

Zinc deficiency *or* hypozincemia is caused by lack of zinc in the diet. The disease is characterized by growth retardation, loss of appetite, and impaired immune function. In more severe cases, zinc deficiency causes hair loss, diarrhea, delayed sexual maturation, impotence, hypogonadism in males, and eye and skin lesions.

Q. How zinc administration decreases development of copper toxicity?

- Zinc induces the synthesis of mucosal metallothioneins in GIT, which bind to copper and prevent Cu absorption. Hence, zinc supplementation decreases the development of copper toxicity.

Q. How zinc deficiency is caused?

- Much of the zinc consumed in the diet is not absorbed and leads to zinc deficiency. A diet high in fiber and phytates (present in whole-grain bread, bran, beans, soybeans, other legumes, and nuts), various disorders, alcoholism, and use of diuretics reduces zinc absorption.

Q. What is the cure for zinc deficiency?
- Zinc deficiency can be treated by taking dietary zinc supplements or by eating foods that are rich and fortified with zinc.

3.11   Manganese

Q.2. Describe the toxic potential of manganese (Mn).
- Despite its essentiality, Mn overexposure can cause a variety of toxic effects in humans and animals. Mn has been linked to a peculiar extrapyramidal syndrome in occupational workers since 1837 (Mn induced Parkinsonism). Clinical investigations include bradykinesia, rigidity, masked face diminished blinking, impaired dexterity, gait abnormalities, hypophonia, and micrographia. Long-term exposure to excess levels may cause kidney failure, hallucinations, as well as diseases of the central nervous system, and reproductive and developmental effects.

Q. What is the role of manganese in the body?
- Manganese is an activator of enzyme reactions concerned with carbohydrate, protein, and lipid metabolism.

3.12   Selenium

Q. What are different forms of selenium?
- Selenium occurs in nature and biological systems as selenate (Se6+), selenite (Se4+), selenide (Se2+), and elemental selenium (Se0).

Q. Why selenium toxicity is more commonly seen in arid and semiarid climatic zones?
- In arid and semiarid climatic zones, due to less rainfall, selenium is not leached from the top layers of the soil. Hence, chances of selenium accumulation are more common.

Q. Why cracked and overgrown hooves are seen in selenium poisoning?
- Selenium replaces sulfur in sulfur-containing amino acids such as cysteine and methionine, which leads to structural abnormalities in proteins. Hence, overgrown and cracked hooves are seen.

Q. What is selenium toxicity?
- Selenium is a non-metal that functions as both toxicant and an essential element. Selenium poisoning occurs when animals ingest excessive amounts of selenium. In its most severe form, it causes blindness and staggering. It can also cause cracked hooves and lameness.
  Subacute toxicity is called blind staggers and caused by the accumulation of 2–5 ppm of selenium in dry matter content.

3.13   Phosphorus

Q. Do you recommend use of administration of oil or fat in phosphorus poisoning? Give reasons.
- No. Oral administration of oil, fat, egg, etc. is not recommended because phosphorus is soluble in these agents and would enhance its absorption.

Q. Name the non-metal toxicity that could occur during some festivals and in war zones?
  It is phosphorus because yellow phosphorus is used in the manufacture of fire crackers and military ammunition.

Q. Why burns due to phosphorus causes higher mortality than other agents?
- The absorption of phosphorus through raw burnt surface leads to multi-organ failure. Hence, burns due to phosphorus are more dangerous than other burns.

Q. Why oily purgatives such as mineral oils are contraindicated in phosphorus poisoning?
- Oils increase the absorption of phosphorus and hence are contraindicated in phosphorus poisoning.

Q. What is phossy jaw?
- Phossy jaw, formally phosphorus necrosis of the jaw, is an occupational disease of those who work with white phosphorus, also known as yellow phosphorus, without proper safeguards. It was most commonly seen in workers in the match industry in the nineteenth and early twentieth century.

Q. What are different forms of phosphorus and
  name their common derivatives?

  • Phosphorus exists in two forms—white or
    yellow and red phosphorus. Derivatives of
    phosphorus include aluminum phosphide,
    zinc phosphide, and phosphine gas.

3.14   Iodine

Q. What are main postmortem findings in iodine
  poisoning?

  • They are brownish stains of skin and
    mucosa, characteristic iodine odor, and
    congestion of all the viscera. Stomach may
    slow blue content if starchy food is present.
    The heart and liver may show fatty degen-
    eration and kidneys glomerular/tubular
    necrosis.

Q. What is the antidote of iodine poisoning?

  • Sodium thiosulfate solution (1–5%) orally,
    in iodism, liberal intake of sodium chloride
    or sodium bicarbonate is useful.

3.15   Sulfur

Q. What are different compounds of sulfur?

  • Sulfur can react with all metals except gold
    and platinum, forming sulfide. It also forms
    compounds with several nonmetallic ele-
    ments. It forms compounds in oxidation
    states: −2 (sulfide, S^{2-}), +4 (sulfite, SO_3^{2-}),
    and +6 (sulfate, SO_4^{2-}). Millions of tons of
    sulfur are produced each year, mostly for
    the manufacture of sulfuric acid, which is
    widely used in industry.

Q. Is sulfur important for our body, if so how?

  • Yes. The "beauty mineral," sulfur, is neces-
    sary for healthy skin, hair, and nails. It is
    also an important element of body detoxifi-
    cation: as a part of detox enzymes and
    sulfur-containing amino acids cysteine and
    methionine, it binds to toxic heavy metal
    contaminants—especially   aluminum—
    making its elimination much easier. Sulfur
    also helps regeneration of joint cartilage,
    both by helping it rebuild and by suppress-
    ing copper, whose high levels promote

joint degeneration. Sulfur is useful in
reducing allergic reactions and parasitic
infections.

Sulfur is also a component of insulin and
thus necessary for proper metabolism of
carbohydrates. Thus low sulfur levels can
aggravate symptoms of diabetes.

Q. What are the symptoms of inorganic sulfur
  compound toxicity?

  • Inorganic (not carbon-bonded) sulfur com-
    pounds, such as those found in fossil fuels
    and their emissions, pesticides, industrial
    compounds, food additives, and drugs, can
    aggravate allergies, chemical sensitivities,
    and symptoms of diabetes, impair immune
    system's antibody response, and, possibly,
    even alter the DNA/RNA function.

Q. What are short-term and long-term effects of
  high sulfur supplementation?

  • Short-term effects of high sulfur supple-
    mentation can cause digestive disturbance,
    while long-term exposure can result in low-
    ering body levels of potassium and
    calcium.

    Some serious chronic diseases—like
    Crohn's and Lou-Gehrig—are further
    aggravated by sulfur intake. On the other
    hand, extra sulfur intake helps with
    Alzheimer's, as well as chronic toxicity
    caused by heavy metals.

3.16   Fluoride

Q. How fluoride excess affects teeth and bones
  of animals and human beings?

  • Chronic excess fluoride ingestion affects
    the teeth and bones of affected animals and
    human beings. Fluoride substitutes for
    hydroxyl groups in the hydroxyapatite of
    the bone matrix which alters the mineral-
    ization and crystal structure of the bone.
    Bone changes induced by excess fluoride
    ingestion, termed skeletal fluorosis or
    osteofluorosis, include the interference of
    the normal sequences of osteogenesis and bone
    remodeling with the resulting production of
    abnormal bone or the resorption of normal
    bone. The fluoride content of the bone can

increase over a period of time without other noticeable changes in the bone structure or function.

Q. Why fluorine is not available in free form?
- Fluorine is the most reactive non-metal (due to high electron gravity) and hence is not available in free form. It is seen in combination with other elements as fluorides.

Q. What is fluorosis?
- Fluorosis is a chronic condition caused by excessive intake of fluorine compounds, marked by mottling and staining of the teeth, and, if severe, calcification of the ligaments and abnormalities of the skeleton are observed.

3.17 Molybdenum

Q. What is molybdenum poisoning in animals?
- It is caused by imbalance in copper/molybdenum ratios in soil. Ruminants, especially young cattle, are most susceptible.

Q. Why molybdate salts are given as supportive therapy in copper poisoning in animals?
- Molybdenum has inverse relationship with copper, increasing its elimination. Hence, molybdate salts are used in copper poisoning.

Q. How you can reverse the adverse effects of excess molybdenum?
- Treatment with supplemental copper can often reverse the adverse effects of excess molybdenum. Conversely, treatment of Wilson disease with molybdenum compounds is used to reduce copper burden. Molybdenum treatment may also be beneficial for angiogenesis, inflammation, and other disorders associated with excess copper.

3.18 Metals Related to Medical Therapy

Q. Which metals are related to medical therapy?
A number of metals that are related to treat a number of human illnesses, including aluminum, bismuth, gold, lithium, and platinum, exert some toxicity.

Aluminum

Q. Which form of aluminum is toxic?
- Aluminum (Al) is the third most abundant element that occurs naturally in the earth's crust. Poisoning in human beings and animals by Al is rare. Among all Al compounds, Al phosphide is of major concern to animals, because at a low stomach pH, phosphide converts to toxic phosphine (PH3) gas.

Q. Define in brief toxicity of aluminum.
- Toxicity of Al depends on its chemical form, route of exposure, and animal species. The central nervous system (CNS) and skeletal system appear to be the two major target organs for Al toxicity. It has been known for a while that Al is involved in neurodegenerative diseases like Alzheimer's, encephalopathy, and amyotrophic sclerosis.

Q. What is the source of exposure to lithium?
Lithium is used in batteries, alloys, catalysts, photographic materials, and the space industry. Lithium hydride produces hydrogen on contact with water and is used in manufacturing electronic tubes, in ceramics, and in chemical analysis. Groundwater contamination with lithium from man-made waste disposal could be a risk factor for the aquatic environment. Lithium carbonate and lithium citrate are widely used for mania and bipolar disorders.

Q. What are symptoms of exposure to platinum?
Platinum can produce profound hypersensitivity reactions in susceptible individuals. The signs of hypersensitivity include urticaria, contact dermatitis to the skin, and respiratory distress, ranging from irritation to an asthmatic syndrome, following exposure to platinum dust.

4   Sample MCQ's

Q.1. Exposure to fumes of which of the following metals is most likely to cause acute chemical pneumonitis and pulmonary edema?

A. Lead
B. Zinc
C. Cadmium
D. Copper
E. Magnesium

Q.2. Deficiency of which element in the sow predisposes baby pigs to toxicosis by injectable iron preparations?

A. Copper
B. Chromium
C. Magnesium
D. Selenium
E. Zinc

Q.3. Which of the following is *not* commonly associated with mercury vapor poisoning?

A. Acute, corrosive bronchitis
B. Interstitial pneumonitis
C. Tremor
D. Increased excitability
E. Vomiting and bloody diarrhea

Q.4. Which form of mercury was the predominant cause of Minamata Bay disease?

A. Metallic mercury
B. Mercuric salts
C. Mercurous salts
D. Organic mercury compounds
E. Mercury was not the causative agent

Q.5. Which is the only arsenical that can cause blindness?

A. Arsenic trioxide
B. Arsenic pentoxide
C. Arsine
D. Arsanilic acid

Q.6. Copper has inverse interrelationship with the following element(s)

A. Iron
B. Molybdenum
C. Sulfur
D. Both B and C

Q.7. In lead poisoning, basophilic stipplings (BS) are commonly seen in which species?

A. Cattle
B. Sheep
C. Dog
D. Horse

Q.8. Which of the following chelating agent(s) that is/are used for treating mercury poisoning?

A. Dimercaprol (BAL)
B. D-Penicillamine
C. DMSA (Succimer)
D. Na-thiosulfate
E. All the above

Q.9. Which of the following nutrient(s) can counteract toxicity of organic mercurial?

A. Vitamin A
B. Vitamin D
C. Vitamin E
D. Selenium

Q.10. Fluoride inhibits pyruvic acid synthesis by inhibiting an enzyme-

A. Enolase
B. Transaminase
C. Phosphatase
D. Phosphodiesterase

Q.11. Which of the following forms of Hg is more toxic?

A. Elemental
B. Monovalent
C. Divalent
D. Organic

Q.12. Mercury can cross the following barriers in the body through ----

A. Blood–brain barrier (BBB)
B. Placental barrier (PB)
C. Both
D. No barrier

Q.13. The following properties can be attributed to methyl mercury (organic Hg) ---

A. Mutagenic
B. Carcinogenic
C. Embryotoxic
D. Teratogenic
E. All the above

Q.14. Which of the following is *not* a major excretory pathway of metals?

A. Sweat
B. Urine
C. Respiration
D. Feces
E. Hair

Q.15. Which of the following conditions represents a manifestation of moderate chronic fluoride toxicity?

A. Osteomalacia
B. Osteosclerosis
C. Osteopetrosis
D. OsteopeniaE
E. Osteolysis

Q.16. Inorganic arsenic toxicosis is manifested clinically as ------

A. Icterus, anemia, and hemoglobinuria
B. Anurosis, incoordination, and constipation
C. Cardiomyopathy, hydrothorax, and ascites
D. Photosensitization, dermatitis, and hair loss
E. Vomiting, gastroenteritis, diarrhea, and dehydration

Q.17. Which combination of mineral additives is most useful in preventing chronic copper toxicosis in sheep?

A. Selenium and molybdenum
B. Selenium and sulfate
C. Zinc and molybdenum
D. Sulfate and molybdenum
E. Arsenic and sulfate

Q.18. Which of the following form of phosphorus is toxic?

A. White
B. Red
C. Yellow
D. Black

Answers
1. C.   2. D.   3. E.   4. D.   5. D.   6. C.
7. C.   8. E.   9. C and D.   10. A.   11. D.
12. C.   13. E.   14. C.   15. B.   16. E.
17. D.   18. A and C.

Further Reading

Gupta PK (1988) Veterinary toxicology. Cosmo Publications, New Delhi
Gupta PK (2010) Modern toxicology: adverse effects of xenobiotics, vol 2, 2nd reprint. PharmaMed Press, Hyderabad
Gupta PK (2014) Essential concepts in toxicology. PharmaMed Press (A Unit of BSP Books Pvt. Ltd, Hyderabad
Gupta PK (2016) Fundamentals of toxicology: essential concepts and applications, 1st edn. BSP/Elsevier, San Diego
Gupta PK (2018) Illustrative toxicology, 1st edn. Elsevier, San Diego
Gupta RC (2018) Veterinary toxicology: basic and clinical principles, 3rd edn. Academic Press/Elsevier, San Diego
Gupta PK (2019) Concepts and applications in veterinary toxicology: an interactive guide, 1st edn. Springer-Nature, Switzerland
Gupta PK (2020) Brainstorming questions in toxicology. Francis and Taylor CRC Press, Boca Raton
Klaassen CD (ed) (2019) Casarett & Doull's toxicology: the basic science of poisons, 9th edn. McGraw-Hill, New York
Klaassen CD, Watkins JB III (eds) (2015) Casarett & Doull's essentials of toxicology, 3rd edn. McGraw-Hill, New York

Solvents, Gasses, and Vapors

13

Abstract

This chapter deals with toxicologic hazards of solvents (alcohols, glycols and petroleum), toxic gases and vapors (carbon monoxide, hydrogen sulfide, oxides of nitrogen, cyanide gas, gaseous ammonia, smoke inhalation, phosphine gas etc.), organic compounds, brominated flame retardants, perfluorinated agents, persistent halogenated aromatic products, coat tar products, pentachlorophenols, and household products (chlorine bleaches, detergents, soaps and shampoos etc.). Hydrogen sulfide (H2S; "sewer gas," "swamp gas," "sour gas," and "stink damp") is most commonly encountered as a byproduct of the decomposition of sulfur-containing organic material. In general, the toxic effects of multiple solvents are additive; solvents may also interact synergistically or antagonistically. The chapter briefly describes the overview, key points, and relevant text that are in the format of problem-solving study questions followed by multiple-choice questions (MCQs) along with their answers.

Keywords

Vapors · Solvents · Gases · Inhalants · MCQs · Toxicity · Solvent abuse · Carbon disulfide · Automobile gasoline · Question and answer bank

1 Introduction

Solvents have variable lipophilicity and volatility, small molecular size, and lack of charge. Absorption of inhaled volatile organic compounds occurs in the alveoli, with almost instantaneous equilibration with the blood in the pulmonary capillaries. Adverse effects of vapors, solvents, and gases such as trichloroethylene chloride, carbon tetrachloride, benzene, toluene, xylene and ethylene, alcohols, glycols, petroleum products, inhalants, solvent abuse, carbon disulfide, and automobile gasoline are briefly discussed along with an overview, key points, and relevant text that are in the format of problem-solving study questions followed by multiple-choice questions (MCQ's) and their answers.

2 Overview

Solvents are frequently complex mixtures and may include nitrogen- or sulfur-containing organics—gasoline, and other oil-based products. Vapor can be condensed to a liquid by increasing the pressure on it without reducing the temperature. A vapor is different from an aerosol. An aerosol is a suspension of tiny particles of liquid, solid, or both within a gas. Solvents can be (a) *aliphatic hydrocarbons*, such as hexane; (b) *halogenated aliphatic hydrocarbons*, such as methylene dichloride, chloroform, and carbon tetrachloride; (c) *aliphatic alcohols*, such as methanol and ethanol; (d) *glycols and glycol ethers such as e*thylene and propylene glycols; and (e) *aromatic hydrocarbons such as* benzene and toluene. Inhalants are a broad range of intoxicative drugs whose gases or volatile vapors are breathed in via the nose or mouth. They are taken by room temperature volatilization or from a pressurized container (e.g., nitrous oxide), and do not include drugs that are sniffed after burning or heating. For example, amyl nitrite and toluene—the solvent used in contact cement and model airplane glue—are considered inhalants, but tobacco, cannabis, and crack are not, even though the latter are also inhaled (as smoke). Assumption is frequently made that the toxic effects of multiple solvents are additive and solvents may also interact synergistically or antagonistically. Although some solvents are less hazardous than others, all solvents can cause toxic effects. Most have the potential to induce narcosis and cause respiratory and mucous membrane irritation. The Occupational Safety and Health Administration (OSHA) has established legally enforceable permissible exposure limits (PELs) for solvents.

Key Points

- A solvent is a liquid organic chemical that has the ability to dissolve, suspend, or extract other materials, without chemical change to the material or solvent.
- Solvents have variable lipophilicity and volatility, small molecular size, and lack of charge.
- Absorption of inhaled volatile organic compounds occurs in the alveoli, with almost instantaneous equilibration with the blood in the pulmonary capillaries.
- Solvents are readily absorbed from the gastrointestinal tract and across the skin.
- Most solvents produce some degree of CNS depression.

- Subtle differences in chemical structure can translate into dramatic differences in solvent toxicity.
- Nearly everyone is exposed to solvents during normal daily activities.
- Environmental exposures to solvents in air and groundwater use multiple exposure pathways.
- A vapor represents the gas phase of components from substances that are either solid or liquid at standard temperatures and pressures.
- Gas is a state of matter consisting of particles that have neither a defined volume nor a defined shape at standard temperatures and pressures.

3   Problem-Solving Study Questions

3.1   Solvents

Q. What are common routes of exposure of solvents?
   A. Oral
   B. Inhalation (major)
   C. Skin
Q. What are the main dangers of solvents?
   A. Toxic effects
   B. Corrosive effects
   C. Flammable effects
   D. Reactive nature-incompatible chemicals
Q. What are the properties of solvents?
   Solvent chemicals have variable lipophilicity and volatility. These properties, coupled with small molecular size and lack of charge, make inhalation the major route of solvent exposure and provide for ready absorption across the lung, gastrointestinal (GI) tract, and skin.
Q. What are the uses of solvents?
   Solvents are so widely used in the modern world as to be ubiquitous and are employed in paints, pharmaceuticals, degreasants, adhesives, printing inks, pesticides, cosmetics, and household cleaners. The largest end user

is the coatings industry where solvents play an important role in the quality and durability of paints and varnishes.

Q. How solvents are absorbed?

The majority of systemic absorption of inhaled volatile organic compounds (VOCs) occurs in the alveoli, although limited absorption has been demonstrated to occur in the upper respiratory tract. Gases in the alveoli are thought to equilibrate almost instantaneously with the blood in the pulmonary capillaries.

Q. What are the commonly used solvents?

The commonly used solvents include isopropanol, toluene, xylene, and solvent mixtures such as white spirits and the chlorinated solvents, methylene chloride, trichloroethylene (TCE), and perchloroethylene. In the recent past, 1-bromopropane has been introduced, to replace ozone-depleting agents such as 1,1,1-trichloroethane (methyl chloroform).

Q. Define factors which govern toxicity from solvent exposure.

A. Solvent exposure is dependent on several factors:

B. Toxicity of the solvent

C. Exposure route

D. Amount or rate of exposure

E. Duration of exposure

F. Individual susceptibility

G. Interactions

Q. What is a painter's syndrome?

The painter's syndrome was first described in Scandinavia in the late 1970s and became a recognized occupational disease in these countries. The cluster of symptoms includes headache, fatigue, sleep disorders, personality changes, and emotional instability, which progress to impaired intellectual function and ultimately, dementia. Early symptoms are often reversible if exposure is stopped.

Q. List possible ways global warming could change the climate and ecology of our planet and alter toxic effects of chemicals.

A. Global warming melts the polar ice caps and reduces the size of ice fields; this increases sea levels, affecting the world's coastline.

B. Local changes—Marshlands will become flooded; lakes and rivers increase in size; and human settlements become flooded. Increased evaporation in dry areas increases desert.

Q. What is Kaposi's sarcoma (KS)?

Amyl and butyl nitrites have been associated with Kaposi's sarcoma (KS), the most common cancer reported among AIDS patients.

Chlorinated Hydrocarbons

Q. How trichloroethylene (TCE) is released into the atmosphere?

TCE is a widely used solvent identified so far. It is released into the atmosphere from vapor degreasing operations; however, direct discharges to surface waters and groundwater from disposal operations have been the frequent occurrences. As a result, TCE can be released to indoor air by vapor intrusion through underground walls and floors and by volatilization from the water supply.

Q. What is the source of exposure to tetrachloroethylene?

Tetrachloroethylene (perchloroethylene) is commonly used as a dry cleaner, fabric finisher, degreaser, rug and upholstery cleaner, paint and stain remover, solvent, and chemical intermediate. The highest exposures usually occur in occupational settings via inhalation.

Q. What are the toxic effects of tetrachloroethylene?

The chemical is well absorbed from the lungs and GI tract and distributed to tissues according to their lipid content. Dry-cleaning workers exposed to these chemicals show modest changes in a few indices of liver or kidney cell functions. More effects may occur in humans exposed for longer periods. Moderate-to-high doses of TCE, as with other halocarbons, are associated with a number of non-cancer toxicities. TCE has been implicated in the development of autoimmune disorders and immune system dysfunction and has been investigated for its potential as a male reproductive toxicant. Several studies indicate that TCE can cause cancer.

Q. How carbon tetrachloride (CC14) is released into the atmosphere?

CC14 has widespread use as a solvent, cleaning agent, fire extinguisher, synthetic intermediate, grain fumigant, and human anthelmintic. Nevertheless, CC14 appears to be ubiquitous in ambient air in the United States, and it is still found in groundwater from some wells and waste sites.

Q. What are hazards and risks of carbon tetrachloride?

A. Carbon tetrachloride is an effective fat solvent, easily ingested, and attacks the liver and the brain and nervous system, causing loss of control and anesthesia.

B. Removes natural oils from the skin, causing blistering.

C. Dissolves sealants in plumbing systems.

D. Liver damage may lead to liver cancer.

E. Not flammable.

Q. Describe in brief toxicity of chloroform (CHCl3).

The primary use of CHCl3 (trichloromethane) is in the production of the refrigerant chlorodifluoromethane (Freon 22), but this use is expected to diminish as chlorine-containing fluorocarbons are phased out under the Montreal Protocol. CHCl3 was among the first inhalation anesthetics, but it was replaced by safer compounds after about 1940. The reproductive and developmental toxicities of CHCl3 are unremarkable. Inhalation of 100–300 ppm CHCl3 by pregnant rats caused a high incidence of fetal resorption, retardation of fetal development, and a low incidence of fetal anomalies. Under certain conditions CHCl3 is hepatotoxic and nephrotoxic. These toxicities are potentiated by aliphatic alcohols, ketones, and dichloroacetate (DCA) and trichloroacetic acid (TCA). The status of CHCl3 as a rodent carcinogen is indisputable. It causes liver and kidney tumors that are species-, strain-, sex-, and route or exposure-dependent.

Q. What are the hazards and risks of chloroform?

A. Effective fat solvent, easily ingested, attacks the liver and the brain and nervous system, causing loss of control and anesthesia.

B. Removes natural oils from the skin, causing blistering.

C. Dissolves sealants in plumbing systems.

D. Vapors are poisonous and affect the nervous system: not flammable

Q. List three most commonly used organic solvents that can cause hazards and risks.

A. Chloroform

B. Carbon tetrachloride

C. Ethanol

Aromatic Hydrocarbons

Q. What is the source of exposure to benzene?

Benzene produced commercially in the United States is derived primarily from petroleum. Benzene has been utilized as a general-purpose solvent, but it is now used principally in the synthesis of other chemicals. The percentage by volume of benzene in gasoline is 1–2%. Benzene plays an important role in unleaded gasoline due to its antiknock properties. Inhalation is the primary route of exposure in industrial and in everyday settings. Cigarette smoke is the major source of benzene in the home.

Q. What are the toxic effects of benzene?

The most important adverse effect of benzene is hematopoietic toxicity. Chronic exposure to benzene can lead to bone marrow damage, which may be manifest initially as anemia, leukopenia, thrombocytopenia, or a combination of these. Bone marrow depression appears to be dose dependent in both laboratory animals and humans. Continued exposure may result in marrow aplasia and pancytopenia, an often fatal outcome. Survivors of aplastic anemia frequently exhibit a preneoplastic state, termed myelodysplasia, which may progress to myelogenous leukemia.

Q. What is the source of exposure to toluene?

Toluene is present in paints, lacquers, thinners, cleaning agents, glues, and many other products. Toluene is also used in the production of other chemicals. Gasoline, which contains 5–7% toluene by weight, is the largest source of atmospheric emissions and exposure of the general populace. Inhalation is the primary route of exposure, though skin contact occurs frequently. Toluene is a favorite of solvent abusers, who intentionally inhale high concentrations to achieve a euphoric effect. Large amounts of toluene enter the environment each year by volatilization. Relatively small amounts are released into industrial wastewater. Toluene is frequently found in water, soil, and air at hazardous waste.

Q. What are the toxic effects of toluene?

The central nervous system (CNS) is the primary target organ of toluene and other alkylbenzenes. Manifestations of acute exposure range from slight dizziness and headache to unconsciousness, respiratory depression, and death. Occupational inhalation exposure guidelines are established to prevent significant decrements in psychomotor functions. Acute encephalopathic effects are rapidly reversible upon cessation of exposure. Subtle neurological effects have been described in some groups of occupationally exposed individuals. Exposure to approximately 100 ppm toluene for years may result in subclinical effects.

Q. What is the source of exposure to xylenes and ethylbenzene?

Xylenes and ethylbenzene, like benzene and toluene, are the major components of gasoline and fuel oil. The primary uses of xylenes industrially are as solvents and synthetic intermediates. Most of these aromatics that are released into the environment evaporate into the atmosphere. They may also enter groundwater from oil and gasoline spills, leakage of storage tanks, and migration from waste sites. The toxicokinetics and acute toxicity of toluene, xylenes, and other aromatic solvents are quite similar. They are well absorbed from the lungs and GI tract, distributed to tissues according to tissue blood flow and lipid content, and exhaled unchanged to some extent.

Q. What are the toxic effects of xylenes and ethylbenzene?

Xylenes and ethylbenzene appear to have very limited capacity to adversely affect organs other than the CNS. Mild, transient liver and/or kidney toxicity has occasionally been reported in humans exposed to high vapor concentrations of xylenes.

Alcohols

Q. Which types of alcohols are most commonly responsible for toxicosis?

Alcohols comprise a class of organic compounds composed of a hydrocarbon chain and a hydroxyl group. Alcohols that have one hydroxyl group are called monohydric, which include methanol, ethanol, and isopropanol. These three alcohols are most commonly responsible for alcohol toxicosis. Alcohols are also classified as primary, secondary, or tertiary, according to the number of carbon atoms bonded to the carbon atom to which the hydroxyl group is bonded. Ethanol and methanol are primary alcohols, and isopropanol is a secondary alcohol.

Q. Describe in brief toxicity of ethanol.

Many humans experience greater exposure to ethanol (ethyl alcohol and alcohol) than to any other solvent. Not only is ethyl alcohol used as an additive in gasoline, as a solvent in industry, in many household products, and in pharmaceuticals, but it is also heavily consumed in intoxicating beverages. Frank toxic effects are less important occupationally than injuries resulting from psychomotor impairment. Driving under the influence of alcohol is, of course, the major cause of fatal auto accidents. In many states in the United States, a blood alcohol level of 80 mg/100 mL blood (80 mg%) is prima facie evidence of "driving while intoxicated." Gender differences in responses to ethanol are well recognized. Women are more sensitive to alcohol and exhibit higher mortality at lower levels of consumption than men. Alcohol-induced hepatotoxicity is postulated to be caused by elevation of endotoxin in the bloodstream. Endotoxin, released by the action of ethanol on gram-negative bacteria in the gut, is believed to be taken up by Kupffer cells, causing the release of inflammatory mediators that are cytotoxic to hepatocytes and chemoattractants for neutrophils. These mediators include interleukins, prostaglandins, free radicals, and tumor necrosis factor-α (TNF-α). Proinflammatory cytokines and oxidative stress stimulate collagen synthesis by hepatic stellate cells, leading to alcoholic fibrosis. There is a concern about the role of ethyl alcohol in carcinogenesis, due to the frequent consumption of alcoholic beverages by millions of people.

Q. What are hazards and risks of ethanol?
A. Effective fat solvent, after ingestion, attacks the liver and the brain and nervous system, causing loss of control and anesthesia.
B. Dissolves natural oils from the skin.
C. Vapors are poisonous and affect the nervous system.
D. Flammable.

Q. What information should appear on a chemical safety card for ethanol?
A. Highly flammable
B. Intoxication if inhaled or ingested
C. Causes drying of the skin or mucous tissues
D. Causes damage to the eyes
E. Is miscible with water

Q. What is the source of exposure to methanol? Describe in brief toxicity of methanol.
Methanol (methyl alcohol, wood alcohol, and CH3OH) is primarily used as a starting material for the synthesis of chemicals such as formaldehyde, acetic acid, methacrylates, ethylene glycol (EG), and methyl tertiary-butyl ether. CH3OH is found in windshield washer fluid, carburetor cleaners, antifreeze, and copy machine toner and serves as fuel for Sterno heaters, model airplanes, and Indianapolis 500 race cars. It also functions as a denaturant for some ethyl and isopropyl alcohols, rendering them unfit for consumption.

Q. What are the toxic effects of methanol?
Ingested methanol is absorbed quickly from the GI tract, and peak methanol concentrations occur within 30–60 minutes following ingestion. Toxicosis has also been reported

following inhalation or dermal absorption. Methanol is much more toxic to human beings and nonhuman primates than it is to other mammals. Methanol is metabolized by alcohol dehydrogenase (ADH) to formaldehyde, which is oxidized to formic acid by formaldehyde dehydrogenase. Formic acid is responsible for ocular and CNS lesions in primates as a result of inhibition of cytochrome oxidase. Blindness and permanent neurological abnormalities are common sequel in primates.

Q. Describe in brief toxicity of isopropanol.
Isopropanol (isopropyl alcohol) has the structural formula CH3CH(OH) CH3; a molecular weight of 60 Da; and is found in rubbing alcohol (70%), antifreeze, detergents, window-cleaning products, and disinfectants. Ingestion is the usual cause of poisoning in humans, although toxicity from inhalation and topical absorption has been reported. Isopropanol toxicosis is rare in domestic animals, possibly due to its bitter taste. Isopropanol is approximately twofold more toxic than ethanol. It is rapidly absorbed from the GI tract, and approximately 80% is metabolized to acetone, which is also a CNS depressant, but acetone has a much longer half-life (16–20 hours) than does alcohol.

Glycols

Q. What is the source of exposure to ethylene glycol (EG)?
EG (1,2-dihydroxyethane) is a constituent of antifreeze, deicers, hydraulic fluids, drying agents, and inks and is used to make plastics and polyester fibers. Workers may be exposed dermally or by inhalation when solutions containing EG are heated or sprayed.

Q. What are the toxic effects of ethylene glycol?
The most important exposure route is ingestion, as EG may be accidentally swallowed, taken deliberately in suicide attempts, or used as a cheap substitute for ethanol. "Antifreeze" poisoning occurs frequently in cats and dogs that find its taste appealing. Acute poisoning

entails three clinical stages after an asymptomatic period, during which EG is metabolized:

1. A period of inebriation, the duration, and degree depending on dose.
2. The cardiopulmonary stage 12–24 hours after exposure, characterized by tachycardia and tachypnea, which may progress to cardiac failure and pulmonary edema.
3. The renal toxicity stage 24–72 hours post exposure.

Metabolic acidosis, due largely to glyoxylic acid (GA) accumulation, can develop and become progressively more severe during stages 2 and 3. Hypocalcemia can result from Ca_{21} chelation by oxalic acid (OA) to form Ca_{21} oxalate monohydrate crystals. Deposition of these crystals in kidney tubules is associated with organ damage and potentially acute renal failure. Nephrotoxicity appears to be an acute, high-dose phenomenon, as no demonstrable kidney damage has been reported in occupational studies of groups.

Q. Describe in brief toxicity of diethylene glycol (DEG).

DEGs use as an excipient in a liquid sulfanilamide preparation resulted in 105 deaths in the United States in 1937. This incident prompted the passage of the Federal Food, Drug, and Cosmetic Act of 1938. Use of DEG-contaminated PG or glycerin in various pharmaceuticals has caused multiple fatalities from renal failure in Nigeria, Bangladesh, India, and Haiti. In the Haitian incident, 109 cases of acute renal failure (with 88 deaths) were identified in children who received locally manufactured acetaminophen syrup containing DEG-contaminated glycerin. Renal failure was the "hallmark" finding in these cases, but hepatitis, pancreatitis, and severe neurological manifestations (e.g., encephalopathy, optic neuritis with retinal edema, and unilateral facial paralysis) were frequently seen.

Q. Describe in brief toxicity of propylene glycol (PG).

PG is used as an intermediate in the synthesis of polyester fibers and resins, as a component of automotive antifreeze/coolants and as a deicing fluid for aircraft. As PG is "generally recognized as safe" by the Food and Drug Administration (FDA), it is a constituent of many cosmetics, processed foods, and tobacco products and serves as a diluent for oral, dermal, and IV drug preparations. The most important routes of exposure in the general population are ingestion and dermal contact with products containing the compound. The acute oral toxicity of propylene glycol is very low, and large quantities are required to cause perceptible health effects in humans; in fact, propylene glycol is three times less toxic than ethanol.

Petroleum Products

Q. Describe in brief toxicity of petroleum.

Health effects from exposure to petroleum products vary depending on the concentration of the substance and the length of time that one is exposed. Breathing petroleum vapors can cause nervous system effects (such as headache, nausea, and dizziness) and respiratory irritation. Very high exposure can cause coma and death. Liquid petroleum products which come in contact with the skin can cause irritation, and some can be absorbed through the skin. Chronic exposure to petroleum products may affect the nervous system, blood, and kidneys. Gasoline contains small amounts of benzene, a known human carcinogen. Animals exposed to high levels of some petroleum products have developed liver and kidney tumors. Whether specific petroleum products can cause cancer in humans is not known; however, there is evidence that occupationally exposed people in the petroleum refining industry have an increased risk of skin cancer and leukemia. Petroleum toxicity is more common in domestic and wild animals. Crude petroleum can be released into the environment during well blowouts, leaks at wellheads, pipeline leaks, land and sea shipping disasters, and other events and activities. Emissions can be from venting storage

tanks, blowouts of gas wells, burning petroleum that has been spilled, or burning
unwanted gaseous material. In general, chemicals associated with petroleum intoxication
in cattle are the gaseous, liquid, and solid
crude petroleum that contain natural gas,
crude oil, and bitumen. Natural gas contains
H2S, other sulfur compounds, methane, and
other petroleum hydrocarbons and is known
as sour gas. Sour gas is extremely irritating to
the eyes and respiratory tract. Many of the
chemicals used have limited toxicological
information, and the toxicology of chemical
mixtures is unknown.

3.2   Automotive Gasoline and Additives

Q. What is gasoline?
   Gasoline is a mixture of hundreds of hydrocarbons predominantly in the range of C4 to
   C12. Because its composition varies with the
   crude oil from which it is refined, the refining
   process, and the use of specific additives,
   generalizations regarding the toxicity of gasoline must be made carefully.
Q. What are gasoline additives?
   The types of additives include oxygenates,
   ethers, antioxidants (stabilizers), antiknock
   agents, fuel dyes, metal deactivators, corrosion inhibitors, and some that can't be catego-
   rized. Oxygenates are fuels infused with
   oxygen. They reduce the carbon monoxide
   emissions created when burning fuel.
Q. What are the toxic effects of gasoline?
   Acute gasoline exposure can cause transient
   CNS excitation followed by CNS depression.
   Confusion, giddiness, nausea, headache,
   blurred vision, dizziness, and weakness can
   occur. In massive exposures, rapid CNS
   depression, respiratory depression, seizures,
   loss of consciousness, coma, and death have
   been reported.

3.3   Carbon Disulfide

Q. What are the uses of carbon disulfide?
   The major uses of CS2 are in the production
   of rayon fiber, cellophane, and CCl4 and as a
   solubilizer for waxes and oils. Human exposure is predominantly occupational.
Q. What are metabolic pathways for CS2?
   There are two metabolic pathways:
   (a) The direct interaction of CS2 with free
       amine and sulfhydryl groups of amino
       acids and polypeptides to form dithiocar-
       bamates and trithiocarbonates
   (b) Microsomal metabolism of CS2 to reac-
       tive sulfur intermediates capable of cova-
       lently binding tissue macromolecules
   The conjugation of CS2 with sulfhydryl of
   cysteine or GSH results in the formation of
   2-thiothiazolidine-4-carboxylic acid (TTCA),
   which is excreted in urine and has been frequently used as a biomarker of CS2
   exposure.
Q. What is the toxic effect of carbon disulfide?
   Carbon disulfide is severely irritating to the
   eyes, mucous membranes, and skin. Acute
   neurological effects may result from all routes
   of exposure and may include headache, confusion, psychosis, and coma. Acute exposure
   to extremely high levels of carbon disulfide
   may result in respiratory failure and death.

3.4   Solvent Abuse

Q. What are inhalants?
   Inhalants are a broad range of intoxicative
   drugs whose gases or volatile vapors are
   breathed in via the nose or mouth. They are
   taken by room temperature volatilization or
   from a pressurized container (e.g., nitrous
   oxide), and do not include drugs that are
   sniffed after burning or heating. For example,
   amyl nitrite and toluene—the solvent used in
   contact cement and model airplane glue—are

considered inhalants, but tobacco, cannabis, and crack are not, even though the latter are also inhaled (as smoke).

Q. What are short-term effects of solvent abuse that are inhaled by kids?

Within seconds of inhalation, the user experiences intoxication along with other effects similar to those produced by alcohol. Alcohol-like effects may include slurred speech, an inability to coordinate movements, dizziness, confusion, and delirium. Nausea and vomiting are other common side effects.

Q. What physical damages inhalants cause in the short term?

There may be drowsiness, and individuals are unable to stop smiling or laughing. The substances also disrupt thinking. Some people experience hallucinations and delusions. They also feel side effects similar to those of alcohol, such as slurred speech, coordination loss, dizziness, poor coordination, loss of sensations, confusion and delirium, nausea and vomiting, unconsciousness, and sudden death.

Q. What effects do inhalants have on the body?

People who use inhalants breathe them in through the mouth (huffing) or nose. Most inhalants affect the central nervous system and slow down brain activity. Short-term health effects include slurred or distorted speech, lack of coordination, euphoria (feeling "high"), dizziness, and hallucinations. After heavy use of inhalants, abusers may feel drowsy for several hours and experience a lingering headache. Because intoxication lasts only a few minutes, abusers frequently seek to prolong their high by continuing to inhale repeatedly over the course of several hours. By doing this, abusers can suffer loss of consciousness and death.

Q. Give some examples of the irreversible effects caused by inhaling specific solvents.

- Hearing loss—toluene (paint sprays, glues, dewaxers) and TCE (cleaning fluids, correction fluids)
- Peripheral neuropathies or limb spasms—hexane (glues, gasoline) and nitrous oxide (whipping cream, gas cylinders)

- CNS or brain damage—toluene (paint sprays, glues, dewaxers)
- Bone marrow damage—benzene (gasoline)

Q. What is sudden sniffing death syndrome (SSDS)?

SSDS is the most common killer of inhalant abusers. An especially exciting or frightening hallucination could also trigger SSDS. When the abuser is surprised or startled, he has a sudden surge of the hormone epinephrine.

Explanation: Epinephrine is also called adrenaline. Epinephrine aids in regulating the functions of the body that are beyond a person's conscious control, like heart rate. When a person is highly stimulated (e.g., by fear or challenge), extra amounts of epinephrine are released into the bloodstream to prepare the body for energetic action. Epinephrine increases blood pressure, heart rate, and cardiac output. The presence of the chemical inhalants in the body makes the heart muscle more sensitive to epinephrine. When the surge of epinephrine reaches the heart, the heart suffers an arrhythmia (irregular heart beat). This massive arrhythmia kills the user in seconds.

Q. What adverse effects inhalants have on the CNS and how?

Many of the chemicals found in commonly abused inhalants cause severe and permanent brain and nerve cell damage. Brain scans of inhalant abusers show dramatic shrinkage in the overall size of the brain. Abusers also lose "white matter" in the brain, which is responsible for conducting nerve impulses throughout the body. The white matter is destroyed because each cell is encased in myelin, a lipid, or fat, and many commonly used inhalants are lipid – solvents, i.e., their purpose is to break down lipids. Chronic inhalant abusers suffer massive CNS damage, which results in dementia (lost contact with reality) and loss of cerebellum function. The cerebellum is the portion of the brain that coordinates movements of the voluntary muscles. Abusers lose the ability to think, reason, learn, and remember. Their gait (way of walking) becomes abnormal, and they lose coordination.

Q. How one can know a person has an inhalant abuse?
Some common signs of inhalant abuse include red eyes, runny nose, unusual smelling breath, paint or stains on clothing or face, loss of appetite, drunk appearance, anxiety, sores around mouth, presence of discarded containers of various sprays or gases, and small bottles labeled "incense" (users of butyl nitrite).

Q. What are the four types of inhalants?
Four main types of inhalants are volatile solvents, aerosols, gases, and nitrites.

Q. Why are inhalants so dangerous?
Inhalants are dangerous chemical vapors produced by a range of common, but highly toxic, substances. When inhaled, these chemicals can cause damaging, mind-altering effects, and sudden death. For example, solvents, gases, and nitrates.

Q. Are inhalants legal?
Although inhalants are not regulated under the *Controlled Substances Act*, 38 states in the United States have placed restrictions on the sale and distribution to minors of certain products that are commonly abused as inhalants. Laws also exist in some US states prohibiting the recreational inhalation of nitrous oxide.

Q. Give examples of products containing solvents that are abused by kids?
Products that are abused by kids to get high include:
Model airplane glue, nail polish remover, cleaning fluids, hair spray, gasoline, the propellant in aerosol whipped cream, spray paint, fabric protector, air-conditioner fluid (freon), cooking spray, and correction fluid.

Q. How solvents are misused to get high?
These products are sniffed, snorted, bagged (fumes inhaled from a plastic bag), or "huffed" (inhalant-soaked rag, sock, or roll of toilet paper in the mouth) to achieve a high. Inhalants are also sniffed directly from the container.

4   Sample MCQ's

Q.1. Which of the following statements regarding benzene is *false*?

A. High-level exposure to benzene could result in acute myelogenous leukemia (AML)
B. Gasoline vapor emissions and auto exhaust are the two main contributors to benzene inhalation.
C. Benzene is used as an ingredient in unleaded gasoline.
D. Benzene metabolites covalently bind DNA, RNA, and proteins and interfere with their normal functioning within the cell.
E. Reactive oxygen species can be derived from benzene.

Q.2. Which of the following is *not* a criterion for fetal alcohol syndrome diagnosis?

A. Maternal alcohol consumption during gestation
B. Pre and postnatal growth retardation
C. Microcephaly
D. Ocular toxicity
E. Mental retardation

Q.3. Which of the following is *not* an important enzyme in ethanol metabolism?

A. Alcohol dehydrogenase
B. Formaldehyde dehydrogenase
C. CYP2E1
D. Catalase
E. Acetaldehyde dehydrogenase

Q.4. Which of the following is *not* associated with glycol ether toxicity?

A. Irreversible spermatotoxicity
B. Craniofacial malformations
C. Hematotoxicity
D. Seminiferous tubule atrophy
E. Cleft lip.

Q.5. Which of the following statements regarding chlorinated hydrocarbons is *false*?

A. Toxicities of trichloroethylene (TCE) are mediated mostly by reactive metabolites, not the parent compound.
B. Glutathione conjugation is an important metabolic step of both trichloroethylene (TCE) and perchloroethylene (PERC).
C. Many chlorinated hydrocarbons are used as degreasing agents.
D. Chloroform interferes with intracellular calcium homeostasis.
E. Carbon tetrachloride causes hepatocellular and kidney toxicity.

Q.6. The most serious consequence of crude oil or kerosene ingestion by cattle is -----

A. Liver damage
B. Kidney damage
C. Aspiration pneumonia
D. Central nervous system stimulation
E. Leukemia

Q.7. In regard to chemically induced adverse effects on the eye---

A. No chemical has been shown to cause glaucoma.
B. Nonionic detergents damage the eye more that cationic detergents.
C. 2,4-dinitrophenol, corticosteroids, and naphthalene are known to cause cataracts in humans.
D. Methanol produces blindness by rendering the cornea and lens opaque.
E. Acids usually produce late-appearing ocular toxicity as contrasted to alkalis which produce immediate damage.

Q.8. Which of the following agents would *not* likely produce reactive airways dysfunction syndrome (RADS)?

A. Carbon monoxide
B. Chlorine
C. Ammonia
D. Toluene diisocyanate
E. Acetic acid

Q.9. Huffing gasoline can result in which of the following serious health problems?

A. Renal failure
B. Pneumothorax
C. Hodgkin's disease
D. Encephalopathy
E. Thrombocytopenia

Q.10. Benzene is similar to toluene -----

A. In its metabolism to redox active metabolites
B. Regarding covalent binding of its metabolites to proteins
C. In its ability to produce CNS depression
D. In its ability to produce acute myelogenous leukemia
E. In its ability to be metabolized to benzoquinone

Q.11. Sorbitol and other sugar alcohols have been associated with -----

A. Respiratory distress syndrome
B. Osmotic diarrhea
C. Hepatotoxicity
D. Immediate hypersensitivity reaction
E. CNS depression

Q.12. Chloroform is not -----

A. Central nervous system depressant
B. Hepatotoxic
C. Metabolized to phosgene
D. Peroxisome proliferator
E. Contaminant of chlorinated water

Q.13. Each of the following solvents is paired with a correct target organ of toxicity except---

A. Methanol:retina
B. Ethylene glycol: kidney

C. Ethylene glycol monomethyl ether: kidney

D. Dichloromethane: central nervous system

E. Carbon tetrachloride: liver

Q.14. Which of the following is not associated with spermatotoxicity in rats?

A. Ethylene glycol monomethyl ether

B. Ethylene glycol monoethyl ether

C. Ethoxy acetic acid

D. Methoxy acetic acid

E. Propylene glycol monomethyl ether

Q.15. Methyl bromide (CH3Br) ------

A. Is a liquid used primarily as a fumigant

B. Has essentially no warning properties, even at physiologically hazardous concentrations

C. Is extremely flammable

D. Is of greater concern from its oral toxicity than from its inhalation toxicity

E. Would not be expected to be readily absorbed through the lungs

Q.16. Which of the following statements regarding solvents is *false*?

A. Solvents can be absorbed from the GI tract and through the skin.

B. Equilibration of absorbed solvents/vapors occurs most quickly in the lungs.

C. Solvents are small molecules that lack charge.

D. Volatility of solvents increases with molecular weight.

E. Most solvents are refined from petroleum.

Q.17. What is the route in which most solvents enter the environment?

A. Chemical spills

B. Contamination of drinking water

C. Evaporation

D. Improper waste disposal

E. Wind

Q.18. All of the following statements are true *except* -----

A. Most solvents can pass freely through membranes by diffusion.

B. A solvent's lipophilicity is important in determining its rate of dermal absorption.

C. Hydrophilic solvents have a relatively low blood: air partition coefficient.

D. Biotransformation of a lipophilic solvent can result in the production of a mutagenic compound.

E. Hepatic first-pass metabolism determines the amount of solvent absorbed in the GI tract.

Q.19. Which of the following statements regarding age solvent toxicity is *true*?

A. GI absorption is greater in adults than it is in children.

B. Polar solvents reach higher blood levels in the elderly than they do in children.

C. Children are always more susceptible to solvent toxicity than are adults.

D. Increased alveolar ventilation increases uptake of lipid-soluble solvents to a greater extent than water-soluble solvents.

E. Increased body fat percentage increases clearance of solvent chemicals.

Answers

1. B. 2. D. 3. B 4. A. 5. D. 6. C
7. C. 8. A. 9. D. 10. C. 11. B.
12. D. 13. C. 14. E. 15. B. 16. D.
17. C. 18. C. 19. B.

Further Readings

Cope R (2018) Toxic gases and vapors. In: Gupta RC (ed) Veterinary toxicology: basic and clinical principles, 3rd edn. Academic Press/Elsevier, San Diego, USA, pp 629–646

Coppock RW, Christian RG (2018) Petroleum. In: Gupta RC (ed) Veterinary toxicology: basic and clinical principles, 3rd edn. Academic Press/Elsevier, San Diego, USA, pp 658–674

Gupta PK (2014) Essential concepts in toxicology. Published by PharmaMed Press (A unit of BSP Books Pvt. Ltd), Hyderabad, India

Gupta PK (2016) Fundamental in toxicology: essential concepts and applications in toxicology. Elsevier/BSP, USA

Gupta PK (2018) Illustrative toxicology, 1st edn. Elsevier, San Diego, USA

Gupta PK (2020) Brainstorming questions in toxicology. Francis and Taylor CRC Press, USA

Klaassen CD, Watkins JB III (eds) (2015) Casarett & Doull's essentials of toxicology, 3rd edn. McGraw-Hill, USA

Witschi H (2010) Pulmonary toxicology. In: Gupta PK (ed) Modern toxicology: basis of organ and reproduction toxicity, vol 2, 2nd reprint. PharmaMed Press, Hyderabad, India, pp 277–339

Toxicology of Nanomaterial Particles

14

Abstract

Nanotechnology is the understanding and control of matter at nanoscale dimensions between approximately 1 and 100 nm, where unique phenomena enable novel applications. Due to unique physicochemical characteristics of NPs, inconsistent toxicological data have been generated even from well-established *in vitro* models. The respiratory tract is the major route for humans to exposure of nanomaterials. The chapter briefly describes the overview, key points, and relevant text that are in the format of problem-solving study questions followed by multiple-choice questions (MCQs) along with their answers.

Keywords

Nanomaterials · Nanotoxicology · Engineered nanoparticles · Biologic reactivity · Routes of exposure · MCQs · Question answer bank · Toxicology

1 Introduction

Nanomaterials are currently being widely used in modern technology. However, there is a serious lack of information concerning the human health and environmental implications of manufactured nanomaterials. The chapter briefly describes an overview, key points, and relevant text that is in the format of problem-solving study questions followed by multiple-choice questions (MCQ's) along with their answers.

2 Overview

Nanotechnology is a rapidly growing field having potential applications in many areas. Nanoparticles have been studied for cell toxicity, immunotoxicity, and genotoxicity. So far, NPs have been prepared from metal and non-metal, polymeric materials and bioceramics. The majority of NPs having medical applications are liposomes, polyethylene glycol, and dendrimers. Humans are exposed to various nanoscale materials since childhood, and the new emerging field of nanotechnology has become another threat to human life. Because of their small size, NPs find their way easily to enter the human body and cross the various biological barriers and may reach the most sensitive organs. Scientists have proposed that NPs of size less than 10 nm act similar to a gas and can enter human tissues easily and may disrupt the cell normal biochemical environment. Animals and human studies have shown that after inhalation and through oral

P K Gupta, *Problem Solving Questions in Toxicology*, https://doi.org/10.1007/978-3-030-50409-0_14

exposure, NPs are distributed to the liver, heart, spleen, and brain in addition to lungs and gastrointestinal tract. In order to clear these NPs from the body, the components of the immune system are activated. The estimated half-life of NPs in human lungs is about 700 days posing a consistent threat to respiratory system. During metabolism, some of the NPs are congregated in the liver tissues. NPs are more toxic to human health in comparison with large-sized particles of the same chemical substance, and it is usually suggested that toxicities are inversely proportional to the size of the NPs.

> **Key Points**
>
> - Nanotoxicology is a subspecialty of particle toxicology, and this branch appears to have toxicity effects that are unusual and not seen with larger particles. For example, even inert elements like gold become highly active at nanometer dimensions.
> - Nanotechnology is the understanding and control of matter at nanoscale dimensions between approximately 1 and 100 nm, where unique phenomena enable novel applications.
> - Due to unique physicochemical characteristics of NPs, inconsistent toxicological data have been generated even from well-established in vitro models.
> - The respiratory tract is the major route for humans to exposure of nanomaterials.
> - Surface properties are major determinants of biologic reactivity due to high surface area, surface charge, hydrophobicity and partitioning into lipid membranes, dissolution and release of metal ions, and redox activity.

3 Problem-Solving Study Questions

3.1 Nanomaterial Basics

Q. What do you mean by nano?

Nano is a prefix meaning "extremely small." When quantifiable, it translates to one billionth, as in the nanosecond. Nano comes from the Greek word "nanos," meaning "dwarf."

Q. How small is nano?

In the International System of Units, the prefix "nano" means one billionth, or 10^{-9}; therefore 1 nanometer is one billionth of a meter.

Q. Who is the father of nanotechnology?

Heinrich Rohrer and Binnig were known as the fathers of nanotechnology—the construction and manipulation of extremely small objects—because their device could be used to move atoms around on a surface. *Rohrer* died of natural causes on May 16, 1979 in, Switzerland (Fig. 14.1).

Q. Are nanoparticles toxic?

Materials which by themselves are not very harmful could be toxic if they are inhaled in the form of nanoparticles. The effects of inhaled nanoparticles in the body may include lung inflammation and heart problems.

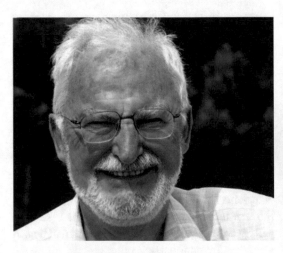

Fig. 14.1 Heinrich Rohrer. (https://www.thefamouspeople.com/profiles/images/heinrich-rohrer-1.jpg)

Q. How are nanoparticles used in everyday life?
Through nanotechnology, nanoparticles can help make materials lighter, more durable, and more reactive. Nanoparticles are applicable in a wide variety of industries and uses, including electronics to make computers faster, memory chips smaller, and screens clearer and brighter.

Q. How do nanoparticles affect human health?
The effects of inhaled nanoparticles in the body may include lung inflammation and heart problems. Studies in humans show that breathing in diesel soot causes a general inflammatory response and alters the system that regulates the involuntary functions in the cardiovascular system, such as control of heart rate.

Q. How do nanoparticles leave the body?
Nanoparticles that are present in the body (i.e., after injection) are largely taken up and eliminated by the reticulohistocytic system (RHS). Particulate materials that are taken up by this system include dead cells, bacteria, viruses, fat particles, and solid particles such as nanoparticles.

Q. Are nanoparticles safe?
Current research indicates that exposure via inhalation and skin contact can result in nanoparticles entering the body. Nanoparticles are tiny particles that can be inhaled or ingested and may pose a possible problem both medically and environmentally.

Q. What is environmental nanotoxicology?
Nanotoxicology is a newer branch of science, and it deals with the study and application of nanomaterials with regard to toxicity in humans and the environment. In environmental systems, nondegradable nanoparticles are ready to deposit in the groundwater, leading to production of environmental pollutants.

Q. Where are nanoparticles found?
Naturally occurring nanoparticles can be found in volcanic ash, ocean spray, fine sand and dust, and even biological matter (e.g., viruses).

Q. What are nanoparticles in food?
Silver (Ag) nanoparticles are used in a variety of applications within the food industry. They have been used as antimicrobial agents in foods and food packaging materials.

Q. Natural sources of ultrafine and nanoparticles.
Natural sources of ultrafine and nanoparticles include gas to particle conversions, forest fires, volcano eruptions, viruses, magnetotactic bacteria, mollusks, arthropods, fish, and birds.

Q. What are unintentional anthropogenic sources?
Unintentional anthropogenic sources include internal combustion engines, power plants, metal fumes from smelting and welding, and heated surfaces.

Q. What are classes of ENMs (engineered nanoparticles)?
Engineered (manufactured) nanomaterials have an enormous range of composition, geometry, and complexity ranging from simple isometric forms (NPs), one-dimensional (1D) forms (fibers or tubes) to two-dimensional (2D) forms (plate-like or disk-like materials).

Q. What properties of nanomaterial are relevant to biologic responses?
The following properties of nanomaterial are relevant to biologic responses:
A. Size (aerodynamic, hydrodynamic)
B. Size distribution
C. Shape
D. Agglomeration/aggregation state
E. Density (material, bulk)
F. Chemical composition and phase
   • Crystallinity
   • Dissolution and toxicant (ion) release
   • Coatings and bioavailable contaminants
   • Bio persistence
G. Surface properties
   • Surface area (external, internal)
   • Electrical charge (zeta potential)
   • Redox activity
   • Hydrophobicity/hydrophilicity
   • Adsorptive capacity for biomolecules
   • Nanoscale quantum and magnetic properties (?)

3.2   Mechanism of Toxicity

Q. What are the most vulnerable in vitro subcellular organelles and physiologic functions
that can be perturbed by exposure to ENPs?

- Damage to cell wall and plasma
membrane
- Interference with electron transport and
aerobic respiration
- Induction of oxidant stress
- Activation of cell signaling pathways
- Perturbed ion homeostasis
- Release of toxic metal ions from internal-
ized nanoparticles
- Disruption of lysosomal membrane
integrity
- Incomplete uptake for frustrated
phagocytosis
- Interference with cytoskeletal unction
- DNA and chromosomal damage

Q. What are the portals of entry of ENM?
The respiratory tract, the gastrointestinal (GI)
tract, and the skin are the main organs of
direct exposure of ENM. For medical application, injection will also be an important
entry route.
Intake via the respiratory tract is the most
prevalent exposure route for occupational
exposures. Additives of ENM to food and
potential contamination of food result in
exposure via GI tract.

4   Sample MCQ's

(choose the correct statement; it may be one, two,
or more or none)

Q1. In contrast to larger particles >500 nm,
nanoparticles ----

A. Are highly likely to enter the body by
dermal absorption
B. Are highly likely to enter the body
through the respiratory tract
C. Are unlikely to adsorb to protein or lipid
D. Are efficiently removed from the lungs
via mucociliary transport

E. Are not likely to undergo uptake and
transport in sensory neurons

Q2. Which of the following statements is *not*
true?

A. Nanomaterials may be classified by
geometry and chemistry.
B. Engineered nanomaterials include quantum dots, C-nanofiber array, and few-
layer grapheme.
C. Agglomerates include primary particles
held together by weak van der Waals
forces.
D. Aggregates include primary particles
held by strong chemical bonds.
E. Hydrodynamic diameter is unimportant
in particle interactions.

Q3. Nanoparticles can exert toxicity by all of the
following mechanisms *except* ------

A. Damage to DNA and chromosomes
B. Induction of oxidant stress
C. Interference with biotransformation
enzyme activities
D. Activation of signaling pathways
E. Release of toxic metal ions from inter-
nalized NPs

Q4. Which of the following is *not* a
nanoparticle?

A. Carbon nanotubes
B. Buckyball
C. Graphene
D. Zinc nanorods
E. Bacteria

Q5. Which of the following answers is *not* true
regarding nanoparticles?

A. NPs can originate from natural sources
including forest fires, volcanoes, and
viruses.
B. NPs can originate from unintentional
sources including internal combustion
engines and electric motors.

C. NPs can originate from unintentional sources including ferritin and magnetotactic bacteria.

D. NPs can originate from intentional sources including carbon nanotubes and metal oxide nanoparticles.

E. NPs can originate from natural and intentional and unintentional anthropogenic sources.

Q6. The goals of nanotoxicology are ----

A. To identify and characterize hazards of engineered nanomaterials

B. To determine "safe" exposure levels

C. To determine biologic and biochemical actions

D. To determine manufacturing procedures and cost

E. To determine preventive exposure guidelines

Q7. Assays to determine the toxicity of manufactured nanoparticles suffer from all of the complications below *except* -----

A. The nanomaterial aggregate may no longer be in the nano-size range

B. Aggregates of the nanoparticle may settle out of solution which may affect exposure dose

C. Alterations in surface chemistry to stabilize suspension may evoke other issues in toxicity assessment

D. Coatings of particles may have their own toxicity

E. Uptake of the nanoparticle into an organism is easily determined

Q8. Biodistribution of nanoparticles may be influenced by --

A. Physicochemical properties such as plasma protein and respiratory tract mucus

B. Physicochemical properties such as surface size and chemistry

C. Physicochemical properties such as the gastrointestinal milieu

D. Body compartment media including surface hydrophobicity

E. Body compartment media including size

Answers

1. B.   2. E.   3. C.   4. E.   5. C.   6. D.
7. E.   8. B.

Further Reading

Dhawan A, Anderson D, Shanker R (2017) Nanotoxicology: experimental and computational perspectives. Royal Chemical Society

Durán N, Guterres SS, Oswaldo L. Alves ed. (2013) Nanotoxicology: materials, methodologies, and assessments. Springer-Verlag New York

Kumar V, Dasgupta N, Ranjan S (eds) (2018) Nanotoxicology: toxicity evaluation, risk assessment and management, 1st edn. Taylor and Francis, CRC Press, USA

Monteiro-Riviere NA, Lang Tran C (eds) (2016) Nanotoxicology: progress toward nanomedicine, 2nd edn. Taylor and Francis, CRC Press, USA

Oberdörster G, Kane AB, Kapler RD, Hurt RH (2015) Nanotoxicology. In: Klaassen CD, Watkins JB III (eds) Casarett & Doull's essentials of toxicology, 3rd edn. McGraw-Hill, USA, pp 411–424

Toxic Effects of Calories

15

Abstract

The human body needs *calories* to survive. *Calorie* consumption that is too low or too high will eventually lead to health problems. It is not only *calories* that are *important*, but also the substance from which the *calories* are taken This chapter deals with biology of eating and digestion, integrated fuel metabolism, and various health impacts of energy imbalance in human beings and briefly describes the overview, key points, and relevant text that are in the format of problem-solving study questions followed by multiple-choice questions (MCQs) along with their answers.

Keywords

Biology of eating · Energy balance · Toxicity · Caloric intake · Obesity · Question bank · MCQs

1 Introduction

Energy in the body is derived from three main nutrient classes: carbohydrates, protein, and fat, which in turn are made up of sugars, amino acids, and free fatty acids, respectively. In this chapter an overview, key points, and relevant text that is in the format of problem-solving study questions of biology of eating and digestion, integrated fuel metabolism, and various health impacts of energy imbalance in human beings have been briefly described followed by multiple-choice questions (MCQ's) along with their answers.

2 Overview

Weight gain is a major effect of eating too many calories. For some people, this is due to something other than dietary intake, such as hormonal disorders. For everyone else, it's the result of taking in too many calories from food and not leading an active enough lifestyle. Not only does excess calorie intake pack on the pounds, but eating too many calories from certain sources causes other health problems. Together, these can cause an avalanche of issues that negatively impact your overall health and well-being. The good news is that taking charge and making the necessary changes effectively reverse these effects or prevent them from progressing in most cases.

P K Gupta, *Problem Solving Questions in Toxicology*, https://doi.org/10.1007/978-3-030-50409-0_15

Key Points

- Energy in the body is derived from three main nutrient classes: carbohydrates, protein, and fat, which in turn are made up of sugars, amino acids, and free fatty acids, respectively.
- In order to maintain a constant weight, one has to balance the number of calories one eats with the number of calories one burns, i.e., Calories in = Calories out.
- Hormonal messages generated by the pancreas, adipose tissue, and GI tract coordinate the elements of a situation to produce a desired effect or multiple responses associated with caloric intake and utilization.
- Food intake and energy expenditure are coordinately regulated in the central nervous system to maintain a relatively constant level of energy reserve and body weight.
- Dieting is defined as the use of a healthy, balanced diet that meets the daily nutritional needs of the body and that reduces caloric intake with increased moderate exercise.

3   Problem-Solving Study Questions

3.1   Toxicity Related to Excess Caloric Intake

Q. How do calories affect our body?

Calories aren't bad for us. Our body needs calories for energy. But eating too many calories—and not burning enough of them off through activity—can lead to weight gain. Most foods and drinks contain calories.

Q. What happens when we eat excess calories?

When we eat, our body uses some of the calories we consume for energy. The rest are stored as fat. Consuming more calories than we burn may cause us to become overweight

or obese. This increases our risk for cancer and other chronic health problems.

Q. What effect does consuming too few calories have on our body?

Too few calories can lead to weight-loss efforts and harm health. One will have risk of going into starvation mode with abnormally low blood pressure and slow heart rate, with rhythm abnormalities.

Q. What's worse sugar or calories?

In general, people feel fats are less harmful than sugar and end up eating far more fat than is healthy, according to the USDA. Because they both add calories to diet, it is important to be aware of both and make an effort to limit solid fats and added sugars as often as possible.

Q. Do fat people burn more calories?

People who are larger or have more muscle burn more calories, even at rest. Men usually have less body fat and more muscle than do women of the same age and weight, which means men burn more calories.

Q. What are signs and symptoms of compulsive overeating?

Signs and symptoms of compulsive overeating include:

- Binge eating, or eating uncontrollably even when not physically hungry
- Eating much more rapidly than normal
- Eating alone due to shame and embarrassment
- Feelings of guilt due to overeating
- Preoccupation with body weight
- Depression or mood swings
- Awareness that eating patterns are abnormal
- History of weight fluctuations
- Withdrawal from activities because of embarrassment about weight
- History of many different unsuccessful diets
- Eating little in public but maintaining a high body weight
- Holding the belief that life will be better if they can lose weight
- Hiding food in strange places (closets, cabinets, suitcases, under the bed)

- Vague or secretive eating patterns
- Self-defeating statements after food consumption
- Holding the belief that food is their only friend
- Weight gain
- Loss of sexual desire or promiscuous relations
- Fatigue

Q. In order to maintain a constant weight, what one should do?

One has to balance the number of calories one eats with the number of calories one burns, i.e.:

$$\text{Calories in} = \text{Calories Out.}$$

Q. What are general calorie factors for the major sources of energy?

The general calorie factors of 4, 9, and 4. For the major sources of energy—carbohydrate, fat, and protein have been widely used.

Q. What is the total energy expenditure or metabolic cost for an average adult?

The total energy expenditure or metabolic cost for an average adult is primarily composed of three components:

1. Basal energy expenditure
2. Thermic effect of food
3. Energy expenditure associated with physical activity

Q. What is basal energy expenditure?

Basal energy expenditure, also called as resting energy expenditure, is the energy expended when the individual is lying down and at complete rest, generally after sleep in the post absorptive state.

Q. What foods have the thermic effect?

Protein-rich foods, such as meat, fish, eggs, dairy, legumes, nuts, and seeds, could help increase your metabolism for a few hours. They do so by requiring your body to use more energy to digest them. This is known as the thermic effect of food (TEF).

Q. What does physical activity consist of?

The energy expenditure from physical activity consists of expenditure related to exercise and non-exercise activity thermogenesis.

Q. Enumerate problems related to excess caloric intake/obesity.

Adaptation of liver and adipose tissue to excess calories as a result of overeating and inadequate physical activity result in toxicity over the long term.

Short-term coordinated changes in metabolic pathways in white adipose tissue in response to overfeeding result in excess energy storage in the form of triglycerides, which leads to increased size of preexisting adipocytes (hypertrophy) and to formation of new adipocytes (hyperplasia).

Under conditions of chronic excess ingested energy, the efficiency of energy storage in adipose tissue is decreased, and the body stores energy in ectopic sites. Triglycerides begin to accumulate in non-adipose tissues such as liver, skeletal muscle, and the pancreas as lipid droplets resulting in insulin resistance, inflammation, and tissue damage.

Adipose tissue from obese individuals releases chemokines and cytokines, the so-called adipokines, which contribute to a state of "metabolic inflammation." Non-esterified fatty acids and the other factors released from adipose tissue contribute to the development of metabolic syndrome in some overweight and obese individuals. This is a cluster of components which lead to insulin resistance, disruptions in lipid homeostasis (dyslipidemia), and elevated blood pressure, all of which substantially increase the risk for development of cardiovascular disease and type 2 diabetes.

3.2   Treatment of Obesity

Treatment of obesity include:
- Drug therapy for weight loss
- Surgical interventions
- Lifestyle modification: dieting and exercise

4   Sample MCQ's

(choose the correct statement; it may be one, two, or more or none)

Q1. Which of the following definitions is *false*?

    A. The set-point hypothesis proposes that food intake and energy expenditure are coordinately regulated by defined regions in the brain that signal to maintain a relatively constant level of energy reserve and body weight.

    B. Hormonal messages generated by the endocrine cells of the pancreas, adipose tissue, and GI tract are involved in orchestration of multiple responses associated with caloric intake and caloric utilization.

    C. Caloric content of foods generally assumes factors of 4, 9, and 4 for carbohydrate, fat, and protein, respectively.

    D. The body mass index (BMI) is an accurate method for assessing body composition.

    E. Liver, adipose, muscle, and other tissues adapt to excess caloric loads.

Q2. Body mass index ----

    A. May be used as an indicator of sufficient caloric and essential nutrient intake

    B. May be defined as body height divided by body weight squared

    C. Has risen insignificantly over the past 30 years in the United States

    D. May not be used in the estimation of cancer risk in humans

    E. May be defined as body weight divided by height squared

Q3. Although dieting may effectively reduce body weight ----

    A. Toxicity may result from stimulation of adipokine release

    B. Toxicity may result from inhibition of drug-metabolizing enzymes

    C. Toxicity may result from a loss of required nutrients

    D. Toxicity may result from extreme mental illness

    E. Toxicity may result from weight cycling

Q4. Excess caloric intake ---

    A. May lead to nonalcoholic steatohepatitis

    B. Is always correlated with obesity and insulin resistance

    C. Is characterized by elevations of serum ALT concentrations in all cases

    D. Leads to hepatic cirrhosis and liver cancer in almost all cases

    E. Is readily reversible by dieting

Q5. Metabolic syndrome is a constellation of actions including ---

    A. Typically results from elevated fasting glucose, increased HDL, and hypertension

    B. Typically results from elevated fasting glucose, increased LDL, and hypertension

    C. Typically results from elevated fasting glucose, hypertriglyceridemia, and hypotension

    D. Typically results from elevated fasting glucose, hypotriglyceridemia, and truncal obesity

    E. Typically results from elevated fasting glucose, hypertriglyceridemia, and truncal obesity

Q6. Excess calories may be -----

    A. Stored as glucose in adipose tissue

    B. Stored as triglycerides in CNS tissue

    C. Stored as glycogen in CNS tissue

    D. Stored as glycogen in the liver

    E. Stored as triglycerides in the GI tract

Q7. Ectopic at deposition includes ------

A. Adipose tissue
B. Skeletal muscle
C. Lungs
D. Heart
E. GI tract

Q8. Body composition may be assessed by -----

A. Electrical impedance because lean mass has more water and greater conductivity than at mass
B. Anthropometric analysis of the body mass index
C. Hydrodensitometry, which uses the density of the whole body and corrects for residual air in the lungs and GI tract to determine relative body fat
D. Nuclear magnetic resonance
E. All of the above

Q9. Neural control of energy balance ----

A. May be defined as the action of leptin on CNS function
B. May be defined as the action of hypothalamic cholinergic control of appetite and hedonic control
C. May involve a balance between food intake and energy expenditure
D. May involve a balance between leptin's action on orexigenic versus anorexigenic peptide expression

E. May involve adrenocortical control of hepatic function

Q10. Humans consume food to provide energy needed to -----

A. Drive cellular functions including digestion, metabolism, pumping blood, nerve activity, and muscle contractions
B. Promote photosynthesis
C. Synthesize oxygen in the lungs
D. Prepare minerals for use in the body
E. Produce carbon dioxide to fuel body functions

Answers
1. D.   2. E.   3. C.   4. A.   5. E.   6. D.
7. B.   8. E.   9. D.   10. A.

Further Reading

Johanna T Dwyer, Kathleen J Melanson, Utchima Sriprachy-Anunt, Paige Cross, and Madelyn Wilson (2015). Dietary treatment of obesity. Endotext [Internet]   https://www.ncbi.nlm.nih.gov/books/NBK278991/

Pritikin M, McGrady PM (1980) The program for diet and exercise. Bantum Books, New York

Ronis MJ, Shankar K, Badger TM (2015) Toxic effects of calories. In: Klaassen CD, Watkins JB III (eds) Casarett & Doull's essentials of toxicology, 3rd edn. McGraw-Hill, USA, pp 401–410

Part VI

Plants, Biotoxins and Food Poisonings

Plant Toxicity

16

Abstract

Some of the common poisonous plants contain various toxic principles such as alkaloids, cyanogenic glycosides, proteinaceous compounds, organic acids, resins, and resinoids. Problems can also occur with animals in ornamental gardens, natural environments, and homes. Poisoning in humans and companion animals from toxic plants also continues to be a significant risk, especially to pets and children. This chapter briefly describes the overview, key points, and relevant text that are in the format of problem-solving study questions followed by multiple-choice questions (MCQs) along with their answers.

Keywords

Poisonous plantsToxicity of plantsPlant toxinsAlkaloids, cyanogenic glycosides, proteinaceous compounds, organic acids, resins and resinoids, alcohols, mechanism of plant toxicity, toxicology question and answer bankMCQs

1 Introduction

A number of plants are known to contain plant defense compounds that primarily defend against consumption by insects and other animals, including humans. The toxic effects of some of the common poisonous plants including mushrooms are due to various toxic principles such as alkaloids, cyanogenic glycosides, proteinaceous compounds, organic acids, resins and resinoids, and alcohols. It is well established that most of the experimental data are available on laboratory animals and reported in veterinary literature. Attempts have been made to summarize information on the toxic effects of plants in animals and human beings exposed to different poisonous plants. The chapter briefly describes an overview, key points, and relevant text that is in the format of problem-solving study questions followed by multiple-choice questions (MCQ's) along with their answers.

2 Overview

The plant kingdom contains potentially 300,000 species, and a number of them are known to contain plant defense compounds that primarily defend against consumption by insects and other animals, including humans. The toxic properties of plants often enhance their ability to survive.

P K Gupta, *Problem Solving Questions in Toxicology*, https://doi.org/10.1007/978-3-030-50409-0_16

Toxic effects on humans can range from simple hay fever caused by exposure to plant pollen all the way to serious systemic reactions caused by ingestion of specific plants. Certain environmental conditions such as climate, type of soil influence, and the age of a plant affect the synthesis of some toxins that can be a major factor in the severity of reaction one will experience on exposure. Plant toxins fall under a number of different chemical structures such as alkaloids, glycosides, proteinaceous compounds, organic acids, alcohols, resins, and resinoids. Poisoning in humans and companion animals from toxic plants also continues to be a significant risk, especially to pets and children. Plant poisoning in small animals is usually accidental. Lack of understanding and increased grazing pressure on these small acreages often contribute to the consumption of toxic plants by animals.

Key Points

- Different portions of the plant (root, stem, leaves, seeds) often contain different concentrations of a toxic substance.
- Certain environmental conditions such as climate, type of soil influence, and the age of a plant affect the synthesis of some toxins.
- Plants contain substances that may exert toxic effects on the skin, lung, cardiovascular system, liver, kidney, bladder, blood, nervous system, bone, and endocrine and reproductive systems.
- Contact dermatitis and photosensitivity are common skin reactions with many plants. Gastrointestinal effects range from local irritation to emesis and/or diarrhea.
- Cardiac glycosides in plants may cause nausea, vomiting, and cardiac arrhythmias in animals and humans.

---

3   Problem-Solving Study Questions

3.1   Mechanism of Plant Toxicity

Q. What are the possible mechanisms of plant that can lead to toxicity?

Possible mechanisms that can lead to toxicity include:

- Blockade of muscarinic cholinoceptors, e.g., *Atropa*, *Datura*, *Hyoscyamus*, *Solanum*
- Inhibition of cellular Na+, K+-ATPase increases contractility, enhanced vagal effect, e.g., *Adenium*, *Digitalis*, *Convallaria*, *Nerium*
- Blockade of gamma-aminobutyric acid (GABA) receptor on the neuronal chloride channel, alteration of acetylcholine homeostasis, mimic excitatory amino acids, sodium channel alteration, and hypoglycemia, e.g., *Anemone*, *Conium*, *Laburnum*, *Nicotiana*, *Ranunculus*
- Gastric acid hydrolysis of cyanogenic glycosides releases cyanide, e.g., *Eriobotrya*, *Hydrangea*, *Prunus*
- Sodium channel activation, e.g., *Aconitum*, *Rhododendron*, *Veratrum*
- Stimulation of nicotinic cholinoceptors, e.g., *Conium*, *Laburnum*, *Lobelia*, *Nicotiana*
- Pyrroles injure endothelium of hepatic or pulmonary vasculature leading to venoocclusive disease and hepatic necrosis, e.g., *Crotalaria*, *Heliotropium*, *Senecia*
- Protein synthesis inhibitors leading to multiple organ system failure, e.g., *Abrus*, *Ricinus*

3.2   Chemical Classification of Plant Toxins

Q. Which plant genera are known to contain alkaloids?

Common plants that are known to contain alkaloids include *Atropa*, *Senecio*, *Nicotiana*,

Coffea, *Papaver*, *Solanum*, and *Aconitum* having, e.g., tropines, pyrrolizidines, pyridines, and purines.

Q. Which plant genera is known to contain glycosides?

Common plants that are known to contain glycosides include *Digitalis* and *Aesculus* that have, e.g., steroids and coumarins.

Q. Which plant genera are known to contain proteinaceous compounds?

Common plants that are known to contain proteinaceous compounds are *Abrus* and *Lathyrus* having, e.g., abrin, ricin, amatoxins, phallotoxins, phalloidin, and aminopropionitrile.

Q. Which plant genera are known to contain organic acids?

Common plants that are known to contain organic acids are *Caladium*, *Dieffenbachia*, and *Rheum*.

Q. Which plant genera are known to contain alcohols?

Common plants that are known to contain alcohols are Cicuta and Eupatorium having, cicutoxin and tremetol.

Q. Which plant genera are known to contain resins and resinoids?

Common plants that are known to contain resins and resinoids include *Cannabis* and *Rhus*. These plants contain tetrahydrocannabinol and urushiol.

3.3 Toxic Effects of Plants

Q. Which plants can lead to cardiovascular problems?

Various plants that contain cardioactive glycosides include *Digitalis purpurea*, squill (*Scilla maritima*), lily of the valley, milkweeds, monkshood, and many other species. The cardiac glycosides inhibit Na+, K+-ATPase.

Q. Name the active toxic principle(s) of *Abrus precatorius*.

Active principles are N-methyl tryptophan, glycyrrhizin (lipolytic enzyme—the active principle of liquorice), abrin (toxalbumin also known as phytotoxin), abrine (amino acid), abralin (glucoside), and abric acid.

Q. Name the active toxic principle(s) of *Croton* plant.

Seed and oil extracted from the seeds are extremely toxic. Seed oil known to have tumor-promoting diesters. Active principles are crotin (toxalbumin) and crotonoside (Glycoside).

Q. What are toxic principles of *Calotropis* plant?

Toxic parts include stem, branches, leaves, and the milky white latex (madar juice). Important toxic principles are uscharin, calotoxin, calotropin, and gigantin.

Q. What are the important toxic principles *Semecarpus anacardium*?

Semicarpol (monohydroxy phenol compound) and bhilawanol (alkaloid)

Q. What are the important principles of *Capsicum annum*?

Capsaicin (8-methyl-*N*-vanillyl-6-nonenamide) is an active component of chili peppers. It is an irritant for mammals, including humans, and produces a sensation of burning in any tissue with which it comes into contact.

Q. What is the toxic principle of *Eucalyptus Globulus* plant?

Eucalyptol (cineole)

Q. What are the important toxic principles of *Colchicum* plant?

Alkaloid colchicine and demecolcine

Q. What are the important oleander plants?

A. *Nerium odourum*: Common names—white/pink oleander, kaner.

B. *Cerbera thevetia*: Common names—yellow oleanders, peela kaner, exile, bastard oleander.

C. *Cerbera odollam*: Common names—Dabur, Dhakur, Pilikibir; all parts of the plant are poisonous, especially fruit with kernels or seeds and the nectar from the flowers, which yields poisonous honey.

Q. What are the toxic principles of *Nerium odourum*?

Nerium odourum has nerin, containing cardiac glycosides: (i) neriodorin, (ii) neriodorein, (iii) karabin, (iv) oleandrin, (v) folinerin, and (vi) rosagerin.

Q. What are the toxic principles of *Cerbera thevetia*?

Cerbera thevetia has glycosides: (i) thevetin (one-eighth as potent as ouabain which is similar in action to digitalis); (ii) thevitoxin, less toxic than thevetin; (iii) nerifolin, which is more potent than thevetin; (iv) peruvoside; (v) ruvoside; and (vi) cerberin.

Q. What are the toxic principles of *Cerbera odollam*?

Cerbera odollam contains glycoside and cerberin.

Q. Describe in brief the mode of action of oleander plants?

Oleanders act like digitalis; toxic doses can produce malignant dysrhythmias and cardiac failure, cardiac arrest, and convulsions. Oleanders are absorbed easily via skin and GI route.

Q. What are the toxic principles of aconite plant?

Toxic principles are triterpene alkaloids known as:

A. Aconitine
B. Misaconitine
C. Hypaconitine

These alkaloids are sparingly soluble in water and considered as most virulent poison with sweetish taste. Other alkaloids present in small quantities in the plant are picraconitine, pseudoaconitine, and aconine.

Q. What is the mode of action of aconite toxins?

Diterpene alkaloids are known as cardiac and neurotoxins that can cause conduction block and paralysis through their action on voltage-sensitive sodium channels in the axons. This can result in initial neurological stimulation, followed by depression of myocardium, smooth and skeletal muscles, CNS, and peripheral nervous system. Aconite is absorbed via skin and oral route. Symptoms generally appear within 30 to 90 min after ingestion of the poison and lasts up to approximately 30 hr.

Q. What are the toxic principles of nicotine plant?

Lobeline is the chief constituent of nicotine plant (Indian tobacco), obtained from the leaves and tops of *Lobelia inflata*, an alkaloid similar to nicotine, but less potent than nicotine, and is used in antismoking tablets and lozenge.

Q. What is the source of strychnine?

Strychnine is a spinal poison caused by *Strychnos nux-vomica*, kuchila plant. It contains alkaloids such as, *strychnine, brucine, and loganin*.

Q. What are invasive plants?

Invasive plants are plant species that can be harmful when introduced to new environments. These plants can reproduce quickly and thrive in different habitats. Invasive plants can grow in natural areas (forests, grasslands, and wetlands), managed areas (cultivated fields, gardens, lawns, and pastures), and areas where the soil and vegetation have been disturbed (ditches, rights of way, and roadsides).

Q. Why are phenothiazine tranquilizers contraindicated in *Datura* intoxication?

In *Datura* intoxication, anticholinergic symptoms are seen. As phenothiazines also possess anticholinergic activity, they are contraindicated for controlling CNS excitation in *Datura* intoxication.

Q. What is prussic acid poisoning?

Prussic acid is also known as hydrocyanic acid (HCN). Prussic acid is not normally present in plants, but under certain conditions, several common plants can accumulate large quantities of cyanogenic glycosides which can convert to prussic acid. It is a potent, rapidly acting poison, which enters the bloodstream of affected animals and is transported through the body. It then inhibits oxygen utilization by the cells so that, in effect, the animal dies from asphyxia.

Q. Which animal species are more susceptible to prussic acid poisoning?

Ruminant animals (cattle and sheep) are more susceptible to prussic acid poisoning than monogastric animals (horses and pigs).

Q. Why are monogastric animals less susceptible to prussic acid poisoning?

The lower pH in the stomach of the monogastric helps to destroy the enzymes that convert cyanogenic glycosides to prussic acid.

Q. What is cyanide poisoning?

Cyanide poisoning is a form of histotoxic hypoxia because the cells of an organism are unable to use oxygen, primarily through the inhibition of cytochrome c oxidase enzyme.

Q. What is the function of cytochrome c oxidase?

Mammalian cytochrome c oxidase (COX) is the terminal complex (complex IV) of the electron transfer chain. It catalyzes the transfer of electrons from ferrocytochrome **c** to molecular oxygen, converting the latter to water.

Q. Why is cytochrome c important?

Cytochrome c is primarily known for its function in the mitochondria as a key participant in the life-supporting function of ATP synthesis. However, when a cell receives an apoptotic stimulus, cytochrome c is released into the cytosol and triggers programmed cell death through apoptosis.

Q. What is the toxic principle of cyanogenic plants?

Cyanogenic glycosides or cyanogens (amygdalin, prunasin, dhurrin, linamarin).

Hydrogen cyanide (HCN) is formed when the glycosides are hydrolyzed by enzymes in plants or by rumen microorganisms.

Q. Why does cyanide have more affinity for cytochrome oxidase than hemoglobin?

Cyanide has more affinity for ferric (Fe3+) form of iron. In hemoglobin, iron is present in ferrous (Fe2+) form, whereas cytochrome oxidase has ferric (Fe3+) iron. Hence, cyanide prefers cytochrome oxidase.

Q. Name the compounds that produce cyanide ions.

A. Hydrogen cyanide gas

B. Crystalline solids such as potassium cyanide and sodium cyanide

Q. How are cyanides produced in nature?

Cyanides are produced by certain bacteria, fungi, and algae and are found in a number of plants. Cyanides are found in substantial amounts in certain seeds and fruit stones, e.g., those of apricots, apples, and peaches. In plants, cyanides are usually bound to sugar molecules in the form of cyanogenic

glycosides and defend the plant against herbivores. Cassava roots (also called manioc), an important potato-like food grown in tropical countries (and the base from which tapioca is made), also contain cyanogenic glycosides.

Q. Is consumption of cassava root responsible for chronic form of cyanide toxicity in humans?

Chronic form of cyanide toxicity is observed in humans due to consumption of cassava root, that is, konzo.

Q. What is the mechanism of cyanide toxicity?

The cyanide ion halts cellular respiration by inhibiting the enzyme cytochrome c oxidase found in the mitochondria. It attaches to the iron within this protein. The binding of cyanide to this enzyme prevents transport of electrons from cytochrome c to oxygen. As a result, the electron transport chain is disrupted, meaning that the cell can no longer aerobically produce ATP for energy. Tissues that depend highly on aerobic respiration, such as the central nervous system and the heart, are particularly affected. This is an example of histotoxic hypoxia.

Q. What is the mode of action of cyanide ions in animal toxicity?

In acute cyanide poisoning, cyanide ions (CN^-) bind to, and inhibit, the ferric (Fe^{3+}) heme moiety form of mitochondrial cytochrome c oxidase. This blocks the fourth step in the mitochondrial electron transport chain (reduction of O2 to H2O), resulting in the arrest of aerobic metabolism and death from histotoxic anoxia. Tissues that heavily depend on aerobic metabolism such as the heart and brain are particularly susceptible to these effects. Cyanide also binds to other heme-containing enzymes, such as members of the cytochrome p450 family and to myoglobin. However, these tissue cyanide "sinks" do not provide sufficient protection from histotoxic anoxia.

Q. Why does chopping, cutting, or chewing plants increase cyanide toxicity?

Cyanogenic glycosides are present in epidermal cells, whereas the enzyme β-glycosidase is present in mesenchymal cells. Hence, chopping, cutting, or chewing ruptures the cells releasing the enzyme which releases HCN.

Q. Why are ruminants more susceptible to cyanogenic glycoside poisoning?

The pH, water content, and microflora of rumen facilitate the release of cyanide from cyanogenic glycosides. Hence, ruminants are more susceptible to cyanogenic glycoside poisoning.

Q. Why are non-ruminants not affected by cyanogenic glycosides?

Acidic pH destroys β-glycosidase enzyme, which is responsible for the release of HCN. Hence, non-ruminants are not affected by cyanogenic glycosides.

Q. What is the lethal dose of cyanide in animals?

The acute lethal dosage of hydrogen cyanide (HCN) in most animal species is ~2 mg/kg. Plant materials containing ≥200 ppm of cyanogenic glycosides are dangerous.

Q. Why do *Halogeton glomeratus* and *Oxalis pes-caprae* commonly cause oxalate poisoning?

The oxalates present in the above plant species are soluble. Hence, these plants cause oxalate poisoning. In H. glomeratus, both sodium and potassium oxalates are present, whereas in *O. pes-caprae*, only potassium oxalates are present.

Q. What are oxalates?

Oxalates belong to a group of substances known as antinutrients. Antinutrients are, as their name would suggest, compounds which prevent the nutritive value of foods from being effective, either by preventing the absorption of nutrients, by being toxic themselves, or by one or more other methods of action.

Q. Name some plants and foods that contain oxalates.

There are several plants and food that contain oxalates, for example, *Dieffenbachia* plant, vegetables, and fruits such as spinach, Swiss chard, rhubarb, soy nuts, plantains, almonds, cashews, sesame seeds, and yucca.

Q. Why are ruminants less susceptible for oxalate poisoning?

Rumen has the ability to convert soluble oxalates into insoluble form. Hence, ruminants are less susceptible for oxalate poisoning. But if the rumen's ability for conversion is exceeded, oxalate poisoning occurs.

Q. How do oxalates damage the body?

These chemicals are present in plants (and some animal foods) that bind with minerals in the body, such as magnesium, potassium, calcium, and sodium, creating oxalate salts. Most of these salts are soluble and pass quickly out of the body. However, oxalates that bind with calcium are practically insoluble, and these crystals solidify in the kidneys (kidney stones) or the urinary tract, causing pain and irritation. These crystals can then easily settle out as sediments from the urine, causing kidney stones.

Q. What is odoratism or osteolathyrism?

The lathyrism resulting from the ingestion of *Lathyrus odoratus* seeds (sweet peas) is often referred to as odoratism or osteolathyrism, which is caused by a different toxin (beta-aminopropionitrile) that affects the linking of collagen, a protein of connective tissues.

Q. What is neurolathyrism?

Neurolathyrism is a neurological disease of humans and domestic animals, caused by long-term feeding/eating of seeds of certain legumes of the genus *Lathyrus*. There is gradual weakness of muscles followed by paralysis leading to death due to respiratory failure.

Q. What is the toxic principle of lathyrism?

Lathyrus grain contains high concentrations of the glutamate analogue neurotoxin β-oxalyl-L-α,β-diaminopropionic acid (ODAP, also known as β-N-oxalyl-amino-L-alanine, or BOAA).

Q. Why does plant accumulate nitrates in toxic proportions?

Plants absorbs nitrates from soil due to physiological requirement. However, any change in environmental conditions that affect the utilization of nitrates leads to nitrate accumulation, for example, lack of rainfall, no leaching of nitrates from soil; low temperature, nitrate reductase activity inhibition; high temperature, excessive absorption from soil; etc.

Q. Why are urinary bladder tumors common in cattle in bracken fern poisoning?

Ptaquiloside is converted into an active carcinogen dienon in alkaline medium. As the urine in cattle is alkaline, the conversion of ptaquiloside to dienon occurs, leading to development of urinary bladder tumors.

Q. Despite the presence of lectins, why is barley nontoxic to animals?

The structure of lectins contains A and B chains linked by two disulfide bonds. The presence of both chains is necessary for producing toxicity. But barley is not toxic due to the presence of only A chain.

Q. What is photodynamic substance?

A substance which absorbs UV light and emits energy while coming to ground state is called photodynamic substance.

Q. What is secondary/hepatogenous photosensitization?

The type of photosensitivity which is produced due to hepatic damage consequent to ingestion of hepatotoxic substances is called secondary/hepatogenous photosensitization.

Q. Name at least three plants that can cause secondary/hepatogenous photosensitization.

A. Pyrrolizidine alkaloid-containing plants—*Senecio* species

B. *Heliotropium* species; *Lantana camara*

C. Mycotoxins, sporodesmins; blue-green algae, *Microcystis* species

Q. Why are lesions in photosensitization seen only in few areas of the body?

Melanin pigment protects the skin from UV light. Hence, in light-pigmented areas or in areas devoid of fur/wool, more UV light is absorbed leading to sunburn lesions. Light-pigmented areas and areas devoid of hair/wool like face, eyelids, muzzle, coronary band, udder, etc. are more prone for photosensitization.

Q. Why is swallowing of seeds of *Abrus* and castors not toxic to animals?

Abrus and castor seeds have tough outer coating which resists digestion and hence are passed through GIT without causing any toxicity. However, crushing or chewing prior to swallowing will produce toxicity.

Q. Why is strychnine least toxic to chicken and pigeons?

In chickens and pigeon, strychnine is absorbed very slowly. Hence, strychnine is least toxic to chicken and pigeons. However, other avian species are easily affected.

3.4 Mushroom Toxicity

Q. Are mushrooms toxic?

Most nonedible mushrooms may cause mild discomfort and are not life-threatening; however, repeated ingestion of the false morel, *Gyromitra esculenta*, has been found to cause hepatitis. Boiling generally inactivates the toxin gyromitrin. Most fatal poisonings related to wild mushrooms are from ingestion of different species within *Amanita*, *Galerina*, and *Lepiota*. *Amanita phalloides* (Fig. 16.1) contains phalloidin and amatoxins. Phalloidin is capable of binding actin in muscle cells; however, it is not readily absorbed during digestion, which limits its harmful effects.

Q. Which amanitins are toxic?

The smaller α-, β-, and γ-amanitins are readily absorbed. Of the amatoxins, α-amanitin is the most toxic as it inhibits protein synthesis in hepatocytes by binding to RNA polymerase II.

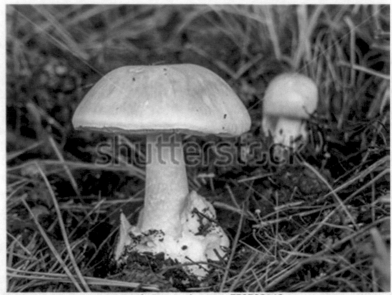

Fig. 16.1 The toxic mushroom *Amanita phalloides*. (https://thumb1.shutterstock.com/display_pic_with_logo/163922440/772763140/stock-photo-death-cap-mushroom-amanita-phalloides-772763140.jpg)

4   Sample MCQ's

(choose the correct statement; it may be one, two, or more or none)

Q.1. Which of the following plants are carcinogenic?

  A. American hellebore
  B. Bracken fern
  C. Buttercup
  D. Tung nut

Q.2. All of the following are true of grayano-toxins *except* -----

  A. They are present in rhododendron
  B. They can contaminate honey
  C. They cause bradycardia
  D. They block the neuromuscular junction

Q.3. Plant molecules that react as bases and usually contain nitrogen in a heterocyclic structure are known as ------

  A. Alkaloids
  B. Terpenes
  C. Resins
  D. Glycosides

Q.4. Plant molecules that are created from iso-prene units with varying functional groups are known as -----

  A. Terpenes
  B. Amines
  C. Alkaloids
  D. Phenols

Q.5. Plant molecules that are hydrolyzed to a sugar and a nonsugar moiety are known as -----

  A. Glycosides
  B. Alkaloids
  C. Resins
  D. Terpene

Q.6. Toxic minerals that may accumulate in plants include all of the following *except* ------

A. Cadmium
B. Magnesium
C. Copper
D. Selenium

Q.7. *Brassica oleracea* (kale) contains ------

A. Cardiac glycoside
B. Cyanogenic glycoside
C. Goitrogenic glycoside
D. Steroid glycoside

Q.8. A plant toxin that can be highly transmitted through milk is -----

A. Oxalate
B. Cyanide
C. Nitrate
D. Tremetol

Q.9. An antidote is available for the toxin present in ------

A. Azalca
B. Pigweed
C. Veratrum
D. Apple seeds

Q.10. Which of the following plant toxins is classified as an alcohol?

A. Nicotine
B. Ranunculus
C. Dogbane
D. Remetol

Q.11. Amygdalin is found in the highest amount in the seeds of ------

A. Bitter almond
B. Tomato
C. Pear
D. Plum

Q.12. Strychnine blocks ------

A. Glycine-gated chloride channel
B. Glutamate receptors
C. GABA receptors
D. Voltage-gated sodium channels

Q.13. The toxin found in species of *Capsicum* has been known to be useful in the therapy of -----

A. Skin cancer
B. Depression
C. Chronic pain
D. Decubitus ulcers

Q.14. All of the following are true of curare *except* -----

A. It was a South American arrow poison.
B. It is a neuromuscular blocking agent.
C. It can be used clinically.
D. It is a CNS toxic.

Q.15. Swainsonine ------

A. Is present in *Vinca* species
B. Is a glycoprotein
C. Causes abortions in livestock
D. None of the above

Q.16. The veratrum and lupine alkaloids are ------

A. Teratogenic
B. Components of marketed pharmaceuticals
C. Used as insecticides
D. Poisons that Socrates drank

Q.17. Which plant caused highest fatalities in the Western United States?

A. Kochia weed
B. Sudan grass
C. Locoweed
D. Sorghum
E. Larkspur

Q.18. What is the difference between larkspur and monkshood?

A. Larkspur contains hollow stems and monkshood does not.
B. Monkshood contains hollow stems and larkspur does not.
C. Larkspur contains woody stems and monkshood does not.

Q.19. What is the treatment for larkspur?

A. Methylene blue
B. Acetyl cholinesterase inhibitor (physostigmine/neostigmine)
C. Sodium thiosulfate
D. All of the above

Q.20. Low energy diet for ruminants may increase susceptibility to _____ poisoning.

A. Nitrite
B. Cardiac glycoside
C. Cyanide
D. Diterpenoid alkaloid
E. Phylloerythrin

Answers
1. B.   2. D.   3. A.   4. A.   5. A.   6. B.
7. C.   8. D.   9. D.   10. D.   11. A.
12. A.   13. C.   14. D.   15. C.   16. A.
17. E.   18. C.   19. B.   20. A.

Further Reading

Gopalakrishnakone P, Carlini CR, Ligabue-Braun R (eds) (2017) Plant toxins. Springer Netherlands

Gupta PK (1988) Veterinary toxicology. Cosmo Publications, New Delhi, India

Gupta PK (2014) Essential concepts in toxicology. BSP Pvt. Ltd, Hyderabad, India

Gupta PK (2016) Fundamental in toxicology: essential concepts and applications in toxicology. Elsevier / BSP, USA

Gupta PK (2018) Illustrative toxicology, 1st edn. Elsevier, San Diego, USA

Gupta PK (2019) Concepts and applications in veterinary toxicology: an interactive guide, 1st edn. Springer Nature, Switzerland

Gupta PK (2020) Brain storming questions in toxicology. Francis and Taylor CRC Press, USA

Klaassen CD, Watkins JB III (eds) (2015) Casarett & Doull's essentials of toxicology, 3rd edn. McGraw-Hill, USA

Panter KE, Welch KD, Gardner DR, Lee ST, Green BT, Pfister JA, Cook D, Davis TZ, Stegelmeier BL (2018) Poisonous plants of the United States. In: Gupta RC (ed) Veterinary toxicology: basic and clinical principles, 3rd edn. Academic Press/Elsevier, San Diego, USA, pp 837–890

Sharma RP, Salunkhe DK (2010) Animal and plant toxins. In: Gupta PK (ed) Modern toxicology: the adverse effects of Xenobiotics, vol 2, 2nd reprint. PharmaMed Press, Hyderabad, India, pp 252–316

Biotoxins and Venomous Organisms

17

Abstract

Poisons are compounds produced in non-specialized tissues as secondary products of metabolism that accumulate in the host animal or that accumulate in predators following ingestion of prey. In contrast, venoms are produced in specialized tissues or glands, and venomous animals have developed a variety of venom apparatuses (stingers, teeth, etc.) to deliver their venom to target animals—a process termed envenomation. Most venoms and poisons are not composed of a single chemical substance but, rather, are mixtures of a variety of chemical compounds that often act synergistically to produce their toxic effects. Typical constituents include peptides, amines, serotonin, quinones, polypeptides, and enzymes. These compounds are collectively termed toxins. Compared to animals, envenomation or poisoning from zootoxins is relatively more in human beings than domestic animals. This chapter briefly describes the overview, key points, and relevant text that are in the format of problem-solving study questions followed by multiple-choice questions (MCQs) along with their answers.

Keywords

Snakes · venomous arthropods · Fish poisoning · Marine bites · Stings · Biotoxins · venomous organisms, poisons, mollusks, question answer bank, MCQs, toxicity

1 Introduction

Toxicity of biotoxins and venomous organisms such as snakes, arthropods, fish, marine animals, and mollusks is very common in animals and human beings. Therefore, the problems of understanding the risks associated with these animal and venomous organisms are very important. The chapter briefly describes an overview, key points, and relevant text that is in the format of problem-solving study questions followed by multiple-choice questions (MCQ's) along with their answers.

2 Overview

The animal kingdom is populated by a vast variety of creatures. In order to survive, they have developed chemical means of defense and/or food procurement. Every phylum within the animal kingdom contains species that produce poisons or venoms. Poisons are compounds produced in nonspecialized tissues as secondary products of metabolism that accumulate in the host animal or that accumulate in predators following ingestion of prey. In contrast, venoms are produced in specialized tissues or glands, and venomous animals have developed a variety of venom apparatuses (stingers, teeth, etc.) to deliver their venom to target animals—a process termed envenomation. Most venoms and poisons are not composed of a

P K Gupta, *Problem Solving Questions in Toxicology*, https://doi.org/10.1007/978-3-030-50409-0_17

single chemical substance but, rather, are mixtures of a variety of chemical compounds that often act synergistically to produce their toxic effects. Typical constituents include peptides, amines, serotonin, quinones, polypeptides, and enzymes. These compounds are collectively termed toxins. Compared to animals, envenomation or poisoning from zootoxins is relatively more in human beings than domestic animals. Clinically significant zootoxins can affect various vital organs, such as nervous, cardiovascular, and reproductive and developmental systems. Bites and stings from arthropods and snakes certainly can occur in any species, and the potential for oral exposure to animals such as poisonous toads, snakes, or insects will vary with the region and environment.

Key Points

- Common poisonous and venomous organisms include snakes, arthropods, fish, and marine animals.
- Poisonous animals are those whose tissues, either in whole or in part, are toxic. Poisoning usually takes place through ingestion.
- Venomous animals produce poison in a developed secretory gland or group of cells and can deliver their toxin during biting or stinging.
- The bioavailability of a venom is determined by its composition, molecular size, amount or concentration gradient, solubility, degree of ionization, and the rate of blood flow into specific tissues.
- The distribution of most venom fractions is rather unequal, being affected by protein binding, variations in pH, and membrane permeability, among other factors.
- A venom may be metabolized in several or many different tissues.
- Because of their protein composition, many toxins produce an antibody response; this response is essential in producing antisera.

---

3   Problem-Solving Study Questions

Q. How one can differentiate toxin, poison, and venom?

Toxins are proteins that lead to immune reaction.

Poisons are chemical substances (not injected by biological vector). i.e., if poison is injected by snake, it becomes venom.

Venoms are biological poisons.

Q. Define tetrodotoxin.

Tetrodotoxin, also known as puffer poison, is found in many species of puffer fish, ocean sunfish, and porcupine fish. It is an amino perhydro-quinazoline compound.

Q. Define saxitoxin.

Some mollusks contain neurotoxins known as saxitoxin which are produced when certain species of algae undergo rapid growth and are ingested by mollusks.

Q. Define hemotoxicity.

Hemotoxicity is related to blood toxicity. It includes coagulopathies, cardiotoxicity, and hemolysis.

Q. What is cytotoxin?

A cytotoxin is any substance that has a toxic effect on cells. Some common examples of cytotoxins include chemical agents and certain snake venoms. Cytotoxins typically attack only a specific type of cell or organ, rather than an entire body.

Q. What are cardiotoxins?

Cardiotoxins are components that are specifically toxic to the heart. They bind to particular sites on the surface of muscle cells and cause depolarization == > the toxin prevents muscle contraction. These toxins may cause the heart to beat irregularly or stop beating, causing death. Example is snakes (mambas and some cobra species).

Q. What are hemotoxins?

Hemotoxins cause hemolysis, the destruction of red blood cells (erythrocytes), or induce blood coagulation (clotting). Example is snakes (most vipers and many cobra species). The tropical rattlesnake *Crotalus durissus* produces convulxin, a coagulant.

Q. What is neurotoxin? Give examples
Neurotoxins are toxins that are poisonous or destructive to nerve tissue (causing neurotoxicity). Neurotoxins are an extensive class of exogenous chemical neurological insults that can adversely affect function in both developing and mature nervous tissue, for example, king cobra (*Ophiophagus hannah*), toxin known as hannahtoxin containing α-neurotoxins; sea snakes (Hydrophiinae), toxin known as erabutoxin); many-banded krait (*Bungarus multicinctus*), toxin known as α-Bungarotoxin; and cobras (Naja species), toxin known as cobratoxin.

Q. What does the word "predator" mean?
An animal that eats other animals

Q. What does the word "prey" mean?
An animal that is eaten by other animals

Q. Who is usually poisonous, the predator or the prey?
The prey

Q. How is a poisonous animal different from a venomous animal?
Poisonous animal is different from a venomous animal because venomous animals inject their poison into its victim. A predator comes in contact with the poison of a poisonous animal if it touches or eats the animal.

Q. What is the difference between poison and venom?
Poison is contained in the tissues and is delivered through eating, e.g., puffer fish—tetradotoxin (poison) must be inhaled, ingested, or delivered via touch—while venom is produced by a specialized gland and is delivered either injected into a wound or through biting or stinging (generally venom won't hurt if delivered in other than this mode, even if one swallows it), e.g., snake, venom.

Q. Describe briefly medically important orders of arthropods.
There are more than a million species of arthropods, generally divided into 25 orders, of which at least 12 are of importance to humans from an economic standpoint. However, medically, the following orders of venomous or poisonous animals are of importance. These include:

A. Arachnids (scorpions, spiders, whip scorpions, solpugids, mites, and ticks)
B. Myriapods (centipedes and millipedes)
C. Insects: Heteroptera (true bugs, water bugs, assassin bugs, and wheel bugs), Hymenoptera (ants, bees, wasps, and hornets), Formicidae (ants), Apidae (bees), Vespidae (wasps), Lepidoptera (caterpillars, moths, and butterflies)
D. Beetles (blister beetles)

Q. What is the difference between poisonous and non-poisonous snakes?
The shape of the head, pupil, fangs, and tail is the biggest and most easily recognizable features that can be used to determine the difference between venomous and nonvenomous snakes.

3.1 Arachnids

Q. Define nature of toxins produced by scorpions.
Many scorpion venoms contain low-molecular-weight proteins, peptides, amino acids, nucleotides, and salts, among other components. Venom (toxalbumin) has two components, a hemolytic and a neurotoxic fraction.

Q. What are the signs and symptoms of scorpion bite/poisoning?
Victim presents with nausea, vomiting, restlessness, and fever followed by convulsions, paralysis, coma, and death (due to respiratory paralysis). Neurotoxic factor can mimic strychnine poisoning. Hemolytic factors can mimic viperine snakebite.

Q. What is the nature of spider venom?
Spider venoms are complex mixtures of low-molecular-weight components, including inorganic ions and salts, free acids, glucose-free amino acids, biogenic amines and neurotransmitters, and polypeptide toxins. Black widow spider venom contains various toxic proteins, alpha-latrotoxin, a labile neurotoxin which is the most important and potent toxin. The venom also contains several other lipoproteins and hyaluronidase. The venom of the

black widow spider is one of the most potent biological toxins and is neurotoxic.

Q. What is tick paralysis?

Tick paralysis (*Dermacentor* species and *Rhipicephalus* species) is the only tick-borne disease that is not caused by an infectious organism. The illness is caused by a neurotoxin produced in the tick's salivary gland.

Q. Which species are associated with tick paralysis?

Potentially 50 species of ticks are associated with clinical paralysis. Tick paralysis is caused by the saliva of certain ticks of the families Ixodidae, Argasidae, and Nuttalliellidae.

Q. What are the signs and symptoms of tick paralysis?

The patient often complains difficulty with gait, followed by paresis and eventually locomotor paresis and paralysis. Problems in speech and respiration may ensue and lead to respiratory paralysis if the tick is not removed.

Q. Which species of mites are commonly associated with bite?

Common mite species that bite and burrow in the skin include *Sarcoptes scabiei*, which cause scabies and *Demodex* mites which cause a scabies-like dermatitis.

3.2   Myriapods

Q. What are myriapods (centipedes, Chilopoda)?

Myriapods are elongated, many-segmented, brownish yellow (gray in print versions) arthropods which have a pair of walking legs on most segments. They are fast-moving, secretive, and nocturnal. They feed on other arthropods and even small vertebrates and birds. Centipede venoms contain high-molecular-weight proteins, proteinases, esterases, 5-hydroxytryptamine, histamine, lipids, and polysaccharides. Such venom contains a heat-labile cardiotoxic protein of 60 kDa that produces, in human, changes associated with acetylcholine release.

Q. How millipedes do protect themselves?

Millipedes protect themselves by oozing sticky droplets when attacked. These droplets are poisonous.

Q. What are the common signs and symptoms of millipede bites?

Usually centipedes can inflict painful bites with erythema, edema, and local lymphangitis.

3.3   Insects

Q. Define in brief nature of toxins of ants.

Fire ant is the common name for several species of ants in the genus *Solenopsis*. Ant venom is any of, or a mixture of, irritants and toxins inflicted by ants. Most ants spray or inject a venom, the main constituent of which is formic acid only in the case of subfamily Formicinae. The ants get a grip and then sting (from the abdomen) and inject a toxic alkaloid venom called solenopsin, a compound from the class of piperidines.

Q. What are the signs and symptoms of toxicity by fire ants?

In human being signs of toxicity include sterile pustules on the body.

Q. Why the stinger is lost due to stinging and results in death of honey bee?

The stinger in honey bees is barbed which gets struck in the victim's skin along with venom sac. Hence, stinger apparatus is lost and results in death of the insect.

Q. Why wasps can sting multiple times?

Wasps can withdraw the stinger as it is not barbed and can sting multiple times.

3.4   Blister Beetle Toxicity

Q. Which animals are susceptible to blister beetle toxicity?

The blister beetle (*Epicauta*) is highly toxic to sheep and cattle but primarily to horses. As little as 4–6 grams of blister beetles can be deadly to an 1100 lb. horse. Blister beetles swarm in alfalfa fields and are drawn into bales by accident.

Q. Which is the principal toxin in blister beetle poisoning?

Cantharidin is the chemical found in blister beetles that causes the damage noticed by the owner and veterinarian. It is a contact irritant and a vesicant (causes blister formation). The tissues most often affected by cantharidin are gastrointestinal mucosa (including the mouth), renal or bladder, and the heart muscle.

3.5   Reptiles

Q. Which are common species of lizards that can cause poisoning?

The Gila monster (*Heloderma suspectum*) and the beaded lizards (*Heloderma horridum*) are the common ones. These large, relatively slow-moving, and largely nocturnal reptiles have few enemies other than humans. They are far less dangerous than is generally believed. Their venom is transferred from venom glands in the lower jaw through ducts that discharge their contents near the base of the larger teeth of the lower jaw. The venom is then drawn up along grooves in the teeth by capillary action.

Q. What is the nature of venom introduced by lizards?

The venom has serotonin and several enzymes having fibrinogeno coagulase activities. The bite can lead to pain, edema, hypotension, nausea, vomiting, weakness, and diaphoresis.

Q. What is the treatment of lizard poisoning?

No antivenin is commercially available. Treatment is supportive.

Q. Classify poisonous snakes.

There are about 3200 species of snakes. Approximately 1300 species are venomous. Venomous snakes are usually defined as those which possess venom glands and specialized venom-conducting fangs, which enable then to inflict serious bites upon their victims. In general, the following are recognized as venomous snakes:

A. The Colubridae, which possess small rear fangs

B. The Elapidae and Hydrophidae, which possess small front fang

C. And the viper group, which consists of the Viperidae and Crotalidae

Venomous snakes are widespread throughout the world. However, they do not occur in several islands such as New Zealand, Ireland, Iceland, the Azores, and Canaries.

Q. What is general nature of snake venom?

Snake venom is highly modified saliva containing zootoxins. It contains more than 20 different compounds, mostly proteins and polypeptides. A complex mixture of proteins, enzymes, and various other substances with toxic and lethal properties serves to immobilize the prey animal. Enzymes play an important role in the digestion of prey, and various other substances are responsible for important but nonlethal biological effects.

Q. Describe mode of action of neurotoxic venomous snakes.

The venoms of different types of venomous snakes are different in composition. Elapidae and Hydrophidae venoms are rich in neurotoxic polypeptides. These venoms are typically fast acting on nerve tissue and neurotransmitters, often degrading neurotransmitters or depolarizing the axonal membrane for long periods of time, thereby preventing nervous impulses from being conducted.

Q. Describe in brief mode of action of viper and crotalid neurotoxic venomous snakes.

The venoms of these snakes are neurotoxins that are not membrane depolarizing but rather are antagonistic to acetylcholine and act as a blocking agent at the neuromuscular junction. Phospholipases, proteases, and lytic factors contained in venom tend to cause hemolytic effects and are largely responsible for the necrosis that follows viper and crotalid bites. Cell metabolism is interrupted by inhibition of oxidative phosphorylation, which leads to an insufficient supply of ATP for the cell. Mitochondrial electron transport is also interrupted as cytochrome C, an electron acceptor protein in the electron transport chain, is denatured.

Q. Describe general symptoms of snakebite.
General symptoms include bloody wound discharge, fang marks or swelling at wound, extreme localized pain, excessive sweating, loss of muscle coordination, blurred vision, numbness or tingling, convulsions, and fainting.

The toxins act like curare affecting mainly the motor nerve cells and results in muscular paralysis. The muscles are affected in the following order:

A. First – muscles of mouth
B. Second – muscles of the throat
C. Finally – muscles of respiration

Q. What are the local actions of neurotoxic snakebite?
Local manifestations of neurotoxic venoms are severe burning at bite site, rapid edema, and inflammatory changes followed by oozing of serum.

Q. What are local actions of hemotoxic venomous snakes?
Systemic actions are due to hemolytic effect on the heart and blood vessels resulting in cardiovascular collapse and death. If the patient survives suppuration, sloughing with infection at the site of bite, hemorrhage from the mucosa of rectum, other natural orifice, etc., and gangrene of the parts involved can occur. The venom acts by cytolysis of endothelium of blood vessels, lysis of red cells and other tissue cells, and coagulation disorders. This can lead to severe swelling with oozing of blood and spreading of cellulitis at bite site. Blood from such patients fails to clot even on adding thrombin, because of very low level of fibrin. This is followed by necrosis of renal tubules and functional disturbances like convulsions, due to intracerebral hemorrhage.

Q. Why alcohol is contraindicated in cleaning the area of snakebite?
Alcohol causes vasodilation promoting the spread of the venom in the body.

Q. What are local actions of myotoxic venomous snakes?

Myotoxic venomous snakes produce minimal swelling and pain.

Q. What are systemic actions of myotoxic venomous snakes?
Myotoxic symptoms are common with Hydrophidae or sea snakes. The venom produces generalized muscular pain, myalgia, muscular stiffness, myoglobinuria, renal tubular necrosis, and death which usually occur due to respiratory failure.

Q. Why snakebite in human beings and dogs is fatal compared to large animals?
Human beings and dogs are relatively smaller in size compared to other large animals like horses and cattle. Hence, the bite is fatal in smaller subjects than the larger ones.

3.6 Fish Poisoning

Q. Define fish poisoning.
Fish poisoning is acute illness resulting from the consumption of fish:

A. Illness due to eating fish that normally contain neurotoxins in their flesh
B. Illness due to eating stale fish either due to histamine or bacterial food poisoning
C. Erysipeloid (dermatitis of the hands due to bacterial infection, occurring mainly among handlers of meat and fish products)

Q. How do we get fish poisoning?
Eating of contaminated fish and sea foods is responsible for fish poisoning. The most common of these is ciguatera poisoning (*Gambierdiscus toxicus*, barracuda fish), scombroid poisoning (mackerel, tuna fish), puffer fish poisoning, and various shellfish poisonings (mussels, clams, oysters, and scallops). For example, ciguatera is a foodborne illness (food poisoning) caused by eating fish that is contaminated by ciguatera toxin. Ciguatera toxin is a heat-stable lipid-soluble compound, produced by dinoflagellates and concentrated in fish organs, that can cause nausea, pain, and cardiac and neurological symptoms in humans when ingested.

Q. What is diarrhetic shellfish poisoning (DSP)?
Diarrhetic shellfish poisoning is caused by chemicals of the okadaic acid family (okadaic acid + 4 related compounds) produced by several species of *Dinophysis* dinoflagellates.

Q. What is ciguatera fish poisoning (CFP)?
Ciguatera fish poisoning is caused by the ciguatoxin family (ciguatoxin + 3 or more related compounds) and produced by several species of dinoflagellates including *Gambierdiscus*, *Prorocentrum*, and *Ostreopsis*.

Q. What are marine bites and stings?
Some marine bites and stings are toxic (Cnidaria, stingrays, mollusks, and sea urchins); all create wounds at risk for infection with marine organisms, most probably *Vibrio* and *Mycobacterium* species. Shark bites result in jagged lacerations with near-total or total amputations.

Q. Why avoiding reef fish consumption is the only way to avoid ciguatera?
The detection of ciguatoxin is difficult as it does not produce any change in organoleptic properties of fish. Further, CTX is not destroyed by temperature or gastric acid. Hence, avoiding eating of reef fish is the only way to prevent ciguatera.

Q. Why puffer fish are resistant to tetradotoxin?
Puffer fish have sodium channels with altered structure due to mutation, which are resistant to tetradotoxin action.

Q. What is amnesic shellfish poisoning (ASP)?
Amnesic shellfish poisoning (ASP) is caused by domoic acid produced by several species of *Pseudo-nitzschia* (planktonic diatom genus).

Q. What is paralytic shellfish poisoning (PSP)?
Paralytic shellfish poisoning (PSP) is caused by the saxitoxin family (saxitoxin + 18 related compounds) produced by several species of *Alexandrium* dinoflagellates.

Q. What is neurotoxic shellfish poisoning (NSP)?
Neurotoxic shellfish poisoning (NSP) is caused by the brevetoxin family including dinoflagellate, *Karenia brevis*, and *Gymnodinium breve*.

3.7 Mollusks

Q. What are mollusks?
Mollusks of human interest are known due to their beautiful patterns on their shells. The genus *Conus* is a group of approximately 500 species of carnivorous predators found in marine habitats that use venom as a weapon for prey capture. The second group is molluscivorous and hunts other gastropods. The final group is piscivorous and has venoms that rapidly immobilize fish. There are probably more than 100 different venom components known as conotoxins, which may be rich in disulfide bonds and conopeptides. Some components have enzymatic activity. Conopeptides also target ligand-gated ion channels that mediate fast synaptic transmission, resulting in poisoning.

4 Sample MCQ's

(Choose the correct statement; it may be one, two, or more or none)

Q.1. Which of the following statements regarding animal toxins is *false*?

A. Animal venoms are strictly metabolized by the liver.
B. The kidneys are responsible for the excretion of metabolized venom.
C. Venoms can be absorbed by facilitated diffusion.
D. Most venom fractions distribute unequally throughout the body.
E. Venom receptor sites exhibit highly variable degrees of sensitivity.

Q.2. Scorpion venoms do *not* ------.

A. Affect potassium channels
B. Affect sodium channels
C. Affect chloride channels
D. Affect calcium channels
E. Affect initial depolarization of the action potential

Q.3. Which of the following statements regarding widow spiders is *true*?

A. Widow spiders are exclusively found in tropical regions.
B. Both male and female widow spiders bite and envenomate humans.
C. The widow spider toxin decreases calcium concentration in the synaptic terminal.
D. Alpha-latrotoxin stimulates increased exocytosis from nerve terminals.
E. A severe alpha-latrotoxin envenomation can result in life-threatening hypotension.

Q.4. Which of the following diseases is caused not commonly by tick envenomation?

A. Rocky Mountain spotted fever
B. Lyme disease
C. Q fever
D. Ehrlichiosis
E. Cat scratch fever

Q.5. Which of the following is *not* characteristic of Lepidoptera envenomation?

A. Increased prothrombin time
B. Decreased fibrinogen levels
C. Decreased partial thromboplastin time
D. Increased risk of hemorrhage
E. Decreased plasminogen levels

Q.6. Which of the following animals has a venom containing histamine and mast cell-degranulating peptide that is known for causing hypersensitivity reactions?

A. Bees
B. Ants
C. Snakes
D. Spiders
E. Reduviidae

Q.7. Which of the following enzymes is *not* typically found in snake venoms?

A. Hyaluronidase
B. Lactate dehydrogenase
C. Collagenase
D. Phosphodiesterase
E. Histaminase

Q.8. Which of the following statements regarding snakes is *false*?

A. Inorganic anions are often found in snake venoms.
B. About 20% of snake species are venomous.
C. Snake venoms often interfere with blood coagulation mechanisms.
D. Proteolytic enzymes are common constituents of snake venoms.
E. Snakebite treatment is often specific for each type of envenomation.

Q.9. Which of the following is false regarding botulism toxin? Please choose only one answer.

A. Acetylcholine release is blocked in the presynaptic neuron resulting in flaccid paralysis.
B. Botulism occurs via ingestion or wound contamination of spores or preformed toxin.
C. Preformed toxin sources are decaying carcasses.
D. For prevention, vaccination against C. botulinum with toxoid
E. Clinical disease signs include "sawhorse stance," muscle rigidity, erect ears, and a reluctance to eat due to "locked jaw."

Q.10. Antivenin (Lycovac) is available and effective for which species toxin?

A. Black widow
B. Brown recluse
C. Hobo spider
D. Tarantula
E. Scorpion

Q.11. Blister beetles cause cantharidin toxicosis which occurs when livestock eat _____.

A. Grain
B. Alfalfa hay
C. Dead chicken carcasses
D. Locoweed
E. Cardenolide

Q.12. Which of the following is *false* regarding *Bufo* toad toxicity?

A. Onset of clinical signs can be rapid and death can occur within 15 minutes.
B. The cardiac glycosides bind and inhibit *Na+/K+-ATPase* resulting in a depressed electrical conduction. Mucous membranes appear pale and tacky.
C. Prognosis is good with most animals with early decontamination and appropriate symptomatic therapy. Majority of animals present with neurologic abnormalities including convulsions, ataxia, nystagmus, stupor, and coma.

Q.13. Which is *false* regarding pit vipers?

A. Most bites are by copperhead snakes.
B. Venom is delivered by the retractable fangs downward and stabbing forward.
C. Echinocytes greatly increase the likelihood that victim has been envenomed.
D. Initial clinical sign is usually marked tissue swelling.
E. Antivenin treatment (CroFab TM) substantially increases the likelihood of survival.

Q.14. How would you identify a female black widow spider?

A. Red, yellow, or orange hourglass on ventral abdomen.

B. The bite causes a "bulls eye "lesion and systemic deletion of clotting factors (vii, ix, and xii).
C. Within 30 min of bite, expanding area of wound will reach up to 15 cm and rupture with serious discharge.
D. Female black widow spiders only build nests in barns housed by talking pigs named Wilbur.
E. The nests will be built on ground level since black widows are poor climbers.

Q.15. Poisoning from these animals is referred to as tegenarism and can generate a wound that takes years to properly heal.

A. Black widow
B. Hobo spider
C. Brown recluse
D. Tarantula
E. Scorpion

Q.16. Which species toxin forms a "bulls eye" lesion?

A. Black widow
B. Brown recluse
C. Hobo dpider
D. Tarantula
E. Scorpion

Answers
1. A.   2. D.   3. D.   4. E.   5. C.   6. A.
7. E.   8. A.   9. E.   10. A.   11. B.
12. C.   13. E.   14. A.   15. B.   16. B.

Further Reading

Gupta PK (1988) Veterinary toxicology. Cosmo Publications, New Delhi, India

Gupta PK (2014) Essential concepts in toxicology. BSP Pvt. Ltd, Hyderabad, India

Gupta PK (2016) Fundamental in toxicology: essential concepts and applications in toxicology. Elsevier/BSP, San Diego, USA

Gupta PK (2018) Illustrative toxicology, 1st edn. Elsevier, San Diego, USA

Gupta PK (2020) Brain storming questions in toxicology. Francis and Taylor CRC Press, USA

Gupta RC (ed) (2018) Veterinary toxicology: basic and clinical principles, 3rd edn. San Diego, USA, Academic Press/Elsevier

Merck Veterinary Manual (2016) Poisonous and venomous animals. Merck Research Laboratories, Merck & Co. Inc, USA, pp 3157–3165

Sharma RP, Salunkhe DK (2010) Animal and plant toxins. In: Gupta PK (ed) Modern toxicology: the adverse effects of xenobiotics, vol 2, 2nd reprint. PharmaMed Press, Hyderabad, India, pp 252–316

Watkins JB III (2015) Toxic effects of plants and animals. In: Klaassen CD, Watkins JB III (eds) Casarett & Doull's essentials of toxicology, 3rd edn. McGraw-Hill, USA, pp 381–400

Poisonous Foods and Food Poisonings

18

Abstract

Food is an exceedingly complex mixture of nutrient and non-nutrient substances. The vast majority of food-borne illnesses in developed countries are attributable to microbiologic contamination of food. Many disorders cause sudden vomiting and diarrhea due to inflammation of the digestive tract (gastroenteritis). Sometimes people loosely refer to all of these disorders as "food poisoning." However, most vomiting and diarrhea is caused by a digestive tract infection from a virus or bacteria. Only gastroenteritis caused by a toxin that was eaten is true food poisoning. For example, bacteria in contaminated food can produce such toxins (see Staphylococcal Food Poisoning). Also, although many poisonous plants, mushrooms, and seafood affect the digestive tract, some affect other organs. This chapter briefly describes the overview, key points, and relevant text that are in the format of problem-solving study questions followed by multiple-choice questions (MCQs) along with their answers.

Keywords

Food poisoning · Microbial toxins · Mycotoxins · Mushroom · Algal toxicity · Question and answer bank · Ttoxicity · MCQs

1 Introduction

Poisonous foods and food poisonings and their hazards are caused by microbial toxins, mycotoxins, mushroom, and algal toxicity. The chapter briefly describes an overview, key points, and relevant text that is in the format of problem-solving study questions followed by multiple-choice questions (MCQ's) along with their answers.

2 Overview

Food poisoning results from eating a plant or animal or ingestion of infected food that contains a toxin such as poisonous species of mushrooms or plants or contaminated fish or shellfish or infections. Foods most commonly associated with food poisoning include chicken, eggs, ready-to-eat foods (i.e., processed meat, soft cheese), shellfish, unpasteurized milk, untreated water, etc. Common foodborne illnesses include bacterial gastroenteritis cause by *Salmonella*, *Campylobacter*, *E. coli*, *Shigella*, *Listeria*, and *Staphylococcus aureus* food poisoning. Food poisoning remains a fairly common illness affecting about one in three people each year. It is particularly prevalent in the summer months when foods have been left out of the fridge for some time. The mass production of food has increased the opportunity for food poisons to

P K Gupta, *Problem Solving Questions in Toxicology*, https://doi.org/10.1007/978-3-030-50409-0_18

infect large populations. It is now possible for food to become contaminated in one country and cause outbreaks of food poisoning in another. It is believed there are 9.4 million cases of gastro-intestinal illness in England annually. The most common symptoms of poisonings are diarrhea, nausea, and vomiting and sometimes seizures and paralysis. The diagnosis is based on symptoms and examination of the ingested substance. Avoiding wild or unfamiliar mushrooms and plants and contaminated fish reduces the risk of poisoning. Replacing fluids and ridding the stomach of the toxic substance are the best forms of treatment, but some substances are deadly.

Key Points

- Food is an exceedingly complex mixture of nutrient and no nutrient substances.
- A substance listed as generally recognized as safe (GRAS) achieves this determination on the adequacy of safety, as shown through scientific procedures or through experience based on common use.
- An estimated daily intake (EDI) is based on two factors: the daily intake of the food in which the substance will be used and the concentration of the substance in that food.
- Food hypersensitivity (allergy) refers to a reaction involving an immune-mediated response, including cutaneous reactions, systemic effects, and even anaphylaxis.
- The vast majority of foodborne illnesses in developed countries are attributable to microbiologic contamination of food.

---

3   Problem-Solving Study Questions

Q. What is food poisoning?

Food poisoning is a vague term. It includes illnesses resulting from ingestion of all foods containing nonbacterial or bacterial products. The nonbacterial products include poisons delivered from plants and animals and certain naturally occurring toxins. Foods containing such products are, by convention, known as poisonous foods.

Q. What is the source of tetrodotoxin?

Tetrodotoxin (TTX) is a naturally occurring toxin that has been responsible for human intoxications and fatalities. Its usual route of toxicity is via the ingestion of contaminated puffer fish which are a culinary delicacy, especially in Japan.

Q. Describe mode of action of tetrodotoxin.

Tetrodotoxin causes paralysis by affecting the sodium ion transport in both the central and peripheral nervous systems. A low dose of tetrodotoxin produces tingling sensations and numbness around the mouth, fingers, and toes. Higher doses produce nausea, vomiting, respiratory failure, difficulty walking, extensive paralysis, and death.

Q. List four methods by which chemicals enter our food, and give an example of each.

A. Packaging materials: Substances such as plasticizers, stabilizers, and inks can enter our food through migration from the packaging, for example, antimony from chipped enamel container, cadmium from trays and containers, and lead from the solder of metal containers and cans.

B. Agricultural application of pesticides and fertilizers: Organochlorides, such as DDT, which is used to control insects and fungi.

C. Food additives for preservation and coloring: MSG to enhance flavor in Chinese food, nitrates which give meat their taste and color, and colorings, i.e., Red dye No.2 which may be a carcinogen.

D. Industrial processes: Mercury, as a by-product of many processes, is an acute toxin which causes neurological complications and birth defects and polychlorinated biphenyls (PCBs).

Q. Describe at least five items in diet and food processing that are responsible for foodborne pathogens.
   A. Processing of milk has caused a decrease in certain competitive bacteria, thereby increasing the chances of survival for *Salmonella* and *Campylobacter*.
   B. Water polluted with raw sewage and manure, carrying harmful microbes, comes in contact with food.
   C. Abuse of antibiotics has allowed some bacteria to acquire antibiotic resistance.
   D. Increase in demand for packaged food supports anaerobic pathogens such as Clostridia.
   E. Ready-to-eat foods that only require minimal heating increases the survivability of bacteria by not destroying the pathogen.

Q. Describe the life cycle of the pork tapeworm and *Taenia solium*.
   A pig becomes infested when it ingests food that is contaminated with human fecal matter that contains tapeworm eggs. The larvae excyst in the intestine and migrate through the bloodstream where they encyst in the muscles. Here they develop into cysterici which contain a scolex or inverted head of the worm. Humans then ingest undercooked pork, and the larvae excyst in the intestine where the scolex attaches to the intestine wall. Here it grows and produces a chain of proglottids. Each mature proglottid produces eggs, which are carried in human fecal matter. If a person ingests the eggs from infected person, the eggs can then enter the bloodstream and migrate throughout the body to the brain, eyes, and muscles of the human.

Q. List at least five factors commonly found to be the cause of foodborne illness, which are largely preventable.
   A. Improperly refrigerated food
   B. Improperly heated or cooked food
   C. Food handlers with poor hygiene
   D. Lapse of time (more than a day) between preparing and serving food
   E. Improper storage of foods at temperatures ideal for bacteria growth

Q. How does food poisoning spread?
   A. The food can be contaminated during growth, production, processing, shipping, and preparation; this preparation can include slaughtering of the animal, cutting into small parts which can become contaminated by the feces of the animal.
   B. There could also be "cross-contamination," a situation in which the platform used for cutting poultry, for example, is used for cutting vegetables and fruits without thorough cleansing first.
   C. Food can be contaminated by flies, by infected food handlers, or by food handlers whose hands became contaminated by touching items previously handled by infected persons and forgetting to wash their hands thoroughly with soap and watetr.

Q. What is "cross-contamination"?
   The process by which bacteria or other microorganisms are unintentionally transferred from one substance or object to another, with harmful effect, is known as cross-contamination. Cross-contamination between raw and cooked food is the cause of most infections.

Q. When do you suspect you may have food poisoning?
   One can suspect food poisoning if:
   A. One develops vomiting and/or diarrhea with severe abdominal pains a few hours after eating at a gathering foods such as vegetable salads, fairly cooked meat/poultry, or canned food
   B. If the stooling and/or vomiting is severe

Q. What can put you at risk of food poisoning?
   The following can put you at risk:
   A. Age (more severe and commoner in old age and childhood)
   B. Pregnancy
   C. Chronic diseases with reduced immunity

Q. How can you prevent food poisoning?
   You can prevent food poisoning by:
   A. Being careful about what you eat at parties and avoiding salads.

B. Preparing your food hygienically
C. Cooking your meat/poultry thoroughly and eating your food while hot
D. Always washing your hands with soap and water before preparing food
E. Covering your food if not ready to eat
F. Reading carefully the label on canned food
G. Cleaning your work top after dealing with animal products (meat, poultry) before preparing vegetables and fruits
H. Always boiling your milk before consumption

Q. Only a large amount of harmful bacteria can cause food poisoning. Write whether statement is right or wrong; give explanation.
Wrong. Some food poisonings can be caused by very tiny amounts of bacteria in the food.

Q. Is it possible to get food poisoning from ice cubes?
Yes. Deep freezing or freezing does not even nearly kill all harmful microbes in food or water even though some microbes may die. If there are harmful microbes in an ice machine or in water being used in ice cubes, they may also appear in the ice cubes and possibly cause food poisoning.

Q. Does temperature affect the reproduction of microbes?
Temperature is one of the factors affecting the reproduction of microbes. The reproduction of microbes becomes more effective when the temperature is favorable for them.

Q. What do you mean by chemical poisoning?
Chemical food poisoning is caused by eating plant or animals that contain a naturally occurring toxin-containing chemicals such as acetylcholine, alkaloids, serotonin, histamines, sulfur, lipids, phenols, glycosides, etc. Chemical food poisoning often involves mushrooms, poisonous plants, or marine animals.

Q. List the seven key principles of HACCP (Hazard Critical Control Point).
A. Assessing hazards
B. Identify critical control points (CCPís)
C. Setting up procedures and standards for CCPís
D. Monitoring CCPís
E. Take corrective actions
F. Set up record-keeping system
G. Verifying that system works

Q. For a pesticide based on toxicity studies, a NOAEL of 2 mg/kg bw/day in mice is derived. Calculate the maximal acceptable concentration in potatoes (if 200 g potatoes per day are eaten for a person weighing 60 kg).
NOAEL = 2 mg/kg bw/day
ADI = 2/100 = 0.02 mg/kg bw/dayADI
ADI for 60 kg bw = 1.2 mg/day
1.2 mg/day is allowed in 200 g potatoes per day.
Therefore, in 1000 g (1 kg) potatoes
$1.2 \times 1000/200 = 6$ mg/kg of the product

3.1   Microbial Food Poisoning

Q. What are microbial toxins?
Microbial toxins are toxins produced by microorganisms, including bacteria and fungi. Microbial toxins promote infection and disease by directly damaging host tissues and by disabling the immune system. Some bacterial toxins, such as botulinum neurotoxins, are the most potent natural toxins known.

Q. Name at least four toxins and bacteria involved in food poisoning.

Name of toxin	Bacteria involved
A. Botulinum toxin	*Clostridium botulinum*
B. Tetanus toxin	*Clostridium tetani*
C. Diphtheria toxin (Dtx)	*Corynebacterium diphtheriae*
D. Exotoxin A	*Pseudomonas aeruginosa*

Q. Define bacterial toxins.
Bacteria generate toxins which can be classified as either exotoxins or endotoxins.
A. Exotoxins are generated and actively secreted.
B. Endotoxins remain part of the bacteria. Usually, an endotoxin is part of the bacterial outer membrane, and it is not released until the bacterium is killed by the immune system. The body's response

to an endotoxin can involve severe inflammation. In general, the inflammation process is usually considered beneficial to the infected host, but if the reaction is severe enough, it can lead to sepsis.

Q. What is toxinosis?

Toxinosis is pathogenesis caused by the bacterial toxin alone, not necessarily involving bacterial infection (e.g., when the bacteria have died, but have already produced toxin, which are ingested). It can be caused by *Staphylococcus aureus* toxins.

Q. What is the source of botulinum toxin?

Botulinum toxin (BTX) is a neurotoxic protein produced by the bacterium *Clostridium botulinum* and related species.

Q. What is mode of action of botulinum?

It prevents the release of the neurotransmitter acetylcholine from axon endings at the neuromuscular junction and thus causes flaccid paralysis. Infection with the bacterium causes the disease botulism.

Q. What are three important types of food poisonings?

Microbial food poisoning is of three types:
A. Infectious type
B. Toxic type
C. Botulism

Q. What is infectious type of food poisoning?

In infectious type, the food poisoning results from ingestion of viable microorganisms that multiply in GI tract producing a true infection, for example, *Salmonella* and *Shigella* group of organisms, etc.

Q. What is toxic type of food poisoning?

In toxic type, the food poisoning results from poisonous substances produced by multiplying organisms that have gained access to the prepared food, for example, enterotoxin produced by the *Staphylococcus*.

Q. What is botulism type of food poisoning?

In botulism type, the food poisoning results from the ingestion of preformed botulinum toxin in the preserved food. The toxin is produced by *Clostridium botulinum*.

Q. What is ptomaine poisoning?

Ptomaine poisoning due to advanced decomposition of food is not common. Ptomaine is proteolytic degradation products formed in decomposing carcasses. There are several main bacteria indicated in ptomaine poisoning, when the term is used interchangeably with food poisoning.

Q. Give three examples of bacteria and germs responsible for food poisoning?

Bacteria and germs responsible for food poisoning are *E. coli*, *Salmonella*, and *Listeria*. *E. coli* is probably the most dangerous bacterium, usually caused by eating improperly cooked ground beef. Even a little bit of pink in a hamburger can mean possible exposure to *E. coli*.

Q. What are the symptoms of *E. coli* poisoning?

E. coli tends to cause watery diarrhea with no fever. In about 5% of cases, significant kidney failure can develop. The risk is higher in children under age five. When this kidney failure develops, it can cause death. Those who recover may require kidney transplantation or regular dialysis while waiting for a transplant. This very serious complication, though rare, is reason enough to use caution when cooking, preparing or serving ground beef.

Q. Describe common signs and symptoms of food poisoning.

There is great variation in the susceptibility of individuals to *Salmonella* food poisoning. Hence, while some participants may remain free from symptoms, other may be severely affected. It is usually self-diagnosable. Food poisoning symptoms may include cramping, nausea, vomiting, or diarrhea. Three characteristics that help to differentiate this poisoning with *staphylococcal* enterotoxin are muscular weakness, fever, and very foul smelling persistent diarrhea. Severe poisoning may show convulsions, muscle paralysis, and death.

3.2   Mycotoxin Poisoning

Q. What are common mycotoxins that cause poisoning?
They include:
A. The ergot alkaloids produced by *Claviceps* sp.
B. Aflatoxins and related compounds produced by *Aspergillus* sp.
C. The trichothecenes produced by several genera of fungi imperfecti, primarily *Fusarium* sp.

Q. Describe common name and properties of ergot.
Common name of ergot is mother of rye. Ergot is an alkaloid. It is the sclerotium (mycelium) of a fungus *Claviceps purpurea*, which grows on many cereals like rye, barley, wheat, oat, etc. Fungus gradually replaces the whole grain to a dark purple mass, which on drying yields ergot.

Q. What are the toxic principles of ergot?
The active toxic principles are ergotamine, ergotoxin, and ergometrine. They are known to contract arterioles which can lead to gangrene of the part supplied.

Q. What are acute toxicity signs and symptoms of ergot?
Acute poisoning is very rare. Some of the common symptoms include irritation of throat, dryness, severe thirst, nausea and vomiting, diarrhea, pain in abdomen, tingling in hands and feet, cramps in muscles (all due to contraction of smooth muscles), dizziness, feeling of coldness, etc. Sometimes symptoms of hypoglycemia, anuria, abortion, and hemorrhages in a pregnant woman may be seen. Death is usually slow.

Q. What are chronic toxicity signs and symptoms of ergot?
Chronic poisoning is called ergotism and is quite common.
It occurs in two forms:
A. Convulsive form: *Shows* painful toxic contraction of voluntary muscles followed by drowsiness, headache, giddiness, madness, etc. Victim may complain of feeling of itching/numbness and ant crawling sensation under the skin.
B. Gangrenous form: Begins as pustules and swelling of limbs and feet, followed by intense hot feeling, severe pain, numbness, etc. followed by gangrenous changes (resemble Raynaud's disease). Recovery is possible, if ergot is withheld.

The ergot alkaloids are known to affect the nervous system and cause vasoconstriction. The ergot alkaloids are derivatives of ergotine, the most active being, more specifically, amides of lysergic acid.

Q. How are trichothecenes produced?
Trichothecenes are produced particularly by members of the genera *Fusarium* and *Trichoderma*.

Q. What do you know about *Penicillium* fungi?
Penicillium fungi are often blue. They are responsible for food spoilage and are commonly known as molds. They are excellent at growing in low humidity environments, allowing for them to remain alive in food storage. Many of these species produce toxins that may cause food poisoning. However, *Penicillium* fungi also are of some benefit to humans (besides production of the antibiotic). They are used in the production of certain cheeses, including Roquefort, Brie, Camembert, and Stilton. *Penicillium* spores were among the most prevalent spores in indoor air. The indoor spore levels were higher even than outdoor levels.

Q. How are rubratoxins produced?
Rubratoxins are produced by *Penicillium rubrum*.

Q. Describe in brief three main *Aspergillus* species that are potentially toxic.
Mycotoxins are fungal secondary metabolites that are potentially harmful to animals or humans. The word "aflatoxin" came from "*Aspergillus flavus* toxin." Three predominant species responsible for aflatoxin poisoning are:
A. *A. flavus*
B. *A. parasiticus*
C. *A. fumigatus*

Q. What are aflatoxins?

Aflatoxins are products of species of the genus *Aspergillus*, common fungi found as a contaminant of grain, maize, peanuts, and so on.

Q. What are the main toxic potentials of aflatoxins?

Aflatoxins are extremely potent liver toxins and carcinogens and are considered the most hazardous of all the mycotoxins. The compounds are resistant to destruction by heat, and ingestion can be dangerous since the toxins can build up if ingested regularly.

Q. What are four major aflatoxins and metabolic derivatives?

There are four major aflatoxins: Aflatoxin B1, B2, G1, and G2.

Additionally, there are two metabolic derivatives: Aflatoxin M1 (derivative of B1) and aflatoxin M2 (derivative of B2)

Q. Name the hormone that is inhibited by zearalenone, which is involved in ovarian follicle maturation.

Follicle-stimulating hormone (FSH). Due to this the characteristic symptom of follicular atresia is observed in ovaries.

3.3   Mushroom Poisoning

Q. What do you mean by mushroom toxicity?

Mushrooms are fungi with umbrella-shaped tops and stems, e.g., *Stropharia semeglobata*, *Hypholoma fasciculare*, and *Lactarius vellereus* are among the poisonous varieties of mushrooms. The toxic mushroom *Amanita muscaria* is commonly known as "fly agaric."

Mostly "poisonous" mushrooms effect gastrointestinal tract but usually does not cause any long-term damage. However, there are a number of recognized mushroom toxins with specific, and sometimes deadly, effects.

Q. Describe in brief mushroom poisoning symptoms.

The symptoms usually appear within 20 mint to 4 hour of ingesting the mushrooms and

include nausea, vomiting, cramps, and diarrhea, which normally pass after the irritant had been expelled. Some mushrooms contain psilocybin which may cause hallucinations, tachycardia, and hypertension. Some mushrooms cause muscarinic symptoms such as miosis, diarrhea, and bradycardia. Members of *Amanita* genera cause hypoglycemia and hepatic and renal failure. Severe cases may require hospitalization.

3.4   Algal Poisoning

Q. Define algal toxins.

Algal toxins are broadly defined to represent the chemicals derived from many species of *cyanobacteria* (blue-green bacteria), *dinoflagellates*, and *diatoms*. The toxins produced by these freshwater and marine organisms often accumulate in fish and shellfish inhabiting the surrounding waters, causing both human and animal poisonings, as well as overt fish kills. Unlike many of the microbial toxins, algal toxins are generally heat stable and, therefore, not altered by cooking methods, which increases the likelihood of human exposures and toxicity.

Q. What is cyanobacterial (blue-green bacteria) toxins?

Cyanobacterial (blue-green bacteria) toxins are produced (biotoxins and cytotoxins) by several species of cyanobacteria.

Q. What is Ambush predator toxins?

Ambush predator (*Pfiesteria piscicida* and toxic *Pfiesteria* complex) toxins are produced by several dinoflagellate species.

Q. Define harmful algal bloom (HAB).

Harmful algal blooms or HABs are algal blooms composed of phytoplankton known to naturally produce biotoxins; they can occur when certain types of microscopic algae grow quickly in water, forming visible patches that may harm the health of the environment, plants, or animals

4   Sample MCQ's

(Choose the correct statement; it may be one, two, or more or none)

Q.1. Which of the following is *not* true regarding *Amanita phalloides* mushrooms?

    A. Toxic components are phalloidin and amatoxins.
    B. Produces liver and gastrointestinal toxicity.
    C. Cardiovascular toxicity is responsible for mortality.
    D. Common name is "death cap."
    E. No specific antidotal treatment of poisoning is available.

Q.2. Which of the following feed stuff supports growth of aflatoxins?

    A. Ground nut cake
    B. Soybean cake
    C. Cotton seed meal
    D. All

Q.3. Which of the aflatoxin has the following character(s)?

    A. Carcinogenic
    B. Mutagenic
    C. Teratogenic
    D. Immunosuppressive

Q.4. Which of the following forms of aflatoxicosis is most common?

    A. Per acute
    B. Acute
    C. Subacute
    D. Chronic

Q.5. Rubratoxins are destroyed at the following temperature --------.

    A. Freezing
    B. Room temperature
    C. 50–60 °C
    D. 85–100 °C

Q.6. The site of action of ochratoxins in the nephron is ---------

    A. Proximal convoluted tubule
    B. Loop of Henle
    C. Distal convoluted tubule
    D. Collecting duct

Q.7. Which of the following serotype(s) of botulinum is most commonly implicated in animals and poultry?

    A. A type
    B. B type
    C. C type
    D. D type

Q.8. Which of the following toxicities are infectious?

    A. Botulism
    B. Tetanus

Q.9. The type of skeletal muscle contractions seen in tetanus is -------

    A. Clonic
    B. Tonic
    C. Both
    D. Twitching

Q.10. What is the correct temperature that frozen food should be kept at?

    A. 0 degrees
    B. 15 degrees or lower
    C. 8 degrees or lower
    D. 20 degrees or lower

Q.11. Overheated Teflon-coated frying pans release vapors that are especially toxic to ------.

    A. Cats
    B. Dogs
    C. Gerbils
    D. Parakeets
    E. Reptiles

Q.12. A major mode of transmission of food-borne illnesses is -----------

  A. Via mosquito transmission
  B. Via fecal–oral route
  C. Via person to person contact
  D. Via hypodermic syringes

Q.13. Which of the following is/are economic consequences of foodborne illness?

  A. Medical costs
  B. Investigative costs
  C. Loss of wages
  D. Litigation costs
  E. All of the above

Q.14. Of those listed below, which is not a food-borne pathogen?

  A. Lectins
  B. Nematodes
  C. Bacteria
  D. Protozoans

Q.15. Which of the following chemicals in food can cause significant neurologic complications?

  A. Mercury
  B. Lead
  C. Cadmium
  D. Antimony

Q.16. GRAS substances are those substances added to food that are ----------.

  A. Generally responsible for acute sickness
  B. Government reported assumed safe
  C. General response acidosis sickness
  D. Generally recognized as safe

Q.17. All of the following are gram-negative bacteria *except* ---------.

  A. *Staphylococcus aureus*
  B. *Escherichia coli*

  C. *Salmonella typhimurium*
  D. *Vibrio cholerae*

Q.18. Acidic conditions will leach all but which of the following from packaging material----------.

  A. Lead
  B. Cadmium
  C. Antimony
  D. Mercury

Q.19. *Taenia solium* (pork tapeworm) has more serious consequences than Taenia saginata (beef tapeworm) because-------------.

  A. It has a hooked rostellum that attaches it to the intestine wall.
  B. It can migrate to the brain, eyes, and muscles.
  C. It can be ingested from the waste of another human.
  D. All of the above.

Q.20. Of those listed below, which is *not* a protozoan?

  A. *Cryptosporidium*
  B. *Entamoeba histolytica*
  C. *Penicillium spp.*
  D. *Giardia lamblia*

Answers
1. C. 2. D. 3. D. 4. D. 5. D. 6. A.
7. C & D. 8. B. 9. B. 10. C. 11. D.
12. B. 13. E. 14. A. 15. A & B.
16. D. 17. A. 18. D. 19. D. 20. C.

Further Reading

Cope Rhian B. (2018) Botulinum neurotoxins. In: Veterinary toxicology: basic and clinical principles. Academic Press/Elsevier: San Diego, USA

Coppock RW, Christian RG, Jacobsen BJ (2018) Aflatoxins. In: Gupta RC (ed) Veterinary toxicology: basic and clinical principles, 3rd edn. Academic Press/Elsevier, San Diego, USA, pp 983–994

Gupta PK (2014) Essential concepts in toxicology. BSP Pvt. Ltd., Hyderabad, India

Gupta PK (2016) Fundamental in toxicology: essential concepts and applications in toxicology. Elsevier/BSP, San Diego, USA

Gupta PK (2018) Illustrative toxicology, 1st edn. Elsevier, San Diego, USA

Gupta PK (2019) Concepts and applications in veterinary toxicology: an interactive guide. Springer-Nature, Switzerland

Gupta PK (2020) Brain storming questions in toxicology. Francis and Taylor CRC Press, USA

Klaassen CD, Watkins JB III (eds) (2015) Casarett & Doull's essentials of toxicology, 3rd edn. McGraw-Hill, USA

Klaassen CD (ed) (2019) Casarett & Doull's toxicology: the basic science of poisons, 9th edn. McGraw-Hill, USA

Part VII

Radioactive Materials

Radiation and Radioactive Materials

19

Abstract

The direct or indirect exposure to ionizing radiations produces number of deleterious effects on health of human beings and on animals. Radiations are produced by disintegration of unstable naturally occurring or man-made elements and have been utilized for many beneficial effects. Ionizing radiations can cause different types of damages in mammalian systems including effects on both proliferative and non-proliferative tissues. This chapter briefly describes the overview, key points, and relevant text that are in the format of problem-solving study questions followed by multiple-choice questions (MCQs) along with their answers.

Keywords

Problem-solving study questions,
Electromagnetic radiation · Radiation ·
Ionizing radiations · X-rays · Alpha particles ·
Beta particles · Electrons · Gamma rays ·
Health hazards of radiation · Toxicology
question bank, MCQs

1 Introduction

The direct or indirect exposure to ionizing radiations produces number of deleterious effects on health of human beings and on animals. Radiations are produced by disintegration of unstable naturally occurring or man-made elements and have been utilized for many beneficial effects. Ionizing radiations can cause different types of damages in mammalian systems including effects on both proliferative and non-proliferative tissues. The chapter begins with key points relevant to the topic followed by the text that is in the form of short problem-solving questions and answers, as related to adverse effects that govern the toxic effects of different radiation and radioactive materials that enter the environment.

2 Overview

Ionizing radiation is of two types: particulate and electromagnetic waves. Particulate radiation may either be electrically charged (α, β, proton) or have no charge (neutron). Ionizing radiations such as γ-rays and X-rays are radiations that have sufficient energy to displace electrons from molecules. These freed electrons then have the capability of damaging other molecules and, in particular, DNA. Atoms of the DNA target may be directly ionized or indirectly affected by the creation of a free radical that can interact with the

DNA molecule. In particular, the hydroxyl radical is predominant in DNA damage. Thus, the potential health effects of low levels of radiation are important to understand in order to be able to quantify their effects. Cancer has been the major adverse health effect of ionizing radiation. Radionuclides (i.e., radioactive atoms), being unstable, release both electromagnetic and particulate radiation during their radioactive decay.

Key Points

- The four main types of radiation are due to alpha particles, electrons (negatively charged beta particles or positively charged positrons), gamma rays, and X-rays.
- Alpha particles are helium nuclei (consisting of two protons and two neutrons), with a charge of +2, that are ejected from the nucleus of an atom.
- Beta particle decay occurs when a neutron in the nucleus of an element is effectively transformed into a proton and an electron, which is ejected.
- Gamma-ray emission occurs in combination with alpha, beta, or positron emission or electron capture.
- Whenever the ejected particle does not utilize all the available energy or decay, the excess energy is released by the nucleus as photon or gamma-ray emission coincident with the ejection of the particle.
- The Compton effect occurs when a photon scatters at a small angle from its original path with reduced energy because part of the photon energy is transferred to an electron.
- Ionizing radiation loses energy when passing through matter by producing ion pairs (an electron and a positively charged atom residue).
- Radiation may deposit energy directly in DNA (direct effect) or may ionize other molecules closely associated with DNA, hydrogen, or oxygen, to form free radicals that can damage DNA (indirect effect).

3 Problem-Solving Study Questions

3.1 Radiation Biology

Q. What do you mean by alpha particles?
Alpha particle is an electrically charged (+) particle emitted from the nucleus of some radioactive chemicals, e.g., plutonium. It contains two protons and two neutrons and is the largest of the atomic particles emitted by radioactive chemicals. It can cause ionization.

Q. What do you mean beta particles?
Beta particle is an electrically charged (−) particle emitted from some radioactive chemicals. It has the mass of an electron. Krypton 85, emitted from nuclear power plants, is a strong beta emitter. Beta particles can cause ionization.

Q. What do you mean by the term curie?
The curie is a unit of ionizing radiation (radioactivity), symbolized as Ci and equal to 37 billion (3.7×10^{10}) disintegrations or nuclear transformations per second. This is approximately the amount of radioactivity emitted by 1 gram (1 g) of radium-226. The unit is named after Pierre Curie, a French physicist. Ci is the symbol used.

Q. What is microcurie?
Microcurie: one-millionth of a curie. (3.7×10^4 disintegrations per second. Symbol: μCi, mCi, μc.

Q. What is picocurie?
Picocurie is one-trillionth of a curie). Thus, a picocurie (abbreviated as pCi) represents 2.2 disintegrations per minute. One can also say it is one-millionth of a microcurie (3.7×10^2 disintegrations per second). Symbol: pCi.
For those interested in the numbers, a picocurie is 0.000,000,000,001 (one-trillionth) of a curie, an international measurement unit of radioactivity. One pCi/l means that in 1 liter of air, there will be 2.2 radioactive disintegrations each minute.

Q. Define dose energy.
Dose energy is imparted to matter by nuclear transformations (radioactivity).
Rad = 100 ergs per gram.

1 GRAY = 100 rad = 10,000 ergs per gram.

Rem = rads × Q

where Q is a quality factor which attempts to convert rads from different types of radioactivity into a common scale of biological damage.

100 rad = 1 SIEVERT

Q. What do you mean by gamma rays?

Gamma ray is a short-wavelength electromagnetic radiation released by some nuclear transformations. It is similar to X-ray and through will penetrate the human body. Iodine 131 emits gamma rays. Both gamma and X-rays cause ionization.

Q. What do you mean by biological half-life?

Half-life, biological time required for the body to eliminate one-half of an administered quantity of a radioactive chemical.

Q. What do you mean by half-life (physical)?

Half-life, physical time required for half of a quantity of radioactive material to undergo a nuclear transformation. The chemical resulting from the transformation may be either radioactive or non-radioactive.

Q. How do you classify radiation by its frequency?

It usually refers to electromagnetic radiation, classified by its frequency:

A. Radio
B. Infrared
C. Visible
D. Ultraviolet
E. X-ray
F. Gamma ray
G. And cosmic rays

Q. What is background radiation?

Background radiation includes emissions from radioactive chemicals which occur naturally and those which result from the nuclear fission process.

Q. Define Atomic Bomb Casualty Commission (ABCC).

ABCC is now called Radiation Effects Research Foundation (RERF).

Q. Who discovered X-ray?

In 1895, Wilhelm Conrad Roentgen (Fig. 19.1) discovered X-rays, and in 1901 he was awarded the first Nobel Prize for physics.

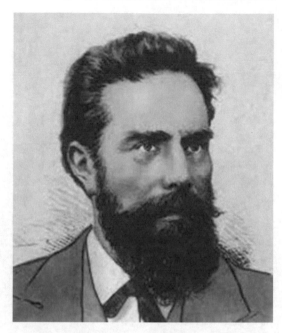

Fig. 19.1 Wilhelm Conrad Roentgen, discoverer of X-rays. (https://encrypted-tbn0.gstatic.com/images?q=tbn:ANd9GcSqQNJ50IrkTkWWN5aJiqCJLkpjtPolgx93uXCXxLJo-3to4cx0&s)

These discoveries led to significant advances in medicine.

Q. Who is Marie Curie and what are her contributions?

In 1903, Marie Curie (Fig. 19.2) and Pierre Curie, along with Henri Becquerel, were awarded the Nobel Prize in physics for their contributions to understanding radioactivity, including the properties of uranium. To this day, the "curie" and the ""Becquerel" are used as units of measure in radiation studies. Subsequently, this knowledge was used to develop the atomic bombs that were dropped on Japan in an effort to end World War II.

Q. Define different types of electromagnetic radiations.

These electromagnetic radiations are broadly of two types. The range of electromagnetic spectrum is summarized as under:

A. Non-ionizing radiation: Non-ionizing radiation includes ultraviolet, visible, infrared, radio and TV, and power transmission. We depend on the sun's radiation for photosynthesis and heat.

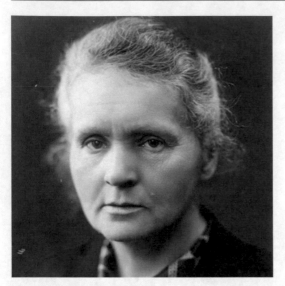

Fig. 19.2 Marie Curie. (https://www.biography.com/. image/t_share/MTE5NTU2MzE2MTkzNzE5ODE5/ marie-curie-9263538-1-402.jpg)

B. Ionizing radiation: Ionizing radiation includes high-energy radiation such as cosmic rays, X-rays, or gamma rays generated by nuclear decay. Ionizing radiation also includes several types of subatomic particles such as beta radiation (high-energy electrons) and alpha radiation (helium ions). Medical X-rays are an example of a common beneficial exposure to ionizing radiation. Nuclear radiation is used to generate electricity and cure disease but is also an important element in military weapons. Uses of nuclear radiation pose serious problems of human exposure and environmental contamination.

Q. What are the uses of non-ionizing radiation?
Uses of non-ionizing radiation include power transmission; TV, radio, and satellite transmissions; radar; light bulbs; heating; cooking; microwave ovens; lasers; photosynthesis (sunlight); mobile phones; Wi-Fi networks; etc.

Q. What are the sources of non-ionizing radiation?
Sourced of non-ionizing radiation include ultraviolet light, visible light, infrared radia-

tion, microwaves, radio and TV, mobile phones, and power transmission.

Q. What is ionizing radiation?
Ionizing radiation is higher-energy radiation, with enough energy to remove an electron from an atom and damage biological material.

Q. What is the source of ionizing radiation?
Source: radon; X-rays; radioactive material producing alpha, beta, and gamma radiation; and cosmic rays from the sun and space.

Q. What are the uses of ionizing radiation?
Uses: nuclear power, medical X-rays, medical diagnostics, scientific research, cancer treatment, and cathode ray tube displays.

Q. What is the recommended daily dose of ionizing radiation?
Recommended daily intake is none (not essential).

Q. How ionizing radiation is absorbed in the body?
Absorption: interaction with atoms of tissue.

Q. What are the main types of ionizing radiation?
The four main types of ionizing radiation are:
A. Alpha particles
B. Beta particles (electrons)
C. Gamma rays,
D. X-rays

Q. What is the mechanism of action of ionizing radiation?
Ionizing radiation has sufficient energy to produce ion pairs as it passes through matter, freeing electrons and leaving the rest of the atoms positively charged. In other words, there is enough energy to remove an electron from an atom. The energy released is also enough to break bonds in DNA, which can lead to significant cellular damage and cancer.

Q. Which radiation is more harmful?
Ionizing radiation is more harmful than non-ionizing radiation because it has enough energy to remove an electron from an atom and thus directly damage biological material. The energy is enough to damage DNA, which can result in cell death or cancer.

Q. What is the nature of alpha particles?

Alpha particles are heavyweight and relatively low-energy emissions from the nucleus of radioactive material. The transfer of energy occurs over a very short distance of about 10 cm in air. A piece of paper or layer of skin will stop an alpha particle. The primary hazard occurs in the case of internal exposure to an alpha-emitting material: cells close to the particle-emitting material will be damaged. Typical sites of accumulation include the bone, kidney, liver, lung, and spleen. Radium is an alpha particle emitter that accumulates in the bone following ingestion, causing a bone sarcoma. Airplane travel increases our exposure to cosmic and solar radiation that is normally blocked by the atmosphere. Radiation intensity is greater across the poles and at higher altitudes; thus individual exposure varies depending on the route of travel. Storms on the sun can produce solar flares that release larger amounts of radiation than normal. For the occasional traveler, this radiation exposure is well below recommended limits established by regulatory authorities.

Q. What is the difference between radiation exposure and irradiation?

In both radiation exposure and irradiation, exposure to radiation occurs. However, in irradiation, contamination with radioactive material does not occur, which prevents post-exposure radiation (e.g., γ-irradiation of syringes; irradiation used for treating cancers, etc.).

Q. Why, in the presence of heavy metals, more free radicals are generated?

Heavy metals (like Fe, Pb, Cd, etc.) have more number of electrons in outer shell. Hence, when a free radical attacks a heavy metal, there will be shower of electrons, which in turn produces more free radicals.

Q. Why are there so many different terms when it comes to radiation? Rem, rad, curie, gray … what are they all for?

One reason for so many different terms is that the United States uses traditional radiation units while the rest of the world uses an International System of Units (very similar to the United States using inches and other countries using centimeters). In the international system, Sievert, gray, Becquerel, and coulombs/kilogram are used, whereas traditional units are rem (= 0.01 Sievert), rad (= 0.01 gray), curie (= 3.7×10^{10} Becquerel), and roentgen (= 2.5×10^{-4} coulombs/kilogram).

Another reason for all the different types of units is our need, as scientists, to be precise and accurate when we are describing radiation interactions and energy left behind.

Q. Can radioactive material affect the body? Explain how.

Yes. Radiation is a "potentially harmful" agent. When radiation interacts with the tissue of our bodies, whether it is from radioactive atoms inside the body or from an external source such as an X-ray machine, it can cause damage to cells. This damage stems from the process of ionization. The radiation from radioactive atoms is called "ionizing radiation" because it causes ionization. Ionization is simply the "knocking off" of electrons from the atoms they are normally said to "orbit." These electrons act as the "glue" that holds atoms together in chemical bonds. So, if some of the electrons get knocked loose by ionizing radiation, some of the chemical bonds get broken. This can result in damage to the cells. Since there is radioactive material in our bodies, this process goes on all the time.

Q. What is uranium?

Uranium is the heaviest metal that occurs in nature. It is an unstable material which gradually breaks apart or "decays" at the atomic level. Any such material is said to be "radioactive."

As uranium slowly decays, it gives off invisible bursts of penetrating energy called "atomic radiation." It also produces more than a dozen other radioactive substances as by-products.

Q. What is radioactivity?

Everything is made of tiny little particles called atoms. They are too small to be seen even under a powerful microscope. When a substance is radioactive, it means that its atoms are exploding (sub-microscopically) and throwing off pieces of themselves with great force. This process is called "radioactive decay." During radioactive decay, two types of tiny electrically charged particles are given off, travelling very fast. They are called alpha and beta particles. Some radioactive materials are alpha emitters, and others are beta emitters. In addition, highly energetic rays called gamma rays are often emitted. Gamma rays are not material particles at all, but a form of pure energy very similar to X-rays, travelling at the speed of light.

Q. How far can atomic radiation penetrate?

Gamma rays penetrate through soft tissue just as light shines through a window. Beta particles have less penetrating power, travelling less than 2 centimeters in soft tissue. Alpha particles have the least penetrating power, travelling just a few micrometers in soft tissue, equivalent to a few cell diameters.

Q. Is radioactivity dangerous?

Alpha particles, beta particles, and gamma rays can do great harm to a living cell by breaking its chemical bonds at random and disrupting the cell's genetic instructions.

Massive exposure to atomic radiation can cause death within a few days or weeks. Smaller doses can cause burns, loss of hair, nausea, loss of fertility, and pronounced changes in the blood. Still smaller doses, too small to cause any immediate visible damage, can result in cancer or leukemia in the person exposed, congenital abnormalities in his or her children (including physical deformities, diseases, and mental retardation), and possible genetic defects in future generations.

Outside the body, alpha emitters are the least harmful, and gamma emitters are more dangerous than beta emitters. Inside the body, however, alpha emitters are the most dangerous. They are about 20 times more damaging than beta emitters or gamma emitters. Thus, although alpha radiation cannot penetrate through a sheet of paper or a dead layer of skin, alpha emitters are extremely hazardous when taken into the body by inhalation or ingestion or through a cut or open sore.

Q. Which ionizing radiation has the least penetrating capacity?

Alpha (α) particles because these particles are large in size (2 protons+2 neutrons = α-particle). Hence, they have least penetration ability. However, due to their high mass, they have high linear energy transfer (LET) ability.

Q. Which ionizing radiation has the highest penetrating capacity?

Gamma (γ) rays because γ-rays are nonparticulate electromagnetic radiation. Hence, they have the highest penetration ability. However, as the mass is least, they have very low linear energy transfer.

Q. How do radioactive elements produce other radioactive elements?

When atoms undergo radioactive decay, they change into new substances, because they have lost something of themselves. These byproducts of radioactive decay are called "decay products" or "progeny." In many cases, the decay products are also radioactive. If so, they too will disintegrate, producing even more decay products and giving off even more atomic radiation.

Q. What is the difference between ionizing radiation and radioactivity?

A radioactive atom is unstable because its nucleus contains extra energy. When this atom decays to a more stable atom, it releases this extra energy as ionizing radiation.

Q. Is there more than one kind of radiation?

Yes, in addition to X-rays, three are common: they are the alpha, beta, and gamma radiations. Alpha rays (the nuclei of helium atom) may be stopped by paper, beta rays (high speed electrons) are stopped less easily, and gamma rays (like X-rays) may need lead or concrete to stop them.

Q. Will these ionizing radiations make any one radioactive?

No, just as light can't make anyone glow in the dark, a chest X-ray will not make anyone radioactive.

Q. If ionizing radiation does not make a thing radioactive, how do items become radioactive in a nuclear reactor?

In a nuclear reactor, there are billions of free nuclear projectiles called neutrons. When absorbed in a material, they make it radioactive, i.e., it emits its own radiation. This is how radioisotopes are made. There are very few free neutrons in the environment.

Q. Where does natural radiation dose come from?

The major part derives from the decay of natural radioactivity in the earth, most of it from uranium and thorium: they give rise to a radioactive gas called radon in the air we breathe. Radon is present in all buildings. Smaller, and roughly equal, parts of everyday radiation come from cosmic rays and from the natural radioactivity of our food and drink. Some other radiations are man-made.

Q. What are the man-made sources of radiation?

Medical uses of ionizing radiation are the major sources. These include the use of X-rays for radiography and computer tomography and radiopharmaceuticals in nuclear medicine.

3.2   Radionuclides

Q. What is natural background radiation?

Natural background radiations are emissions from radioactive chemicals which are not man-made. These chemicals include uranium, radon, potassium, and other trace elements. They are made more hazardous through human activities such as mining and milling, since this makes them more available for uptake in food, air, and water.

Q. Where does natural radiation dose come from?

The major part derives from the decay of natural radioactivity in the earth, most of it from uranium and thorium: they give rise to a radioactive gas called radon in the air we breathe. Radon is present in all buildings. Smaller, and roughly equal, parts of everyday radiation come from cosmic rays and from the natural radioactivity of our food and drink. Some other radiations are man-made.

Q. Name the two elements which are responsible for natural background radiation in earth?

Radon (from uranium) and thoron (from thorium) are responsible for 54% of natural background radiation in earth.

Q. What is radon?

These unstable by-products, having little or no commercial value, are called "uranium decay products." They are discarded as waste when uranium is mined. One of them is a toxic radioactive gas called radon. The others are radioactive solids.

Q. What is radium?

There are 25 isotopes of radium of which four occur naturally (radium 223, 224, 226, and 228); the others are man-made or decay products of man-made radionuclides. Except for radium 228, which is a β emitter, the other three are all α emitters. The different isotopes have been used both occupationally as luminescent paint on watches and instruments (radium 226 and 228) and in medical applications (radium 223 and 224).

Q. What is plutonium?

Plutonium is a radioactive chemical element with the symbol Pu and atomic number 94. It is an actinide metal of silvery-gray appearance that tarnishes when exposed to air and forms a dull coating when oxidized.

Q. For what purpose plutonium is used?

Plutonium is used for nuclear weapon production and in the production of mixed oxide fuels.

Q. What happens if you are exposed to plutonium?

Radioactive plutonium, as it decays, can cause harm. It can linger preferentially in the liver and blood cells, leaching alpha radiation (two protons and neutrons bound together). When inhaled, plutonium can also cause lung cancer.

Q. How exposure to plutonium occurs?
   Most of the exposure to plutonium is to workers involved in the processing of plutonium in
   nuclear weapons (Pu 239) and in nuclear
   power generation (Pu 238). The major exposure to plutonium is by inhalation and is
   retained primarily in the lung and, liver.

Q. What is radioiodine?
   Radioiodine is released from nuclear facilities of fission product radionuclides deposited in the environment as well as internal
   doses from the ingestion of foods containing
   fission products have been the result of the
   Chernobyl and Fukushima accidents.

Q. What is the major observable health effect of
   radioiodine in children?
   The major observable health effect has been
   childhood thyroid cancer resulting from the β
   emitter iodine 131.

4.3. Health Effects of Radiation

Q. Who are the sensitive individuals to ionizing
   radiation?
   Children, developing organisms.

Q. Who are sensitive to non-ionizing radiation?
   Sensitive individuals: variable, e.g., fair-
   skinned children (sunburn).

Q. What are the biological effects of non-
   ionizing radiations?
   Non-ionizing radiation is harmless but, however, at higher levels and longer durations of
   exposure, can be harmful. The classic example is sunlight or solar radiation. Ultraviolet
   radiation from the sun, part of the electromagnetic spectrum with wavelengths less
   than 400 nm, can damage the skin. Sunburn
   (erythema) is the result of excessive exposure
   of our skin to UV radiation when we lack the
   protection of UV-absorbing melanin. Acute
   cellular damage causes an inflammatory-type
   response and increased vascular circulation
   (vasodilation) close to the skin. The increased
   circulation causes the redness and hot feeling
   to the skin. Lightly pressing on the skin
   pushes the blood away and the spot appears
   white. Darker-skinned people have an ongo-
   ing production of melanin, which protects
   them to some extent from UV radiation. In
   lighter-skinned people, UV radiation stimulates the production of melanin, producing a
   tan and protection against UV radiation.
   Extreme exposure can result in blistering and
   severe skin damage. UV radiation can also
   damage cellular DNA, and repeated damage
   can overwhelm the DNA repair mechanism,
   resulting in skin cancer. Skin cancer accounts
   for approximately one-third of all cancers
   diagnosed each year. Thinning of the atmospheric ozone layer, which filters UV radiation, is suspected as being one cause of the
   increased incidence of skin cancer.

Q. What do you know about Hiroshima and
   Nagasaki incidences?
   The US military dropped the first atomic
   bomb on Hiroshima, Japan, on August 6,
   1945, and a second on Nagasaki, Japan, 3
   days later. The bombs used two different
   types of radioactive material, 235 U in the
   first bomb {(uranium 235 (^{235}U)} and 239 Pu
   (plutonium 239) in the second. It is estimated
   that 64,000 people died from the initial blasts
   and radiation exposure. Approximately
   100,000 survivors were enrolled in follow-up
   studies.

Q. What are the lessons learned from Hiroshima
   and Nagasaki incidences?
   These incidences indicated that the greater
   the dose, the greater the likelihood of developing cancer. The second lesson was that
   there could be a very long delay in the onset
   of the cancer, from 10 to 40 years. This con-
   firmed an increased incidence of cancer. It is
   estimated that 1 in 100 cancers are the result
   of this background exposure.

Q. What are the health benefits from radiation?
   All life is dependent on small doses of electromagnetic radiation. Radiations are produced by disintegration of unstable naturally
   occurring or man-made elements. Radiations
   have been utilized for many beneficial effects.
   For example, use of radiation-emitting
   devices helps us to use many devices such as
   cell phones and radios, from medical X-rays
   to the electricity that powers our homes.
   X-rays were also used to treat disease such as
   ringworm in children. Subsequently during
   the 1950s, X-rays were used to treat a
   degenerative bone disease called ankylosing
   spondylitis.

Q. What are the main adverse health effects/hazards of electromagnetic radiation?

Direct or indirect exposure to ionizing radiations produces number of deleterious effects on health of human beings as well as on animals. Ionizing radiations can cause different types of damages in mammalian systems including effects on both proliferative and non-proliferative tissues.

Q. Will radiation build up in the body until it gets to a point where it kills you?

No, ionizing radiation does not build up in the body. All radiation will eventually disperse. However, radiation effect may appear, following exposure to a high intensity of radiation, just as you may get sunburn from overexposure to sunlight.

Q. When radiation does not build up in the body, how does it harm a person?

All radiation carries energy that may damage living cells. This damage may cause cells either to die or to change their structure and function.

Q. If anyone gets a dose of radiation, will he die?

Very unlikely, since it would take a very large dose to kill sufficient numbers of your cells to cause death.

Q. Why cornea of the eye gets affected by dielectric heating from mobile phones during usage?

Cornea of the eye lacks temperature-regulating mechanism and hence could be affected by dielectric heating from mobile phones during usage

---

4 Sample MCQ's

(Choose the correct statement; it may be one, two, or more or none)

Q.1. Which of the following ionizing radiations has the shortest range (i.e., travels the shortest distance in tissue) for the same initial energy?

A. Alpha particle
B. Beta particle
C. Gamma ray
D. X-ray
E. Cosmic ray

Q.2. An individual exposed to 10 rads (0.1 Gy) of whole body x-irradiation would be expected to -----.

A. Have a severe bone marrow depression
B. Die
C. Be permanently sterilized
D. Exhibit no symptoms
E. Vomit

Q.3. The cellular component, which is affected during radiation damage, is -----.

A. Lipid
B. DNA
C. RNA
D. Sugar

Q.4. Molecules with unpaired electrons in the outer shells are known as ----.

A. Free radicals
B. Sulfur
C. Nitrogen
D. Carbon

Q.5. Cells are more susceptible for radiation in the following stage(s) of cell cycle -------.

A. M phase (mitosis)
B. Early G phase
C. Late G phase
D. S phase

Q.6. The following organ is resistant to radiation -------.

A. Endocrine glands
B. Kidney
C. Bone marrow
D. Germinal cells

Q.7. More than 99% of the energy from the sun is within the spectral range of ___ to ____ nanometers.

A. 150–4000
B. 700–4000
C. 140–400
D. 400–700

Q.8. Which of the following inversions is short-lived?

A. Radiation
B. Subsidence

Q.9. The most common type of free radicals produced in the body are ------.

A. NO
B. O2
C. SO2
D. Reactive oxygen species (ROS)

Q.10. The part of the head, which can be affected by the heating effects of mobile phone, is ----.

A. Ears
B. Nose
C. Tongue
D. Cornea

Q.11. Which of the following is *not* a main type of radiation?

A. Alpha particles
B. Microwaves
C. Beta particles
D. Gamma rays
E. X-rays

Q.12. Which of the following statements regarding alpha particles is *false*?

A. Alpha particles are ejected from the nucleus of an atom.
B. The atomic number decreases by two after emission of an alpha particle.

C. The atomic weight decreases by two after emission of an alpha particle.
D. Energies of most alpha particles range between 4 and 8 MeV.
E. Alpha particles are helium nuclei.

Q.13. Which of the following types of radiation is likely the *most* energetic?

A. Alpha particles
B. Beta particles
C. Positron emission
D. Electron capture
E. Photon emission

Q.14. Pair production and the Compton effect characterize which type of radiation's interaction with matter?

A. Alpha particles
B. Beta particles
C. Positron emission
D. Electron capture
E. Photon emission

Q.15. Which of the following statements regarding radiation DNA damage is *false*?

A. Ionizing radiation slows down by forming ion pairs.
B. A main form of radiation DNA damage occurs by the production of free radicals.
C. High-LET radiation causes more ionizations than does low-LET radiation.
D. Most DNA damage caused by radiation happens directly.
E. Direct and indirect ionization causes similar damage to DNA.

Q.16. Low-LET radiation -----.

A. Causes large-scale ionizations throughout the cell
B. Results from alpha particle emission
C. Causes damage that is readily repaired by cellular enzymes

D. Is also known as densely ionizing radiation

E. Usually causes irreparable cell damage

Q.17. What is the most common type of DNA damage caused by low-LET radiation exposure?

A. Base damage
B. DNA protein crosslinks
C. Single-strand breaks
D. Double-strand breaks
E. Thymine dimer formation

Q.18. Which of the following statements regarding radon exposure is *false*?

A. Miners are exposed to increased environmental radon levels.
B. Radon exposure has been linked to the development of lung cancer.
C. Smokers are at a higher risk from radon exposure.
D. Radon levels are relatively higher in urban areas than in rural areas.
E. The use of open frames indoors increases radon exposure.

Q.19. The largest dose of radiation is received from which of the following sources?

A. Inhalation
B. In body
C. Cosmic

D. Cosmogenic
E. Terrestrial

Q.20. The largest contributor to the effective dose of radiation in the US population is which of the following?

A. Nuclear medicine
B. Medical X-rays
C. Terrestrial
D. Internal
E. Radon

Answers
1. A.   2. D.   3. B.   4. A   5. A and B.
6. A.   7. A.   8. A.   9. D.   10. D.
11. B.   12. C.   13. A.   14. E.   15. D.
16. C.   17. C.   18. D.   19. A.   20. E.

Further Reading

Gupta PK (2016) Fundamental in toxicology: essential concepts and applications in toxicology. Elsevier/BSP, USA

Gupta PK (2018) Illustrative toxicology, 1st edn. Elsevier, San Diego, USA

Gupta PK (2020) Brain storming questions in toxicology. Francis and Taylor CRC Press, USA

Henriksen T, Maillie DH (2003) Radiation and health. Taylor and Francis, USA

Hoel David G (2015) Toxic effects of radiation and radioactive materials. In: Klaassen CD, Watkins JB III (eds) Casarett & Doull's essentials of toxicology, 3rd edn. McGraw-Hill, USA, pp 373–380

Lisa M (2018) Ionizing radiation in veterinary medicine. In: Gupta RC (ed) Veterinary toxicology: basic and clinical principles, 2nd edn. Academic Press/Elsevier, San Diego, USA, pp 327–338

Part VIII

Applications of Toxicology

Food Toxicology

20

Abstract

An unknown number of naturally occurring contaminants find their way into food. The most ominous are products of mold growth called mycotoxins, which include the carcinogenic aflatoxins. On the other hand, more than 2500 chemical substances are added to foods to modify or impart flavor, color, stability, and texture, to fortify or enrich nutritive value, or to reduce cost. In addition, an estimated 12,000 substances are used in such a way that they may unintentionally enter the food supply. This chapter briefly describes the overview, key points relevant to food and nutritional toxic responses, toxic effects of specific food toxicants, mechanisms of action, food allergies versus food toxicants, mechanisms for interactions between multiple food compounds and/or drugs, and problem-solving study questions followed by multiple-choice questions (MCQs) along with their answers.

Keywords

Food toxicology · Nutritional toxic responses · Allergies · Interactions · Xenobiotics · Toxic responses · MCQs · Question answer bank · Toxicity

1 Introduction

An unknown number of naturally occurring contaminants find their way into food. The most ominous are products of mold growth called mycotoxins, which include the carcinogenic aflatoxins. On the other hand, more than 2500 chemical substances are added to foods to modify or impart flavor, color, stability, and texture, to fortify or enrich nutritive value, or to reduce cost. In addition, an estimated 12,000 substances are used in such a way that they may unintentionally enter the food supply. The chapter briefly describe an overview, key points relevant to food and nutritional toxic responses, toxic effects of specific food toxicants, mechanisms of action, food allergies versus food toxicants, mechanisms for interactions between multiple food compounds and/or drugs, and problem-solving study questions followed by multiple-choice questions (MCQ's) along with their answers.

2 Overview

Food toxicology is the study of the nature, properties, effects, and detection of toxic substances in food and their disease manifestation in humans. An unknown number of naturally occurring

P K Gupta, *Problem Solving Questions in Toxicology*, https://doi.org/10.1007/978-3-030-50409-0_20

contaminants find their way into food. The most ominous are products of mold growth called mycotoxins, which include the carcinogenic aflatoxins. On the other hand, more than 2500 chemical substances are added to foods to modify or impart flavor, color, stability, and texture, to fortify or enrich nutritive value, or to reduce cost. In addition, an estimated 12,000 substances are used in such a way that they may unintentionally enter the food supply. This field is therefore devoted to studying the complexity of the chemicals in food, particularly those that have the potential of producing adverse health effects. The field includes studies of human health impacts of food containing environmental contaminants or natural toxicants. The field includes investigations of food additives, migration of chemicals from packaging materials into foods, and persistence of feed and food contaminants in food products. Also, the field covers examining the impact of contaminants on nutrient utilization, adverse effects of nutrient excesses, metabolism of food toxicants, and the relationship of the body's biological defense mechanisms to such toxicants. Finally, because the study of food and nutritional toxicology has obvious societal implication, one must examine the risk determination process, how food is regulated to ensure safety, and the current status of regulatory processes.

- Food additives are substances added to a food to preserve it, give it flavor, or improve its taste and/or appearance. Additives such as fiber, vitamins, and minerals can improve the nutrient density of a product and help protect against certain health problems.
- Some foods include plant hormones and naturally occurring pesticides; antinutrients such as lectins, saponins, trypsin, and/or chymotrypsin inhibitors in soybeans; phytates that may bind minerals; antihistamines; and frankly toxic constituents such as tomatine or cycasin.
- Several thousand volatile chemicals have been identified in food.
- The Pure Food and Drugs Act of 1906 made illegal any food found to be adulterated (containing an "added impure or…deleterious ingredient") which may render the food injurious to health.

3   Problem-Solving Study Questions

3.1   Complexities of Food

Q. What is a food toxicology?
Food toxicology is the study of the nature, properties, effects, and detection of toxic substances in food and their disease manifestation in humans.

Q. What is food toxicant?
Food toxicants can be poisonous and they may be man-made or naturally occurring in food. In contrast, a toxin is a poison produced naturally by an organism (e.g., plant, animal, insect).

Q. What is the nature and complexity of food?
Food is an exceedingly complex mixture whether it is consumed in the "natural" (unprocessed) form or as a highly processed "Meal, Ready-to-Eat" (MRE). Nonnutrient substances (substances other than carbohydrates, proteins, fats, or vitamins/minerals)

Key Points

- Food is an exceedingly complex mixture whether it is consumed in the "natural" (unprocessed) form or as a highly processed "Meal, Ready-to-Eat" (MRE).
- Food toxicants can be poisonous, and they may be man-made or naturally occurring in food. In contrast, a toxin is a poison produced naturally by an organism (e.g., plant, animal, insect).
- Nonnutrient substances present in food may be food additives and flavoring ingredients.

may be contributed by food processing, but nature provides the vast majority of nonnutrient constituents.

Q. What types of nonnutrient substances are present in food?

Nonnutrient substances present in food may be food additives; flavoring ingredients; plant hormones and naturally occurring pesticides; antinutrients such as lectins, saponins, trypsin, and/or chymotrypsin inhibitors in soybeans; phytates that may bind minerals; antihistamines; and frankly toxic constituents such as tomatine or cycasin. Several thousand volatile chemicals have been identified in food.

3.2 Food Additives

Q. What is a food additive?

The term "food additive" is a regulatory term that encompasses any functional substance that is normally neither consumed as a food itself but is intentionally added to food (usually in small quantities) to augment its processing or to improve aroma, color, consistency, taste, texture, or shelf life. Additives are not considered "nutritional" even if they possess nutritive value.

Q. What is the role of food additives in the diet?

Food additives are substances added to a food to preserve it, give it flavor, or improve its taste and/or appearance. Additives such as fiber, vitamins, and minerals can improve the nutrient density of a product and help protect against certain health problems.

Q. What is a direct food additive?

Substances added to a food for a specific purpose are direct additives and are identified on the ingredient label of the food to which the ingredient is added. For example, the low-calorie sweetener, aspartame, added to puddings, soft drinks, yogurt, and many other foods is a direct food additive.

Q. What is an indirect food additive?

An indirect additive becomes part of the food in very small amounts during processing, packaging, or storage. Such additives serve valuable technical functions: (1) to maintain the nutritional quality of the food; (2) to enhance keeping quality or stability, with resulting reductions in food wastage; (3) to make food attractive to consumers; and (4) to provide essential aids during processing. At present, there are thousands of additives in the US food supply, most of which are indirect additives. By law, manufacturers must document that the amount of an additive in a food is below the threshold of observable adverse effects.

3.3 Safety Standards for Foods

Q. What was Pure Food and Drugs Act of 1906?

The Pure Food and Drugs Act of 1906 made illegal any food found to be adulterated (containing an "added impure or…deleterious ingredient") which may render the food injurious to health. This act provided regulatory authority to the federal government of the US Department of Agriculture (USDA) and others to launch an initiative known as the "Poison Squad," to address food adulteration.

Q. Why was Federal Food, Drug, and Cosmetic Act (abbreviated as FFDCA, FDCA, or FD&C) passed by Congress in 1938?

The introduction of this act was influenced by the death of more than 100 patients due to a sulfanilamide medication where diethylene glycol was used to dissolve the drug and make a liquid form. It replaced the earlier Pure Food and Drugs Act of 1906.

Q. What are the requirements of Food, Drug, and Cosmetic Act (FDCA) of 1938?

The Food, Drug, and Cosmetic Act (FDCA) of 1938 required manufacturers to demonstrate the safety of a product marketed over state lines and be able to meet three standards: (1) standards (definitions) of identity, (2) standards of quality, and (3) standards regulating the fill of a container.

Q. What is Food Additives Amendment (1958) to the FDCA?

The Food Additives Amendment (1958) to the FDCA subjected food additives to regulatory scrutiny and gave the Food and Drug Administration (FDA) the authority to require information from manufacturers demonstrating that the additive is reasonably free of harm prior to its introduction into the food supply. Since that time, the FDA has delineated the types of toxicity and chemistry studies needed to assess the safety of food additives and generally recognized as safe (GRAS) substances.

Q. What are the safety standards for foods, food ingredients, and contaminants?

The US Federal Food, Drug, and Cosmetic Act (abbreviated as FFDCA, FDCA, or FD&C) is a set of laws passed by Congress in 1938 giving authority to the US Food and Drug Administration (FDA) to oversee the safety of food, drugs, medical devices, and cosmetics. The act requires food should be safe for consumption. The act permits the addition of substances to food to accomplish a specific technical effect if the substance is determined to be generally recognized as safe (GRAS).

Q. What is FCS (indirect food additive) notification?

In 1997, the Food and Drug Administration Modernization Act of 1997 established a food contact notification (FCN) process to allow faster review of nonexempt FCS. FCN, because of similar safety standard to a petition, must contain sufficient scientific information to demonstrate that the FCS is safe for its intended use. Regardless of whether an FCN or petition is submitted, the information is required in addition to relevant information required in a direct food additive.

Q. What is Delaney Clause?

The Delaney Clause, which was introduced into US food safety law in 1958, stipulated that "no additive shall be deemed to be safe if it is found to induce cancer when ingested by man or animal."

Q. What is color additive?

A color additive, as defined by FDA regulations, is any dye, pigment, or other substance that can impart color to a food, drink, pharmaceutical, or cosmetic or to the human body.

Q. Which synthetic colors are permitted to be used in food products?

The Pure Food and Drugs Act of 1906 reduced the permitted list of synthetic colors from 700 to 7: These 7 colors include Ponceau 3R (FD&C red no. 1), amaranth (FD&C red no. 2), erythrosine (FD&C red no. 3), indigotine (FD&C blue no. 2), light green SF (FD&C green no. 2), naphthol yellow 1 (FD&C yellow no. 1), and orange 1 (FD&C orange no. 1).

3.4 Safety Assessment of Food Additives

Q. What is estimated daily intake (EDI)?

The estimated daily intake exposure is most often referred to as an estimated daily intake (EDI). It is based on two factors: the daily intake (DI) of the food in which the substance will be used and the concentration (C) of the substance in that food. In estimates of consumption and/or exposure, one must also consider other sources of consumption for the proposed intended use of the additive if it already is used in other foods for another purpose, occurs naturally in foods, or is used in non-food sources.

Q. What is the differences between estimated daily intake (EDI) and acceptable daily intake (ADI) for food additives?

Estimated daily intake (EDI) is less than acceptable daily intake (ADI) because the ADI is generally based on results from animal toxicology studies.

Q. How is estimated daily intake (EDI) determined?

The EDI is determined by multiplying the dietary concentration ($[M]$) by the total weight of food consumed by an individual per day (3000 g).

$$EDI(mg / person\, per\, day)$$
$$= 3000\, g / person\, per\, day \times [M] \times CF$$

The *consumption factor* (CF depends upon package category as per FDA) is used to describe that portion of the diet likely to contact specific packaging materials. The FDA defines the CF as the ratio of the weight of food containing the specific packaging material to the weight of all goods packaged with that material. Examples of CF values used by the agency for different packaging categories are variable and are specified by the company.

The EDI is used together with information on exposure from all other uses of the indirect additive to establish the CEDI (cumulative estimated daily intake) which is used to establish the level of toxicological testing recommended.

3.5 Toxicological Studies

The extent and types of toxicological studies required to support the safety of either direct or indirect food additives are dependent on both the EDI and the expected nature and potential for toxicity of the additive.

Q. What are short-term genetic in vitro tests used for food additives toxicity?

A modified battery including *Salmonella typhimurium* reverses mutation assay, in vitro mutagenicity in mammalian cells, and in vivo cytogenetics.

Q. What type of acute oral studies is carried out for food additives toxicity?

The focus of acute oral studies is not on the number of animals that die at a given dose or LD50 determination but rather the toxic effects on organ systems and the potential recovery of the animals from the administration of high doses of the test compound. Results of acute oral toxicity study will provide information on the type of toxicity (e.g., neurotoxicity and cardiotoxicity), identity target organ(s), and dose levels for longer-term toxicity studies.

Q. What type of short-term feeding studies is carried out for food additives toxicity?

Short-term studies generally last 28 days in duration, with multiple-dose groups of animals exposed repeatedly to the chemical in their diets. This type of study is required for Concern Level I (CL I) compounds and is useful for identifying the toxic characteristics and target organ(s) of an additive and as a range-finding study for subchronic and chronic studies to help set doses for these studies. Animals should be observed daily for overt signs of toxicity and necropsies are performed typically on all animals, including those that die during the course of the study.

Explanation: A compound is assigned a level of expected toxicity based on its molecular structure into one of the three categories: A (low toxicity), B (moderate toxicity), or C (high toxicity). Category assignments are based on a decision tree (Redbook II) related to the additive's (1) chemical structure, (2) number and amount of unidentified components in the additive, and (3) predicted metabolites. If fewer than 90% of the components of the additive have been structurally characterized, the additive is automatically placed into the highest toxicity category C. Examples of compounds in category A include simple aliphatic, acyclic, and monocyclic hydrocarbons; fats; fatty acids; simple aliphatic and noncyclic (saturated) mono-functional alcohols; ketones; aldehydes; acids; esters; ethers; and normal human metabolites of carbohydrates and lipids. Category B compounds include non-conjugated olefins (excluding unsaturated fatty acids and fats); inorganic salts of iron, copper, zinc, and tin; amino acids; polypeptides; and proteins. Category C compounds are structurally varied and include organic halides; amides and imines; conjugated alkenes; polycyclic aromatic hydrocarbons; and compounds with nitro, N-nitroso, azide, and purine groups. An additive with a higher CL (CL III) is more likely to be dangerous than one with a lower CL (CL I). Once the CL is established, a specific test battery is prescribed.

Q. What type of subchronic feeding studies is carried out for food additives toxicity?

Subchronic feeding studies are required for CL II compounds and examine the toxicity (target organs, potency, etc.) of a compound in greater detail after repeated dosing of at least three dose groups of 20 rodents or 4 dogs/gender/group, generally for a period of 90 days. Blood and urine sampling is performed periodically throughout the studies for determination of insidious toxicity and to aid in target organ identification. At termination of the study, detailed necropsies and histopathology are performed on representative test (high dose) and control animals. The tests are designed to mimic human exposure and may involve administration in the diet, through drinking water, in tablets, or by gavage. Redbook II recommends that screening for neurotoxicity and immunotoxicity be performed and that rodents be single caged. For a CL III compound, the subchronic study helps dose selection for chronic study. For substances in CLs I and II, data from subchronic tests are often used for the ultimate determination of safety and NOAEL.

Q. What type of reproductive and developmental studies is carried out for food additives toxicity?

Reproductive and developmental toxicity (DART) testing is required for compounds of CLs II and III and are conducted by exposing male and female rodents (20/gender/group) orally to the additive to determine its effects on a variety of end points including male and female gonadal function, estrous cycles, mating behavior, conception, parturition, lactation, weaning, and growth and development of the offspring. The studies are continued to see the effect on multigeneration and to a teratogenicity phase.

Q. What type of teratogenicity studies is carried out for food additives toxicity?

In a teratogenicity phase of any multigeneration study, the test substance must be administered during in utero development. Multiple-dose groups are included as well as a control. The dams are killed 1 day before parturition. The uterus is removed and examined for embryonic or fetal deaths, live fetuses, and any evidence of malformations of skeletal or soft tissues. Ovaries are examined for the number of corpora lutea. Live fetuses are weighed, sexed, and examined for external abnormalities. A selected number of fetuses are examined for soft tissue malformations, usually by random selection of one-third of the group. The remaining two-thirds of the fetuses are examined for skeletal defects.

Q. What type of chronic toxicity and carcinogenicity studies is carried out for food additives toxicity?

Chronic toxicity and carcinogenicity studies are required for a CL III food additive and are often combined into a single study. The studies are of lifetime duration in two rodent species lasting typically 104 weeks. The studies are usually designed to include several satellite groups for interim kills at 3, 6, and 12 months to determine the compound-related effects that are not due to aging. In this study, 50 animals/sex/group, single housing of rodents, periodic observation of the animals for signs of onset and progression of toxic effects, hematological and organ function tests, and clinical examinations for neurological and ocular changes are observed. Histopathology is performed on all animals in the study.

3.6 Food Allergies/Reactions

Q. What is food hypersensitivity?

Food hypersensitivity (allergy) refers to a reaction involving an immune-mediated response. An allergic reaction may be manifested by one or more of the symptoms such as cutaneous reactions and anaphylaxis which are the most common symptoms associated with food allergy. Any protein in food may act as an allergen, for example, casein, β-lactoglobulin, α-lactalbumin, ovomucoid, ovalbumin, β-conglycinin (7S fraction), glycinin (11S fraction), and Kunitz trypsin inhibitor.

Q. What is food idiosyncrasy?
Food idiosyncrasies are generally defined as quantitatively abnormal responses to a food substance or additive. They may resemble hypersensitivity, but do not involve immune mechanisms. Examples of such foods include fava beans, beets, and choline- and carnitine-containing foods.

Q. What are anaphylactoid reactions?
Anaphylactoid reactions are historically thought of as reactions mimicking anaphylaxis (and other "allergic-type" responses) through direct application of histamine. Ingestion of some types of fish that have been acted upon by certain microorganisms to produce histamine may result in an anaphylactoid reaction also called "scombrotoxicosis," for example, tuna, albacore, mackerel, bonito, mahi-mahi, and blue fish.

Q. What are metabolic food reactions?
Metabolic food reactions differ from other categories of adverse reactions in that the foods are more or less commonly eaten and demonstrate toxic effects only when eaten in excess or improperly processed. The susceptible population exists as a result of its own behavior, that is, the "voluntary" consumption of food as a result of a limited food supply or an abnormal craving for a specific food. For example, lima beans, cassava roots, millet, rapeseed, polar bear and chicken liver, cycads (cycad flour) are known to cause metabolic reactions to some individuals.

3.7 Toxic Substances in Food

Q. Which chemicals or substances are likely to present in food as contaminants?
Metals (lead, cadmium, and mercury are familiar as contaminants), hydrocarbons (such as pesticides, solvents, and heat-trans-fer agents), N-nitroso substances, mycotoxins, microbiologic agents, etc., as these substances are unavoidable in food.

Q. Name a few marine organisms responsible for toxicity/poisoning in human beings.
Marine organisms that contain toxins include fish, shellfish, turtles, etc. Toxins are known to cause gastrointestinal disorders, neurologic symptoms, or death.

Q. What is bovine spongiform encephalopathy (BSE)?
Bovine spongiform encephalopathy (BSE, or mad cow disease) is transmitted by an infectious protein called a prion. Present in diseased cows, prions are transmitted to humans in meat that is improperly handled. BSE manifests clinically as neurologic deterioration leading to death.

4 Sample MCQ's

Q.1. Which of the following wheat proteins is famous for being allergenic?
  A. Casein
  B. Ovalbumin
  C. Livetin
  D. Gluten
  E. Glycinin

Q.2. Which of the following foods contains a chemical that causes hypertension by acting as a noradrenergic stimulant?

  A. Cheese
  B. Peanuts
  C. Shrimp
  D. Chocolate
  E. Beets

Q.3. What is the mechanism of saxitoxin, found in shellfish?

  A. Interference with ion channels
  B. Direct neurotoxicity
  C. Interference with DNA replication
  D. Binding to hemoglobin
  E. Interference with a stimulatory G protein

Q.4. Which of the following foods can cause a reaction that mimics iodine deficiency?

A. Chocolate
B. Shellfish
C. Peanuts
D. Fava beans
E. Cabbage

Q.5. Improperly canned foods can be contaminated with which of the following bacteria, causing respiratory paralysis?

A. *C. perfringens*
B. *R. rickettsii*
C. *S. aureus*
D. *C. botulinum*
E. *E. coli*

Q.6. Which of the following statements regarding food complexity is *false*?

A. Many flavor additives are nonnutrient substances.
B. Foods are subjected to environmental forces that alter their chemical composition.
C. There are more nonnutrient chemicals in food than nutrient chemicals.
D. A majority of nonnutrient chemicals are added to food by humans.
E. Food is more variable and complex than most other substances to which humans are exposed.

Q.7. Which of the following foods contains the most nonnutrient chemicals?

A. Bee
B. Banana
C. Tomato
D. Orange juice
E. Cheddar cheese

Q.8. Which of the following is considered an indirect food additive?

A. Nitrites
B. Plastic
C. Food coloring

D. EDTA
E. Citric acid

Q.9. Estimated daily intake (EDI) is based on which of the following?

A. Metabolic rate
B. Daily intake
C. Substance concentration in a food item
D. Body mass index
E. Concentration of substance in a food item and daily intake

Q.10. Which of the following is *not* characteristic of IgE-mediated food allergies?

A. Urticaria
B. Wheezing
C. Hypertension
D. Nausea
E. Shock

Answers
1. D.   2. D.   3. A.   4. E.   5. D.   6. D.
7. A.   8. B.   9. E.   10. C.

Further Reading

Choudhuri S, Chanderbhan RF, Mattia A (2019) Food toxicology: fundamental and regulatory aspects. In: Klaassen CD (ed) Casarett and Doull's toxicology: the basic science of poisons, 9th edn. McGraw-Hill, New York, pp 1315–1360

Gupta PK (ed) (2010) Modern toxicology: adverse effects of xenobitics, vol 2, 2nd reprint. PharmaMed Press, Hyderabad, India

Gupta PK (2014) Essential concepts in toxicology. BSP Pvt. Ltd, Hyderabad, India

Gupta PK (2016) Fundamental in toxicology: essential concepts and applications in toxicology, 1st edn. Elsevier/BSP, Boston

Gupta PK (2018) Illustrative toxicology, 1st edn. Elsevier, San Diego

Gupta PK (2019) Concepts and applications in veterinary toxicology: an interactive guide, 1st edn. Springer Nature, Switzerland

Gupta PK (2020) Brain storming questions in toxicology. Francis and Taylor CRC Press, Boca Raton

Kotsonis FN, Burdock GA (2015) Food toxicology. In: Klaassen CD, Watkins JB III (eds) Casarett & Doull's essentials of toxicology, 3rd edn. McGraw-Hill, New York, pp 453–462

Ecotoxicology

21

Abstract

Ecotoxicology is a multidisciplinary field, which integrates toxicology and ecology. The ecosystems that are already impacted by pollution ecotoxicological studies can inform as to the best course of action to restore ecosystem services and functions efficiently and effectively. This chapter briefly describes the overview, key points, and relevant text that are in the format of problem-solving study questions followed by multiple-choice questions (MCQs) along with their answers.

Keywords

Terrestrial toxicology · Aquatic toxicology · Chemodynamics · Ecotoxicology · Toxicology · Question bank · MCQs, toxicity

1   Introduction

Ecotoxicology is a multidisciplinary field, which integrates toxicology and ecology. The ecosystems that are already impacted by pollution ecotoxicological studies can inform as to the best course of action to restore ecosystem services and functions efficiently and effectively. The chapter deals with biological, toxicological, risk assessment, an overview, key points, and relevant text that is in the format of problem-solving study questions followed by multiple-choice questions (MCQ's) along with their answers.

2   Overview

The publication in 1962 of Rachel Carson's *Silent Spring* catalyzed the separation of environmental toxicology – and, subsequently, ecotoxicology – from classical toxicology. The revolutionary element in Carson's work was her extrapolation from single-organism effects to effects at the whole ecosystem and the "balance of nature." Ecotoxicology is the study of the effects of toxic chemicals on biological organisms, especially at the population, community, ecosystem, and biosphere levels. Ecotoxicology is a multidisciplinary field, which integrates toxicology and ecology. The ultimate goal of this approach is to be able to reveal and to predict the effects of pollution within the context of all other environmental factors. Based on this knowledge, the most efficient and effective action to prevent or remediate any detrimental effect can be identified. In those ecosystems that are already impacted by pollution, ecotoxicological studies can inform as to the best course of action to restore ecosystem services and functions efficiently and effectively.

P K Gupta, *Problem Solving Questions in Toxicology*, https://doi.org/10.1007/978-3-030-50409-0_21

Ecotoxicology differs from environmental toxicology in that it integrates the effects of stressors across all levels of biological organization from the molecular to whole communities and ecosystems, whereas environmental toxicology focuses upon effects at the level of the individual and below.

Key Points

- Chemodynamics is, in essence, the study of chemical release, distribution, degradation, and fate in the environment.
- A chemical can enter any of the four matrices: the atmosphere by evaporation, the lithosphere by adsorption, the hydrosphere by dissolution, or the biosphere by absorption, inhalation, or ingestion (depending on the species). Once in a matrix, the toxicant can enter another matrix by these methods.
- The biologic availability (or bioavailability) of a chemical is the portion of the total quantity of chemical present that is potentially available or uptake by organisms.
- Pollution may result in a cascade of events, beginning with effects on homeostasis in individuals and extending through populations, communities, ecosystems, and landscapes.
- Terrestrial toxicology is the science of the exposure to and effects of toxic compounds in terrestrial ecosystems.
- Aquatic toxicology is the study of effects of anthropogenic chemicals on organisms in the aquatic environment.
- Ecological risk assessment (EcoRA) involves the assessment of the risks posed by the presence of substances released to the environment by man, in theory, on all living organisms in the variety of ecosystems which make up the environment.

---

3   Problem-Solving Study Questions

3.1   Biological Effects

Q. What are ecotoxicologic effects of chemicals at biologic levels?

One may consider ecotoxicologic effects, in ascending order, at the subcellular (molecular and biochemical), cellular, organismal, population, community, and ecosystem levels of organization. Ecotoxicology deals with, theoretically at least, all species, and in line with other aspects of natural resource management, the primary concern is one of sustainability.

Q. What are molecular and biochemical deleterious effects of toxicants?

Molecular and biochemical effects are associated with the regulation of gene transcription and translation, biotransformation of xenobiotics, and the deleterious biochemical effects of xenobiotics on cellular constituents including proteins, lipids, and DNA.

Q. What are xenoestrogens?

A number of chemicals can serve as ligands for estrogen receptor (ER); in most cases these "xenoestrogens" activate gene transcription acting as receptor agonists.

Q. Give examples of chemicals that act as xenoestrogens.

Examples of xenoestrogens include diethylstilbestrol (DES), DDT, methoxychlor, endosulfan, surfactants (nonylphenol), some PCBs, bisphenol A, and ethinyl E2. Environmental exposures to these chemicals are sufficient to perturb reproduction or development. Moreover, endocrine disruption by environmental xenoestrogens appears to be stronger for wildlife than for humans.

Q. How some environmental pollutants lead to changes in gene transcription?

The aryl hydrocarbon receptor (AhR or AHR or ahr or ahR) is a protein that in humans is encoded by the AhR gene. The aryl hydrocarbon receptor (AhR) is a member of the family of basic helix-loop-helix transcription factors.

AhR binds several exogenous ligands such as natural plant flavonoids, polyphenolics, and indoles, as well as synthetic polycyclic aromatic hydrocarbons and dioxin-like compounds. AhR is a cytosolic transcription factor that is normally inactive, bound to several co-chaperones. Upon ligand binding to chemicals such as 2,3,7,8-tetrachlorodibenzo-*p*-dioxin (TCDD), the chaperones dissociate resulting in AhR translocating into the nucleus and dimerizing with ARNT (*AhR nuclear translocator*), leading to changes in gene transcription.

Q. How do nutrients enter our ecosystem?

- Nutrients, primarily nitrogen (N) and phosphorus (P), enter environments from chemical fertilizers, manure, urine, sewage effluents, burning fossil fuels, fires, decay of plants and animals, and industrial processes such as pulp/paper milling and nitric acid production. Free nutrients are washed into water bodies and enter groundwater and aquifers, some of which feed streams, ponds, lakes, estuaries, bays, and oceans. Agricultural production of plants and animals is the primary source of excess nutrients in the environment.

Q. How do petroleum products enter our ecosystem?

- Petroleum products include a wide array of aliphatic as well as aromatic hydrocarbons. Aromatic hydrocarbons are also present at high concentrations in coal tar and are formed during incomplete combustion of coal, oil, gas, garbage, and other materials. Among the best known polycyclic aromatic hydrocarbons (PAHs) is benzo(*a*) pyrene, which is a component of cigarette smoke.

Q. What is the impact of nutrient pollution on ecosystem?

- Nutrient pollution is the process where too many nutrients, mainly nitrogen and phosphorus, are added to bodies of water and can act like fertilizer, causing excessive growth of algae. Nutrients can run off of land in urban areas where lawn fertilizers

are used. Too much nitrogen and phosphorus in the water can have diverse and far-reaching impacts on public health, the environment, and the ecosystem.

Q. What is the impact of wastes on ecosystem?

- Introduction of vast amounts of cast-off food, chemicals, and other wastes alters the relationship between predators and prey in various environments and ecosystem leading to death of wildlife, birds, fishes, and other species of plants. For example, the Pasión River in Guatemala was declared an ecological disaster after thousands of dead fish surfaced in June as a result of agrochemicals pollution from a nearby palm oil production site.

Explanation: Persistent organic pollutants and semivolatile chemicals, such as organochlorine insecticides, the fungicide hexachlorobenzene, and polychlorinated dibenzodioxins and polychlorinated dibenzofurans, which are toxic by-products of organochlorine, synthesis, and manufacturing processes, such as the kraft paper, and bleaching process, can have serious effects on the immune, nervous, and reproductive systems, especially those of developing organisms. Such compounds can also reduce control of impulsive behaviors, impair learning, cause liver damage, and disrupt reproductive and thyroid hormone functions. Likewise, leakage of acids from coal mines and drainage of hazardous substances, pollutants, or contaminants into the environment lead harm to fish and other aquatic life: If mine waste is acid-generating, the impacts to fish, animals, and plants can be severe (Fig. 21.1).

Q. What are the effects of lead on ecosystems?

Lead is persistent in the environment and can be added to soils and sediments through deposition from sources of lead air pollution. Other sources of lead to ecosystems include direct discharge of waste streams to water bodies and mining. Elevated lead in the environment can result in decreased growth and reproductive rates in plants and animals and neurological effects in vertebrates.

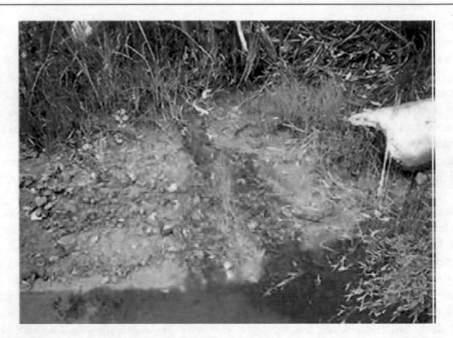

Fig. 21.1   Acid rock drainage (Andalusia coal mines, Spain). Reproduced from US Fish and Wildlife Service

Q. Describe briefly the greenhouse effect.
- Heat energy (infrared) reflected from the Earth may be absorbed by infrared-absorbing gases such as carbon dioxide, chlorofluorocarbons (CFCs), methane, and water vapors. Such gases then trap the warmth and reflect it back to the Earth's atmosphere in a process known as the greenhouse effect. If the greenhouse gases increase in concentration, it is logical that more heat energy will be absorbed and the average annual global temperature may rise causing a global warming trend.

3.2   Toxicity Evaluation

Q. What is the practical approach to characterize chemical effects on biologic systems?

Toxicity tests address the potential direct effects of toxic substances on individual ecosystem components in a controlled and reproducible manner. Ecotoxicology tests feature a wide variety of aquatic (including algae, invertebrates, tadpoles, bivalves, shrimp, and fish), avian (quail and duck), and terrestrial (soil microorganisms, crops, honey bees, earthworms, and wild mammals) species. In acute toxicity testing, single species are exposed to various concentrations of the test agent. The most common end point in acute tests is death. Abnormal behavior and other gross observations are commonly noted, and nonlethal end points occasionally apply. Data from different test concentrations are used to derive concentration–response curves, e.g., LC50, EC50, and IC50 for the test population. Other quantitative values are LOEC and NOEC. In addition, several other short-term, long-term, and reproductive, including more elaborate microcosm and mesocosm, field studies and other studies as per regulation have to be conducted.

3.3   Ecological Risk Assessment

Q. What is ecological risk assessment?

Ecological risk assessment (EcoRA) involves the assessment of the risks posed by the presence of substances released to the environment by man, in theory, on all living organisms in the variety of ecosystems which make up the environment.

Q. What are the components of environmental risk assessment (ERA)?

ERA has two components: human health risk assessment and ecological risk assessment. The stages of doing an ERA include hazard identification and problem formulation, analysis, and risk characterization. The main outputs are the risk management and communication plans.

Q. What is an ecological risk assessment?

An ecological risk assessment is the process for evaluating how likely it is that the environment may be impacted as a result of exposure to one or more environmental stressors such as chemicals, land change, disease, invasive species, and climate change.

Q. What are different phases of ecological risk assessment?

An ecological risk assessment starts with a good plan. Before anything thought there is a need to make judgments early when planning major risk assessments regarding the purpose, scope, and technical approaches that will be used. EPA begins the process of an ecological risk assessment with planning and research. An ecological risk assessment includes three phases (Fig. 21.2).

- *Phase 1—Problem Formulation*
  Information is gathered to help determine what, in terms of plants and animals, is at risk and what needs to be protected.
- *Phase 2—Analysis*
  This is the determination of what plants and animals are exposed and to what degree they are exposed and if that level of exposure is likely or not to cause harmful ecological effects.
- *Phase 3—Risk Characterization*
  Risk characterization includes two major components: risk estimation and risk description. "Risk estimation" combines exposure profiles and exposure effects. "Risk description" provides information important for interpreting the risk results

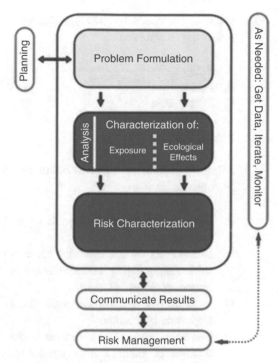

Fig. 21.2 An ecological risk assessment. https://www.epa.gov/sites/production/files/styles/large/public/2014-10/logo_hilight1sm_0.gif

and identifies a level for harmful effects on the plants and animals of concern.

4   Sample MCQ's

(choose the correct statement; it may be one, two, or more or none)

Q.1. Chemodynamics does *not* study ------

A. The fate of chemicals in the environment
B. The rate at which chemicals are metabolized
C. The distribution of chemicals in the environment
D. The effects of toxic substances on the environment
E. The release of chemicals into the environment

Q.2. What is the mode by which a chemical enters the lithosphere?

  A. Evaporation
  B. Adsorption
  C. Dissolution
  D. Absorption
  E. Diffusion

Q.3. All of the following regarding biomarkers are true *except* -------

  A. Dermal absorption is considered an external dose.
  B. Biomarkers of susceptibility are useful in extrapolating wildlife disease to human diseases.
  C. Induction of certain enzymes is an important biomarker.
  D. The biologically effective dose is the amount of internal dose needed to elicit a certain response.
  E. The effects of chemical exposure can be different across species.

Q.4. The bioavailability of contaminants in the hydrosphere is directly related to -------

  A. Chemical concentration
  B. Amount of chemical
  C. Water solubility of chemical
  D. Toxicity of chemical
  E. Molecular size of chemical

Q.5. Which of the following processes is *least* likely to be affected by endocrine-disrupting agents?

  A. Enzyme activity
  B. Transcription
  C. Hormone secretion
  D. Signal transduction
  E. DNA replication

Q.6. Estrogen exposure has been shown to cause all of the following in wildlife species *except* ---------

  A. Sexual imprinting
  B. Altered sex hormone levels
  C. Immune suppression
  D. Gonadal malformations
  E. Sex reversal

Q.7. An important type(s) of compound that is far more toxic in water than in air is/are -------

  A. Organic compounds
  B. Photochemicals
  C. Vapors
  D. Lipid-soluble xenobiotics
  E. Metals

Q.8. Which of the following is *false* regarding terrestrial ecotoxicology?

  A. Terrestrial organisms are generally exposed to contaminants via ingestion.
  B. Predation is an important confounder of measurements in terrestrial toxicology field studies.
  C. Reproductive tests are not important in measuring end points in toxicity tests.
  D. Enclosure studies are better able to control for environmental factors in field studies.
  E. Toxicity tests usually test the effects of an oral chemical dose.

Q.9. Biologic availability is -------

  A. The total amount of chemical within an organism
  B. The concentration of chemical in an environmental reservoir
  C. The threshold concentration of a chemical needed for toxic effect
  D. The concentration of chemical within an organism
  E. The proportion of chemical potentially available for uptake

Q.10. Which of the following are used to record end point toxicity of aquatic toxicity tests?

    A. LD50 and ED50
    B. LC50 and EC50
    C. Reproductive tests
    D. LD50 and LC50
    E. LD50 and EC50

Answers

1. D. 2. B. 3. A. 4. C. 5. E. 6. C.
7. E. 8. C. 9. E. 10. B.

Further Reading

Gupta PK (2018) Illustrative toxicology, 1st edn. Elsevier, San Diego

Gupta PK (2020) Brain storming questions in toxicology. Francis and Taylor CRC Press, USA

Di Giulio R, Newman MC (2015) Ecotoxicology. In: Klaassen CD, Watkins JB III (eds) Casarett & Doull's essentials of toxicology, 3rd edn. McGraw-Hill, USA, pp 441–452

Di Giulio RT, Newman MC (2019) Ecotoxicology. In: Klaassen CD (ed) Casarett & Doull's the basic science of poisons, 9th edn. McGraw-Hill, USA, pp 1433–1464

Environmental Toxicology

22

Abstract

Environment is exposed to various toxicants such as ozone (O2), sulfur dioxide (SO2), particulate matter, oxides of nitrogen (NO2), carbon monoxide (CO), and lead (Pb). These six major air pollutants account for 98% of pollution. This chapter covers various hazards and risks associated with environmental pollution, bioaccumulation, and biomagnification along with unintentional or coincidental exposures to chemicals including identification of hazards and risks, which is a complex one with multiple uncertainties. This chapter briefly describes the overview, key points, and problem-solving study questions followed by multiple-choice questions (MCQs) along with their answers.

Keywords

Exposure · Outdoor ambient air · Particulate matter · Photochemical air pollution · Smog · Toxic gasses · Ozone · Hazardous air pollutants · Pollution · Environmental toxicology · Toxicology question bank · MCQs

1 Introduction

Environmental toxicology is the multidisciplinary study of the effects of man-made and natural chemicals on health and the environment. This includes the study of the effects of chemicals on organisms in their natural environments. This chapter covers various hazards and risks associated with environmental pollution, bioaccumulation, and biomagnification along with unintentional or coincidental exposures to chemicals including identification of hazards and risks, which is a complex one with multiple uncertainties. An overview, key points, and problem-solving study questions followed by multiple-choice questions (MCQ's) along with their answers are briefly discussed.

Key Points

- Environmental toxicology is a multidisciplinary field of science concerned with the study of the harmful effects of various chemical, biological, and physical agents on living organisms, whereas ecotoxicology is a sub-discipline of environmental toxicology concerned with studying the harmful effects of toxicants at the population and ecosystem levels.

- Environment is exposed to various toxicants such as ozone (O2), sulfur dioxide (SO2), particulate matter, oxides of nitrogen (NO2), carbon monoxide (CO), and lead (Pb).
- These six major air pollutants account for 98% of pollution.
- Other pollutants include volatile organic compounds, and a myriad of other compounds are considered under the category of hazardous air pollutants in the environment.
- Reducing-type air pollution, characterized by SO2 and smoke, is capable of producing deleterious human health effects.
- Once in a matrix, the toxicant can enter another matrix by these methods.
- The biologic availability (or bioavailability) of a chemical is the portion of the total quantity of chemical present that is potentially available or uptake by organisms.
- Pollution may result in a cascade of events, beginning with effects on homeostasis in individuals and extending through populations, communities, ecosystems, and landscapes.

2   Overview

Environmental pollution is one of the most serious problems facing humanity and other life forms on our planet today. Other issues facing many parts of the developing world tie closely to domestic culture and economy, as well as to the level of technological sophistication. Prime among these problems is exposure to carbon and soot from combustion of biomass in cooking and heating in domestic stoves. Pollutants can be naturally occurring substances or energies, but they are considered contaminants when in excess of natural levels. Any use of natural resources at a rate higher than nature's capacity to restore itself can result in pollution of air, water, and land.

Currently, advanced molecular biology tools along with conventional approaches allow us to rapidly degrade or accumulate hazardous materials from environments. This can help modify microorganisms to gain the ability to sense and degrade hazardous chemicals from contaminated sites, in turn allowing us to grow vegetation and improve crop productivity.

3   Problem-Solving Study Questions

3.1   Common Terms

Q. What is photodegradation?
- Photodegradation is the alteration of materials by light. The process implies reduction in toxicity, or some chemicals may become more toxic to organisms through photoactivation. For example, dechlorination of hexachlordibenzo-p-dioxin may produce lower chlorinated but more toxic dioxin congeners. Typically, the term refers to the combined action of sunlight and air and results in oxidation and hydrolysis.

Q. What is photosynthesis?
- Photosynthesis is the process used by plants, algae, and certain bacteria to harness energy from sunlight into chemical energy.

Q. What is sunburn?
- Sunburn is a form of radiation burn that affects living tissue, such as skin, that results from an overexposure to ultraviolet (UV) radiation, commonly from the sun.

Q. Describe in brief signs and symptoms of sunburn.
- There is initial redness (erythema), followed by varying degrees of pain, proportional in severity to both the duration and intensity of exposure. Other symptoms can include edema, itching, peeling skin, rash, nausea, fever, chills, and syncope. Also, a small amount of heat is given off from the burn, caused by the concentration of blood in the healing process, giving a warm feeling to the affected area. Sunburns may be

classified as superficial or partial thickness burns.

Q. What is biotransformation?

- Biotransformation is the chemical modification (or modifications) made by an organism on a chemical compound. If this modification ends in mineral compounds like CO_2, NH_4^+, or H2O, the biotransformation is called mineralization. Biotransformation occurs not only in animals and plants but also in soil microbes such as fungi and bacteria under aerobic or anaerobic conditions. In vertebrates, microbes within digestive tracts can also greatly influence the biotransformation of environmental contaminants. Metabolism and conjugation of xenobiotics often reduce toxicity and enhance the ability of the animal to eliminate the agent from the body.

Q. What is bioactivation?

- Bioactivation is the process where enzymes or other biologically active molecules acquire the ability to perform their biological function, such as inactive proenzymes being converted into active enzymes that are able to catalyze their substrates into products to produce (by definition) metabolites that are more toxic than their parent compounds. For example, *the organochlorine pesticide DDT is not itself highly toxic to birds, but its metabolite p, p'-DDE can cause thinning of eggshells due to disruption of calcium metabolism.*

Q. What is biomagnification?

- Biomagnification, also known as bioamplification or biological magnification, is the increasing concentration of a substance, such as a toxic chemical, in the tissues of organisms at successively higher levels in a food chain.

3.2 Exposure of Toxicants

Q. What are the different steps involved from exposure to toxic substance at concentrations that are harmful to the environment?

(a) Release of pollutant into the environment.

(b) Transport and fate into biota (with/without chemical transformation).

(c) Exposure to biological and ecological system.

(d) Understanding responses and/or effects (molecular to ecological systems).

(e) Design remediation, minimization, conservation, and risk assessment plans to eliminate, prevent, or predict environmental and human health pollution situations.

The study involves air pollution that includes the earth, air, water, living environments, and social components. In addition, it also involves ecotoxicology (ecology + toxicology) that want to protect many individuals, populations, communities, and ecosystems from exposure to toxic substance at concentration that are harmful.

Q. What is the source of environmental contamination?

- Environmental contamination can emanate from:

(a) Industries

(b) Mines

(c) Refineries

(d) Coal-burning power plants

(e) Sewage treatment plants

Nonpoint sources include pesticides washed from large areas of land after precipitation, effluents from the tailpipes of myriad motor vehicles, or semivolatile pollutants that circle the globe after evaporation from the soils of agricultural and urban environments.

3.3 Hazards of Outdoor Exposure

Q. What is Donora Smog?

The Donora smog was a historic air inversion in Pennsylvania that killed 20 people and sickened 7000 or more in 1948.

Q. What is Great Smog of London?

In 1952, Great Smog occurred over 5 days in London. During this period more than normal coal emissions mixed with fog in a temperature inversion resulted in thousands of deaths and tens of thousands of hospitalizations.

Q. What is nitrogen cycle?

- The nitrogen cycle is a model that explains how nitrogen is recycled. It includes a series of processes by which nitrogen and its compounds are interconverted in the environment and in living organisms, including nitrogen fixation and decomposition.

Q. What is the importance of nitrogen?

Nitrogen is essential for the formation of amino acids in proteins. There's lot of nitrogen in air— about 78% of the air is nitrogen. Because nitrogen is so unreactive, it cannot be used directly by plants to make protein. Nitrogen is converted to nitrates in the soil. Plants absorb nitrates from the soil and use these to build up proteins.

Q. How nitrogen gas is converted to nitrate compounds?

Nitrogen gas is converted to nitrate compounds by nitrogen-fixing bacteria in soil or root nodules. Lightning also converts nitrogen gas to nitrate compounds. The Haber process converts nitrogen gas into ammonia used in fertilizers. Ammonia is converted to nitrates by nitrifying bacteria in the soil.

Q. What is carbon dioxide cycle?

(a) The first step is carbon enters the atmosphere as carbon dioxide from respiration and combustion.

(b) The second step is carbon dioxide is absorbed by producers to make carbohydrates in photosynthesis.

(c) The third step is animals feed on the plant passing the carbon compounds along the food chain. Most of the carbon they consume is exhaled as carbon dioxide formed during respiration. The animals and plants eventually die.

(d) The dead organisms are eaten by decomposers, and the carbon in their bodies is returned to the atmosphere as carbon dioxide. In some conditions decomposition is blocked. The plant and animal material may then be available as fossil fuel in the future for combustion.

Q. What are major pollutants in the air?

(a) Ozone (O_3)

(b) Sulfur dioxide (SO_2)

(c) Oxides of nitrogen (NO_2)

(d) Carbon monoxide (CO)

(e) Particulate matter (PM)

(f) Lead (Pb)

Six major air pollutants account for 98% of pollution.

Others include volatile organic compounds (VOCs), and a myriad of other compounds are considered under the category of hazardous air pollutants (HAPs).

Q. What is the effect of stratosphere ozone depletion?

- Ozone in the stratosphere protects us from the harmful effects of excess ultraviolet radiation from the sun which, among other things, causes skin cancer. CFCs— chlorofluorocarbons (formerly used extensively as refrigerants and solvents)—after entering the stratosphere catalytically reacts with the ozone, thereby reducing the ozone layer leading to harmful effects of excess ultraviolet radiation from the sun which, among other things, causes skin cancer.

Q. What is sulfate aerosols?

- The term sulfate aerosol is used for a suspension of fine solid particles of a sulfate or tiny droplets of a solution of a sulfate or of sulfuric acid (which is not technically a sulfate). They are produced by chemical reactions in the atmosphere from gaseous precursors (with the exception of sea salt sulfate and gypsum dust particles). The two main sulfuric acid precursors are sulfur dioxide (SO2) from anthropogenic sources and volcanoes and dimethyl sulfide (DMS) from biogenic sources, especially marine plankton. These aerosols can cause a cooling effect on earth.

Q. What are health effects of oxides of nitrogen (NO2)?

- NO2 irritates the lungs and promotes respiratory infections. Short-term NO2 exposures, ranging from 30 min to 24 hours, have adverse respiratory effects including airway inflammation. Nitrogen dioxide, like

O3, is a deep lung irritant that can produce pulmonary edema if it is inhaled at high concentrations. It is a much less potent irritant and oxidant than O3, but NO2 can pose clear toxicological problems. Exposure to nitrogen oxides to farmers leads to "silo-filler disease" (a toxic gas-induced pneumonitis and bronchiolitis caused by inhalation of nitrogen oxides in freshly filled grain silos, often coupled with asphyxia).

Q. What are the harmful effects of carbon monoxide (CO)?

- CO is ubiquitous and most commonly produced by incomplete hydrocarbon combustion. A component of CO poisoning is almost always present in cases of smoke inhalation injury. It is a chemical asphyxiant because its toxic action stems from its formation of carboxyhemoglobin, preventing oxygenation of the blood for systemic transport. The normal concentration of carboxyhemoglobin (COHb) in the blood of nonsmokers is about 0.5%. This is attributed to endogenous production of CO from heme catabolism. No overt human health effects have been demonstrated for COHb levels below 2%, while levels above 40% cause fatal asphyxiation.

Q. What do you mean by particulate matter (PM)?

- Atmospheric particulate matter—also known as particulate matter (PM) or particulates—are microscopic solid or liquid matter suspended in the Earth's atmosphere.

Q. What is aerosol?

- The term aerosol commonly refers to the particulate/air mixture, as opposed to the particulate matter alone.

Q. What is particulate matter?

- Particulate matter (PM), also known as particle pollution, is a complex mixture of extremely small particles and liquid droplets that get into the air. Once inhaled, these particles can affect the heart and lungs and cause serious health effects.

Q. What are sources of particulate matter?

- Sources of particulate matter can be man-made or natural. They have impacts on climate and precipitation that adversely affect human health.

Q. What are total suspended particles?

- Total suspended particles include all particles, of whatever size; PM_{10} are particles less than 10 μm (10 microns) in diameter, and $PM_{2.5}$ are particles less than 2.5 μm in diameter; black carbon emissions are based on a chemical speciation of $PM_{2.5}$ emissions.

Q. How soot differs from particulate matter?

- Soot is indicative of poorly (inefficiently) combusted fuel. Particulate matter in the atmosphere can be solid, liquid, or a combination of both with a melange of organic, inorganic, and biological compounds. The compositional matrix of PM can vary significantly depending on the emission source and secondary transformations, many of which involve gas to particle conversions.

Q. What does $PM_{2.5}$ means?

- Particles less than 2.5 micrometers in diameter ($PM_{2.5}$) are referred to as "fine" particles and are believed to pose the greatest health risks. Because of their small size (approximately 1/30th the average width of a human hair), fine particles can lodge deeply into the lungs.

Q. What is nanoparticle?

- In nanotechnology, a particle is defined as a small object that behaves as a whole unit with respect to its transport and properties. Particles are further classified according to diameter.

Nanoparticles are particles between 1 and 100 nanometers (nm) in size with a surrounding interfacial layer. The interfacial layer is an integral part of nanoscale matter, fundamentally affecting all of its properties. The interfacial layer typically consists of ions and inorganic and organic molecules. Organic molecules coating inorganic nanoparticles are known as stabilizers, capping and surface ligands, or passivating agents.

Q. What are hazardous air pollutants?

- Hazardous air pollutants are also known as toxic air pollutants or air toxics. Examples of toxic air pollutants include benzene, which is found in gasoline; perchloroethylene, which is emitted from some dry cleaning facilities; and methylene chloride, which is used as a solvent and paint stripper by a number of industries. Examples of other listed air toxics include dioxin, asbestos, toluene, pesticides, and metals such as cadmium, mercury, chromium, and lead compounds.

Q. What are health and environmental effects of hazardous air pollutants (HAPs)?

- People exposed to toxic air pollutants at sufficient concentrations and durations may have an increased chance of getting cancer or experiencing other serious health effects. These health effects can include damage to the immune system, as well as neurological, reproductive (e.g., reduced fertility), developmental, respiratory, and other health problems. In addition to exposure from breathing air toxics, some toxic air pollutants such as mercury can deposit onto soils or surface waters, where they are taken up by plants and ingested by animals and are eventually magnified up through the food chain. Like humans, animals may experience health problems if exposed to sufficient quantities of air toxics over time.

Q. Describe gas–particle interactions

- These interactions can be extremely complex involving multiple components of the particles, gases/vapors, and sunlight. In view of several components together with those focusing on irritancy and infectivity, raise the question of realistic exposure scenarios of gaseous and particulate pollutants that can interact through either chemical or physiologic mechanisms to enhance health risks of complex polluted atmospheres.

Q. What is the size of ultrafine carbonaceous matter?

- Particles that are less than 100 nm in diameter are commonly *defined* as *ultrafine*. This matter typically results from high-temperature oxidation or as the product of the atmospheric transformation involving organic vapors and sunlight.

Q. What is smog?

- Combination of smoke and fog is smog which considerably reduces visibility.

Q. What are the adverse effects of smog?

- Smog is made up of a combination of air pollutants that can injure health, harm the environment, and cause property damage. Smog causes health problems such as difficulty in breathing, asthma, reduced resistance to lung infections and colds, and eye irritation. The ozone in smog also inhibits plant growth and can cause widespread damage to crops and forest, and the haze reduces visibility. The smog or haze is particularly noticeable from mountains and other beautiful vistas, such as those in national parks.

Q. What is photochemical smog?

- Haze in the atmosphere accompanied by high levels of ozone and nitrogen oxides, caused by the action of sunlight on pollutants, is called photochemical smog. It is short lived because of their reaction with co-pollutants. Peroxyacetyl nitrate (PAN) is thought to be responsible for much of the eye stinging activity of smog. It is more soluble and reactive than O3 and hence rapidly decomposes in mucous membranes before it can penetrate into the respiratory tract. The cornea is a sensitive target and is prominent in the burning/stinging discomfort often associated with oxidant smog.

Q. Describe what happens during an asthma attack.

- The beginning signs of an attack include wheezing, coughing, and difficulty breathing. As the problem persists, the airways begin to spasm. During a spasm, the muscles in the bronchi and bronchioles contract, and membranes swell. Mucus forms in the airways, and this narrowing of the airway makes it difficult to breath. With an extended attack, the person sweats, the pulse becomes rapid, the skin turns blue, and the arms and legs become chilled or cold.

Q. Describe the nature of a subsidence inversion.

- Subsidence refers to the descent of air masses. Cool air masses (anticyclones) associated with Hadley cells descend causing air molecules to compress in a layer above the ground. This layer becomes warmed by compression while the air at ground level remains unchanged and often cooler than the air above, producing an inversion layer at distances of 500 to 1000 meters above the ground. Such inversions may occur frequently along coastal areas such as California which has documented inversions more than 300 days of the year. Such subsidence inversions occur most often during the fall and winter months and are particularly troublesome since they may persist for days.

Q. Discuss the impact of acid rain on plant life.

- Acidic deposition at levels of pH 4.0 to 5.0 is most common and does not appear to cause widespread adverse effects on forest ecosystems. However, acid clouds (as low as pH 2.2) can have the following adverse effects:
  (a) Damage leaves
  (b) Mobilize toxic metals in soil such as aluminum, which adversely affects roots
  (c) Leach nutrients from soil
  (d) Over-stimulate plants from excess nitrates which aggravate deficiencies of other nutrients
- These factors may combine to increase forest susceptibility to insect and fungal pathogens.

Q. List some of the indicators of indoor air pollution.

- Signs of indoor air pollution may include physical or health signs or both.
- Physical symptoms may include:
  (a) Heating or cooling equipment that is dirty and/or moldy
  (b) Moisture condensation on walls and windows
  (c) Air that has a stuffy or has an unpleasant odor

(d) Signs of water leakage anywhere in the building with the growth of molds

Health indicators of indoor air pollution may include immediate or acute effects such as eye irritation, dry throat, headaches, fatigue, sinus congestion, shortness of breath, cough dizziness, nausea, sneezing, and nose irritation.

Q. What are the possible toxic effects of environmental chemicals?
  (a) Produce reversible or irreversible bodily injury
  (b) Have the capacity to cause tumors, neoplastic effects, or cancer
  (c) Cause reproductive errors including mutations and teratogenic effects
  (d) Produce irritation and sensitization of mucous membranes
  (e) Cause a reduction in motivation, mental alertness, or capability
  (f) Alter behavior or cause death of the organism

Q. List the variety of processes of absorption including their characteristics.
  (a) Diffusion: molecules move from areas of high concentration to low concentration.
  (b) Facilitated diffusion: require specialized carrier proteins, no high energy phosphate bonds are required.
  (c) Active transport: ATP is required in conjunction with special carrier proteins to move molecules through a membrane against a concentration gradient.
  (d) Endocytosis: particles and large molecules that might otherwise be restricted from crossing a plasma membrane can be brought in or removed by this process.

Q. How do toxic substances enter the body?
  - There are several ways in which toxic substances can enter the body. They may enter through:
    (a) Lungs by inhalation
    (b) Skin
    (c) Oral
    (d) Mucous membranes or eyes by absorption

Q. What are the major functions of the skin?
- The skin can help to:
  (a) Regulate body temperature through sweat glands
  (b) Provide a physical barrier to dehydration, microbial invasion, and some chemical insults
  (c) Excrete salts, water, and organic compounds
  (d) Serve as a sensory organ for touch, temperature, pressure, and pain
  (e) Provide some important components of immunity

Q. What are the three major mechanisms for the harmful effects of environmental toxins?
  (a) The toxins' influence on enzymes
  (b) Direct chemical combination of the toxin with a cell constituent
  (c) Secondary action as a result of the toxins' presence in the system

Q. List the four major types of hypersensitivity reactions of environmental pollutants.
  (a) Cytotoxic
  (b) Cell-mediated
  (c) Immune complex
  (d) Anaphylactic

Q. What are the messages given through the public media about toxic chemicals?
  (a) Exposure to toxic chemicals have dramatically increased the risk of cancer;
  (b) Common household and agricultural chemicals are causing many human diseases and death.
  (c) Polluted air and water are major sources of disease risk.
  (d) Environmental chemicals are interfering with the reproductive process in humans and producing harmful effects in the fetus and young children.

Q. What are the major mechanisms for chemical injury?
  (a) Interfere with enzyme activity
  (b) Directly combine with some cell component other than enzymes
  (c) Produce a secondary action in which a chemical causes the release or formation of a more harmful substance

Q. What is environmental disease and its external causal factors?
- Environmental disease refers to any pathologic process having a characteristic set of signs and symptoms which are detrimental to the well-being of the individual and are the consequence of external factors, including exposure to physical or chemical agents, poor nutrition, and social or cultural behaviors.

Q. What are the differences between DNA and mRNA?
- Messenger RNA is quite similar to its DNA counterpart except it is single stranded and contains the nucleotide base uracil instead of thymine and the sugar D-ribose instead of 2-deoxyribose in the four mononucleotides.

Q. What are the health consequences of air pollution?
- Air pollution increases the risk of respiratory and heart disease in the population. Both short- and long-term exposure to air pollutants has been associated to health impacts. More severe impacts affect people who are already ill. Children, the elderly, and poor people are more susceptible.

Q. How bad is air pollution?
- Air pollution is a major environmental health problem affecting everyone. It is a problem from exhaust fumes from cars, domestic combustion, or factory smoke. Worldwide there are risks to health from exposure to particulate matter (PM) and ozone (O3) in many cities of developed and developing countries alike.

Q. What are the most polluted cities in the world?
- Unfortunately, there is no comprehensive, worldwide data base allowing precise answer to this question. Nevertheless, the available data indicate that air pollution is very high in a number of Asian cities (Karachi, New Delhi, Katmandu, Beijing), in Latin American cities (Lima, Arequipa), and in Africa (Cairo).

Q. In which regions of the world/countries and cities are particulate matter concentrations particularly high?

- As often is the case, the biggest air pollution-related burden to health is observed in developing countries. The lack of knowledge of the health impacts from pollution is a big obstacle in defining the actions and mobilizing local and international resources.

Q. Have there been any new guidelines or other significant, relevant documents since 2005 about the health impact of air pollution?

- The 2005 global guidelines are the most up to date providing the latest scientific evidence. They set targets for air quality which would protect the large majority of individuals from the effects of air pollution on health.

Q. Which effects can be expected of long-term exposure to levels of PM observed currently in Europe (include both clinical and pre-clinical effects, e.g., development of respiratory system)?

- Long-term exposure to current ambient PM concentrations may lead to a marked reduction in life expectancy. The reduction in life expectancy is primarily due to increased cardiopulmonary and lung cancer mortality. Increases are likely in lower respiratory symptoms and reduced lung function in children and chronic obstructive pulmonary disease and reduced lung function in adults.

Q. Is there a threshold below which no effects on health of PM are expected to occur in all people?

- Epidemiological studies on large populations have been unable to identify a threshold concentration below which ambient PM has no effect on health. It is likely that within any large human population, there is such a wide range in susceptibility that some subjects are at risk even at the lowest end of the concentration range.

Q. Are effects of the pollutant dependent upon the subjects' characteristics such as age, gender, underlying disease, smoking status, atopy, education, etc.? What are the critical characteristics?

- In short-term studies, elderly subjects and subjects with preexisting heart and lung disease were found to be more susceptible to effects of ambient PM on mortality and morbidity. In panel studies, asthmatics have also been shown to respond to ambient PM with more symptoms, larger lung function changes, and increased medication use than non-asthmatics. In long-term studies, it has been suggested that socially disadvantaged and poorly educated populations respond more strongly in terms of mortality. PM also is related to reduced lung growth in children. No consistent differences have been found between men and women and between smokers and nonsmokers in PM responses in the cohort studies.

Q. To what extent is mortality being accelerated by long- and short-term exposure to the pollutant (harvesting)?

- Cohort studies have suggested that life expectancy is decreased by long-term exposure to PM. This is supported by new analyses of time-series studies that have shown death being advanced by periods of at least a few months, for causes of death such as cardiovascular and chronic pulmonary disease.

Q. For PM which of the physical and chemical characteristics of particulate air pollution are responsible for health effects?

- There is strong evidence to conclude that fine particles (< 2.5 µm, PM2.5) are more hazardous than larger ones (coarse particles) in terms of mortality and cardiovascular and respiratory end points in panel studies. This does not imply that the coarse fraction of PM10 is innocuous. In toxicological and controlled human exposure studies, several physical, biological, and chemical characteristics of particles have been found to elicit cardiopulmonary responses. Among the characteristics found to be contributing to toxicity in epidemiological and controlled exposure studies are metal content, presence of PAHs, other organic components, endo-toxin, and both small (<2.5 μm) and extremely small size (<100 nm).

Q. What is the evidence of synergy/interaction of the pollutant with other air pollutants?

- Few epidemiological studies have addressed interactions of PM with other pollutants. Toxicological and controlled human exposure studies have shown additive and, in some cases, more than additive effects, especially for combinations of PM and ozone and of PM (especially diesel particles) and allergens. Finally, studies of atmospheric chemistry demonstrate that PM interacts with gases to alter its composition and hence its toxicity.

Q. What is the relationship between ambient levels and personal exposure to the pollutant over short term and long term (including exposures indoors)? Can the differences influence the results of studies?

- Whereas personal exposure to PM and its components is influenced by indoor sources (such as smoking) in addition to outdoor sources, there is a clear relationship on population level between ambient PM and personal PM of ambient origin over time, especially for fine combustion particles. On a population level, personal PM of ambient origin "tracks" ambient PM over time; thus measurements of PM in ambient air can serve as a reasonable "proxy" for personal exposure in time-series studies. The relationship between long-term average ambient PM concentrations and long-term average personal PM exposure has been studied less. Contributions to personal PM exposure from smoking and occupation need to be taken into account. However, the available data suggest that imperfect relations between ambient and personal PM do not invalidate the results of the long-term studies.

Q. Which effects can be expected of long e-term xposure to levels of O3 observed currently in Europe (both clinical and pre-clinical effects)?

- There are few epidemiological studies on the chronic effects of ozone on human health. Incidence of asthma, a decreased lung function growth, lung cancer, and total mortality are the main outcomes studied. At levels currently observed in Europe, the evidence linking O3 exposure to asthma incidence and prevalence in children and adults is not consistent. Available evidence suggests that long-term O3 exposure reduces lung function growth in children. There is little evidence for an independent long-term O3 effect on lung cancer or total mortality. The plausibility of chronic damage to the human lung from prolonged O3 exposure is supported by the results of a series of chronic animal exposure studies.

Q. Is there a threshold below which ozone has no effects on health are expected to occur in all people?

- There may be different concentration–response curves for individuals in the population response to O3 exposure. There is evidence for a threshold for lung damage and inflammation at about 60 to 80 ppb (120–160 ug/m3) for short-term exposure (6.6 hours) with intermittent moderate exercise. Where there are thresholds, they depend on the individual exercise levels.

Q. What is the evidence of synergy/interaction of O3 with other air pollutants?

- Epidemiological studies show that short-term effects of O3 can be enhanced by particulate matter and vice versa. Experimental evidence from studies at higher O3 concentrations shows synergistic, additive, or antagonistic effects, depending on the experimental design, but their relevance for ambient exposures is unclear. O3 may act as a primer for allergen response.

Q. Are effects of NO2 dependent upon the subjects' characteristics such as age, gender, underlying disease, smoking status, atopy, education, etc.? What are the critical characteristics?

- In general, individuals with asthma are expected to be more responsive to short-term exposure to inhaled agents, when compared to individuals without asthma. Controlled human exposure studies of short-term responses of persons with and without asthma to NO2 have not been carried out. There is limited evidence from epidemiological studies that individuals with asthma show steeper concentration–response relationships. Small-scale human exposure studies have not shown consistent effects of NO2 exposure on airway reactivity in persons with asthma, even at exposure levels higher than typical ambient concentrations. As for other pollutants, children can reasonably be considered to be at increased risk. There is limited evidence for influence of the other listed factors on the effects of NO2.

Q. Is the considered pollutant NO2 per se responsible for effects on health?

- The evidence for acute effects of NO2 comes from controlled human exposure studies to NO_2 alone. For the effects observed in epidemiological studies, a clear answer to the question cannot be given. Effects estimated for NO2 exposure in epidemiological studies may reflect other traffic-related pollutants, for which NO2 is a surrogate. Additionally, there are complex interrelationships among the concentrations of NO2, PM, and O3 in ambient air.

Q. What is the evidence of synergy/interaction of the pollutant NO2 with other air pollutants?

- There have been few controlled human exposure studies on interactions with other chemical pollutants, although several studies show that NO2 exposure enhances responses to inhaled pollens. Some epidemiological studies have explored statistical interactions of NO2 with other pollutants, including particles, but the findings are not readily interpretable.

Q. Which are the critical sources of the pollutant NO2 responsible for health effects?

- In most urban environments in Europe, the principal source of NO2 is NOx from motor vehicles of all types and energy production in some places.

Q. How is ozone produced and destroyed?

- The ozone molecule (O3) contains three atoms of oxygen and is mainly formed by the action of the UV rays of the sun on oxygen molecules (diatomic oxygen, O2) in the upper part of Earth's atmosphere (called the stratosphere). Ozone is also produced locally near Earth's surface from the action of UV radiation on some air pollutants.

Q. What is the relationship between ozone and solar ultraviolet radiation?

- There is an inverse relationship between the concentration of ozone and the amount of harmful UV radiation transmitted through the atmosphere since ozone absorbs some of the UV radiation.

Q. How and why has the situation regarding the ozone layer changed over the past 35 years?

- Stratospheric ozone has decreased over the globe since the 1980s. Averaged over the globe, ozone in the period 1996–2009 is about 4% lower than before 1980. Much larger depletion, up to 40%, occurs over the high latitudes of the Southern Hemisphere in October.

Q. What determines the level of solar UV-B radiation at a specific place?

- The sun is the source of the UV radiation reaching Earth. UV radiation is partly absorbed by the components of Earth's atmosphere. The amount of UV radiation that is absorbed depends mainly on the length of the path of the sunlight through the atmosphere.

Q. What is the solar UV index?

- The solar UV index (UVI) describes the level of solar UV radiation relevant to human sunburn (erythema).

Q. How does the UV index vary with location and time?

- The combination of total ozone, aerosols, clouds, air pollution, altitude, surface reflectivity, and solar zenith angle (that is determined by the geographical position, season, and time of the day) are the main factors resulting in variation in the UV index.

Q. What is the effect of the interaction between UV-B radiation, climate change, and human activity on air pollution?

- Pollutants emitted by human activities can reduce UV-B radiation near the surface, while particles may lead to enhancement by scattering. These processes decrease some exposures to UV while enhancing others. Interactions between UV radiation and pollutants resulting from changes in climate and burning of fossil and plant fuels will worsen the effects of ozone on humans and plants in the lower atmosphere.

Q. What are the effects of exposure to solar UV radiation on the human eye, and how can the eye be protected?

- The effects of UV radiation on the eye can be almost immediate (acute) occurring several hours after a short, intense exposure. They can also be long-term (chronic), following exposure of the eye to levels of UV radiation below those required for the acute effects but occurring repeatedly over a long period of time. The commonest acute effect, photokeratitis (snow blindness), leaves few or no permanent effects, whereas cataract due to chronic exposure is irreversible and ultimately leads to severe loss of vision requiring surgery.

Q. What are the adverse effects of exposure to solar UV-B radiation on human skin?

- Acute overexposure of the skin to solar UV radiation causes sunburn; chronic sunlight exposure can lead to the development of skin cancers.

Q. Do ozone-depleting gases and their substitutes have an effect on climate?

- Stratospheric ozone depletion has an influence on climate change since both ozone and the compounds responsible for its depletion are active greenhouse gases.

Q. Is ozone depletion affected by climate change?

- Climate change affects ozone depletion through changes in atmospheric conditions that affect the chemical production and loss of stratospheric ozone. The interactions are complex. Climate change is expected to decrease temperatures and water vapor abundances in the stratosphere. This will tend to speed up ozone recovery outside polar regions but slow down the recovery in polar regions.

Q. Name at least three things the word climate takes into consideration.

- Temperature, precipitation, humidity, wind velocity and direction, and cloud cover and solar radiation.

Q. Name different phenomena associated with climatic change.

(a) Changes in ocean temperature
(b) Changes in earth 's orbital geometry
(c) Volcanic activity with increased atmosphere dust and reduced sunlight penetration
(d) Variations in solar radiation
(e) Increases in atmospheric gases that absorb heat energy

Q. Which is the most important factor(s) that affect the climate?

- Temperature/the sun.

Q. Give examples of ecosystem.

- The planet, an ant farm, tidal pool, pond, river valley, and garbage can.

Q. Give examples of physical or abiotic components of an ecosystem.

- Water, air, sunlight, and minerals.

Q. By which process green plants and some other organisms use sunlight to synthesize nutrients from carbon dioxide and water.

- Photosynthesis.

Q. What is the term associated with the accumulation of organic material in an ecosystem?

- Biomass.

Q. What term describes the amount of energy stored by a plant to be used as chemical energy?

- Kilocalories.

Q. Give an example of an organism in the first trophic level.

- Plant.

Q. Give examples of primary consumers.

- Caterpillar, grasshopper, cattle, and elephants.

Q. Name macronutrients.

- Sulfur, carbon, oxygen, phosphorus, nitrogen, and hydrogen.

List three sources from which carbon dioxide is released into the atmosphere.

(a) Respiratory process of plants and animals which consume oxygen and release carbon dioxide

(b) Combustion of fossil or organic fuels

(c) Decomposition of organic matter

Q. What part of the carbon cycle do scientists think is contributing to the greenhouse effect?

- The increase of carbon dioxide due to the burning of forests and fossil fuels.

Q. What macronutrient makes up the largest percent of the earth's air?

- Nitrogen.

Q. In which state carbon is found?

- Carbon can be found in three different states:

(a) Gas

(b) Liquid

(c) And solid

Q. Discuss the impact of acid rain on plant life.

- Acidic deposition at levels of pH 4.0 to 5.0, which are most common, does not appear to cause widespread adverse effects on forest ecosystems. However, conifer forests such as Red Spruce on mountain tops in New Hampshire, Vermont, and in the Appalachians have been more than 80 percent decimated at the cloud line. Severe damage is also evidenced in Central Europe in such places as the Czech Republic and Poland where 60 to 70 percent of forests show evidence of damage associated with sulfur and nitrogen disposition. The mechanisms for such destruction are not immediately obvious but may be attributed to combinations of ozone and acid clouds (as low as pH 2.2) which (1) directly damage leaves; (2) mobilize toxic metals in soil such as aluminum, which adversely effects roots; (3) leach nutrients from soil; and (4) over-stimulate plants from excess nitrates which aggravate deficiencies of other nutrients. These factors may combine to increase forest susceptibility to insect and fungal pathogens.

Q. What causes depletion of ozone?

- Scientific evidence indicates that stratospheric ozone is being destroyed by a group of manufactured chemicals, containing chlorine and/or bromine. These chemicals are called "ozone-depleting substances" (ODS).

Q. How do chlorofluorocarbons (CFCs) lead to ozone depletion?

- Because of their relative stability, CFCs rise into the stratosphere where they are eventually broken down by ultraviolet (UV) rays from the sun. This causes them to release free chlorine. The chlorine reacts with oxygen which leads to the chemical process of destroying ozone molecules.

Q. What is causing the depletion of the ozone layer?

- Ozone depletion occurs when chlorofluorocarbons (CFCs)—formerly found in aerosol spray cans and refrigerants—are released into the atmosphere. These gases, through several chemical reactions, cause the ozone molecules to break down, reducing ozone's ultraviolet (UV) radiation-absorbing capacity.

4 Sample MCQ's

(Choose the correct statement; it may be one, two, or more or none)

Q.1. A threshold limit value time weighted average for a chemical represents -------.

A. An airborne concentration of a chemical that can never be exceeded

B. An airborne concentration of a chemical that is believed to cause no adverse health effect to a worker exposed for 8 hours a day, 40 hours a week

C. An airborne concentration of a chemical that cannot be exceeded for longer than 15 minutes a day

D. A value for an acceptable airborne concentration of a chemical established by the Occupational Safety and Health Administration

E. An airborne concentration which cannot be measured using available technology

Q.2. Which of the following is the most significant contributor to air pollution by mass in suburban areas?

A. Manufacturing
B. Transportation
C. Apace heaters
D. Electric power generation
E. Waste disposal

Q.3. The major toxic effect of hydrogen cyanide exposure is -------.

A. Lung damage
B. Hemoglobin alteration
C. Hemolysis of RBCs
D. Inhibition of mitochondrial respiration
E. Lipid peroxidation

Q.4. Which of the following agents would *not* likely produce reactive airway dysfunction syndrome (RADS)?

A. Carbon monoxide
B. Chlorine
C. Ammonia
D. Toluene diisocyanate
E. Acetic acid

Q.5. Benzene is similar to toluene ------.

A. In its metabolism to redox active metabolites
B. Regarding covalent binding of its metabolites to proteins
C. In its ability to produce CNS depression

D. In its ability to produce acute myelogenous leukemia
E. In its ability to be metabolized to benzoquinone

Q.6. Which of the following is *not* a primary pollutant?

A. Carbon monoxide
B. Lead
C. Ozone
D. Nitrogen dioxide

Q.7. Most automobiles emit up to ---- % less pollutants now than in 1960.

A. 80
B. 30
C. 99
D. 50

Q.8. Particulates may cause which of the following health hazards to humans -------.

A. Respiratory distress
B. Damage to nervous system
C. Blindness
D. Learning disabilities

Q.9. Carbon monoxide may produce _____ as one of the symptoms of exposure in humans.

A. Excess urination
B. Headache
C. Throat irritation
D. Hearing loss

Q.10. Tropospheric ozone may cause which of the following effects --------.

A. Grime deposits
B. Reduced visibility
C. Retardation of plant growth
D. Metal corrosion

Q.11. Fine particulates from motor vehicles and power plants are reported to kill about _____ Americans annually.

A. 38,000
B. Two million
C. 9100
D. 64,000

Q.12. _____ may be the primary health problem when a person's bronchial tubes respond to allergens, pollution, etc. resulting in hyperactive airways.

A. Cardiac arrest
B. Asthma
C. Laryngitis
D. Sneezing

Q.13. Signs of an extended asthma attack may include -------

A. Sweating
B. Rapid pulse
C. Skin turning blue
D. All of the above

Q.14. Most adult people spend an average of ____% of their time indoors.

A. 50
B. 25
C. 90
D. 10

Q.15. Which is a potential source of indoor air pollution?

A. Moisture
B. Room air fresheners
C. Personal care products
D. All of the above

Q.16. A smoker is exposed to nearly _____ compounds in main stream cigarette smoke.

A. 4700
B. 320
C. 9400
D. 560

Q.17. Building related illnesses (BRI) refers to -------.

A. Well-defined illnesses occurring in a building that can be traced to specific building problems.
B. The display of acute symptoms by a number of people in a building without a particular pattern and the varied symptoms cannot be associated with a particular pattern.
C. Well-defined illnesses occurring in a building that cannot be traced to specific building problems.
D. The display of acute symptoms by a number of people in a building with a specific pattern of disease associated with a particular pattern.

Q.18. Biological contaminants are most likely aggravated by what problem?

A. Auto exhaust
B. Unvented gas stove
C. Moisture
D. Household chemicals

Q.19. Air that is drawn into the home by cracks in the foundation is known as -------

A. Natural ventilation
B. Infiltration
C. Mechanical filtration
D. Foundation suction

Q.20. When considering the contribution of all greenhouse gases, carbon monoxide contributes approximately ____% to global warming?

A. 24
B. 6
C. 55
D. 15

Answers

1. B.   2. B.   3. D.   4. A.   5. C.   6. C.
7. A.   8. A.   9. B.   10. C.   11. D.
12. B.   13. D.   14. C.   15. D.   16. A.
17. A.   18. C.   19. B.   20. C.

Further Reading

Costa DL, Gordon T (2015) Air pollution. In: Klaassen CD, Watkins JB III (eds) Casarett & Doull's essentials of toxicology, 3rd edn. McGraw-Hill, USA, pp 425–440

Dixon Robert L (2010) Environmental Toxicology. In: Gupta PK (ed) Modern toxicology: the adverse effects of xenobiotics, vol 2., 2nd reprint. PharmaMed Press, Hyderabad, India, pp 398–446

Gupta PK (2018) Illustrative toxicology, 1st edn. Elsevier, San Diego

Gupta PK (2020) Brain storming questions in toxicology. Francis and Taylor CRC Press, USA

Laws EA (2013) Environmental toxicology USA ISBN: 978-1-4614-5763-3 (Print) 978–1–4614-5764-0 (Online) Springer, USA

Analytical and Clinical Toxicology

23

Abstract

Analytical toxicology is important for the qualitative and/or quantitative estimation of chemicals that may exert adverse effects on living organisms. Clinical toxicology includes application of knowledge of medical toxicology, applicd toxicology, and clinical poison information. It plays an important role in case of acute poisoning, which may be intentional, accidental, or during occupation exposure. Principles of diagnosis include clinical history, physical examination, and analytical evidence. This is followed by general management of poisoning of the patients including methods of removal of poisons from the body. This chapter briefly describes the overview, key points, and relevant text that are in the format of problem-solving study questions followed by multiple-choice questions (MCQs) along with their answers.

Keywords

Clinical toxicology · Analytical toxicology poisoning · Treatment of poisoning · Principles of diagnosis · Management of poisoning · Medical toxicology · MCQs · Question and answers bank

1 Introduction

Analytical toxicology is important for the qualitative and/or quantitative estimation of chemicals that may exert adverse effects on living organisms. Clinical toxicology includes application of knowledge of medical toxicology, applied toxicology, and clinical poison information. It plays an important role in the case of acute poisoning, which may be intentional, accidental, or during occupation exposure. Principles of diagnosis include clinical history, physical examination, and analytical evidence. This is followed by general management of poisoning of the patients including methods of removal of poisons from the body. The chapter briefly describes an overview, key points, and relevant text that is in the format of problem-solving study questions followed by multiple-choice questions (MCQ's) along with their answers.

2 Overview

Clinical toxicology includes physicians and scientists involved with the understanding of the diagnosis and treatment of poisoning. Some clinical toxicologists work with poisoned patients through poison control (and poison information and treatment), while others are in a university, hospital, government agency, or industry. The function of clinical analytic toxicology (also called clinical chemistry in toxicology) is to provide, via laboratory analysis of tissues and fluids, evaluations of the qualitative and quantitative characteristics of (1) specific endogenous and potentially adverse exogenous chemical components present in samples of blood, urine, feces, spinal fluid, and tissues, (2) changes in the formed elements of the blood and their function, and (3) histological changes in tissues and the components of the blood. The purpose is to help identify abnormal or pathological changes or their causes in organ system functions. The provision of services for the management of poisoned patients varies greatly, from specialized treatment units to, more commonly, general emergency medicine. Analytical toxicology services, which provide support for the diagnosis, prognosis, and management of poisoning, are also variable and dependent on local arrangements. Treatment should focus on supportive measures, with the addition of further interventions to reduce absorption and increase elimination, and where appropriate administration of an appropriate antidote.

Key Points

- Analytical toxicology is important for the qualitative and/or quantitative estimation of chemicals that may exert adverse effects on living organisms.
- Clinical toxicology includes application of knowledge of medical toxicology, applied toxicology, and clinical poison information.
- Clinical toxicology encompasses the expertise in the specialties of medical toxicology, applied toxicology. The toxicologic investigation of a poison death involves (1) obtaining the case history in as much detail as possible and gathering suitable specimens, (2) conducting suitable toxicologic analyses based on the available specimens, and (3) the interpretation of the analytic findings.

- Important components of the initial clinical encounter with a poisoned patient include stabilization of the patient, clinical evaluation (history, physical, laboratory, and radiology), prevention of further toxin absorption, enhancement of toxin elimination, administration of antidote, and supportive care.
- The toxicologist as an expert witness may provide two objectives: testimony and opinion. Objective testimony usually involves a description of analytic methods and findings. When a toxicologist testifies as to the interpretation of analytic results, that toxicologist is offering an "opinion" of follow-up.

3 Problem-Solving Study Questions

3.1 Analytical Toxicology

Q. What is analytical protocol in toxicology?
Analytical toxicology is the detection, identification, and measurement of foreign compounds (xenobiotics) in biological and other specimens. Analytical methods are available for a very wide range of compounds: these may be gases, volatile substances, corrosive agents, metals, anions and non-metals, nonvolatile organic substances, chemicals, pesticides, pharmaceuticals, drugs of abuse, and natural toxins.

Q. What is included in a toxicology test?
A toxicology test ("tox screen") checks for drugs or other chemicals in the blood, urine, or saliva. These may include prescription medicines, nonprescription medicines (such as aspirin), vitamins, supplements, alcohol, and illegal drugs, such as cocaine and heroin.

Q. Describe the steps to be followed in an analytical toxicological investigation.

The steps to be followed in an analytical toxicological investigation are given below:

Step 1 Based on circumstantial evidence—biochemical and blood investigation

Step 2 Based on medical history—decide priorities for the analysis

Step 3 Analytical phase

Step 4 Interpretation of the results

Step 5 Perform additional analysis on the original samples or on further samples from the patient, if necessary

Q. What are general precautions to be followed by any investigator in toxicology laboratory?

1. Strong acids or alkalis should always be added to water and not vice versa.
2. Strong acids and alkalis should never be preserved together.
3. Organic solvents should not be heated over a naked flame but in water bath.
4. Use fume cupboards/hoods when organic solvents are heated.

3.2 Case History and Poisonings

Q. What type of information should be collected about the intoxicated/poisoned patient?

The age, sex, weight, medical history, and occupation of the decedent, as well as any treatment administered before death, the gross autopsy findings, the drugs available to the decedent, and the interval of the onset of symptoms, etc., should be noted.

Q. What are the objectives of clinical toxicology?

In brief clinical toxicology includes DIMPLE which means:

(a) Diagnosis (D)
(b) Identification of poisons (I)
(c) Management and treatment of poisoning (M)
(d) Prognosis (P)
(e) Law enforcement (L)
(f) Education and research (E)

All the six indications mentioned above can be remembered by the mnemonic DIMPLE.

Q. What are the most common poisons in children?

1. Cosmetics and personal care products
2. Cleaning substances and laundry products
3. Pain medicines
4. Foreign bodies such as toys, coins, and thermometers
5. Topical preparations
6. Vitamins
7. Antihistamines
8. Pesticides
9. Plants
10. Antimicrobials

Q. Which are the most common poisons in adults?

1. Pain killer medicines
2. Sedatives, hypnotics, and antipsychotics
3. Antidepressants
4. Cardiovascular drugs
5. Cleaning substances (household)
6. Alcohols
7. Pesticides
8. Bites and envenomations (ticks, spiders, bees, snakes)
9. Anticonvulsants
10. Cosmetics and personal care products

Q. Which are the most common routes of poisoning?

Substances can enter the body in three ways:

1. Ingestion (swallowing)
2. Inhalation (breathing in)
3. Exposure of body surfaces (e.g., skin, eye, and mucous membrane)

Q. How does carbon monoxide cause normal appearing or pink-colored skin?

• Carbon monoxide causes normal appearing or pink-colored skin due to its ability to increase hemoglobin's affinity for oxygen, resulting in hyper-oxygenated red blood cells.

Q. List groups of chemicals which are non-naturally produced toxicants:

(a) Pesticides
(b) Pharmaceuticals
(c) Food additives
(d) Solvents
(e) Environment contaminants

Q. Give four examples of naturally produced toxicants.
  (a) Plants (plant toxins)
  (b) Fungus (mycotoxins)
  (c) Bacterial (exotoxins)
  (d) Animal/insects (venoms)
Q. What are top four causes of poisonings for animal or human control centers?
  • Pesticides >plants> household products >medicines
Q. In which season toxicant exposures have highest incidence?
  • In summer -----   May–August
    In December ---- (young and adult dogs)
Q. Name top three toxicant exposure agents causing death.
  (a) Organophosphate insecticides
  (b) Ethylene glycol (antifreeze)
  (c) Anticoagulant rodenticides
Q. Indicate the circumstances under which activated charcoal should not be administered.
  • It is ineffective in cases of heavy metal or corrosive chemical poisoning.
Q. Indicate the circumstances under which iso-osmotic laxative should not be administered.
  • Suspected or proven obstruction or perforation of the bowel.
Q. Indicate the circumstances under which penicillamine should not be administered.
  • A person with a hypersensitivity to penicillamine.
Q. A delayed toxicity can include....
  (a) Development of cancer (by carcinogens)
  (b) Damage to the CNS by organophosphorus insecticides
  (c) Toxic damage to the liver which can be reversible
Q. To manage unconscious poisoned patients, what can you do?
  (a) Administer oxygenation during cardiac arrest/cardiopulmonary resuscitation (CPR).
  (b) Transfer the patient to clinical facilities.
  (c) Do not remove stomach contents by emesis.
Q. Name three major systems that are required for monitoring in the poisoned patients?

  (a) Cardiovascular
  (b) Respiratory
  (c) CNS

3.3 Diagnosis

Q. What are the basics of diagnosis?
  1. Medical history
  2. Physical examination
  3. Differential diagnosis
  4. Investigation and final diagnosis
Q. When conducting an investigation, what type of question (s) is to be asked?
  These include:
  1. What was the route of administration?
  2. What was the administered dose?
  3. Is concentration enough to have caused death or injury or altered the victim's behavior enough to cause death or injury?
Q. Respiratory breath that smells of bitter almond is indicative of -------?
  • Intoxication with cyanide.
Q. What is the characteristic odor associated with different poisonings?
  Characteristic odor associated with different poisoning is summarized in Table 23.1.
Q. Give at least a few examples of some poisonous drugs showing pupillary manifestations such as miosis, mydriasis, and nystagmus.
  Chemicals/drugs that are responsible for pupillary manifestations such as miosis,

Table 23.1 Characteristic odor and potential poisons

Odor	Potential poison
Bitter	Almonds, cyanide
Rotten eggs	Hydrogen sulfide, mercaptans
Garlic	As, organophosphates, DMSO, thallium
Mothballs	Naphthalene, camphor
Vinyl	Ethchlorvynol
Winter green	Methyl salicylate
	Phenol and phenolic disinfectants
Phenolic	Nicotine
Stale tobacco	Nitrobenzene
Shoe polish	Chloroform and other halogenated hydrocarbons
Sweet	

Table 23.2 Examples of some poisonous drugs showing pupillary manifestations

Miosis (papillary constriction)	Mydriasis (papillary dilatation)	Nystagmus
Barbiturates	Alcohol (constricted in coma)	Alcohol
Caffeine	Amphetamines	Barbiturates
Carbamate	Antihistamines	Carbamazepine
Carbolic acid (phenol)	Carbon monoxide	Phencyclidine
Clonidine	Cocaine	Phenytoin
Methyl dopa	Cyanide	
Nicotine	Datura	
Opiates	Ephedrine	
Organophosphates		
Parasympathomimetics		

Table 23.3 Selected drugs showing common symptoms with drug poisoning

Respiratory depression	Diazepam, opioids
Irregular pulse	Salbutamol, quinine, antimuscarinics, tricyclic antidepressants
Hypothermia	Alcohol, barbiturates, benzodiazepines (BZD)
Hyperthermia	Antimuscarinics, antidepressants, (MAO inhibitors, cocaine, amphetamine, opioids, alcohol, BZD
Coma	Hypoglycemic agents, aminophylline
Constricted pupils	Opioids, antipsychotics (haloperidol, quetiapine, olanzapine, organophosphates
Dilated pupil	Anticholinergic drugs (atropine, hyoscine, scopolamine, LSD)

Table 23.4 Color of urine versus toxin

Urine color	Toxin /substance
Green or blue	Methylene blue
Grey- black	Phenols or cresols
Opaque appearance which settles on standing	Primidone, cresols
Orange or orange-red	Rifampicin, iron (especially after giving desferrioxamine

mydriasis, and nystagmus are summarized in Table 23.2.

Q. Give examples of some common symptoms observed with drug poisonings.

Selected drugs showing common symptoms with drug poisoning are summarized in Table 23.3.

Q. Give some examples of urine color versus toxin substance.

Observation of the urine passed may also give some clue about the type of poison ingested by the patient. Color of urine versus toxin is summarized in Table 23.4.

3.4   Clinical Strategy for the Treatment

Q. What are the basic principles of therapy?
There are four basic principles:
(a) Prevention of further poison absorption
(b) Enhancement of poison elimination
(c) Supportive treatment
(d) Specific antidote

Q. Before starting treatment, what type of information is essential and helpful from poisoned patients?
The information should include:
1. The presence of preexisting conditions or allergies
2. Whether the patient is currently using any medications or substances of any kind
3. Whether the patient is pregnant, in the case of female
4. Historical information obtained from family, friends, law enforcement and medical personnel, and any observers.

Q. In cases of poisoning, what is the aim of treatment?
The aim is to decrease the slope of ascending phase (AP) and increasing slope of descending phase (DP). When the slope of AP is decreased, it takes longer time for the toxicant

Fig 23.1 Time vs concentration curve of toxicant in body during treatment

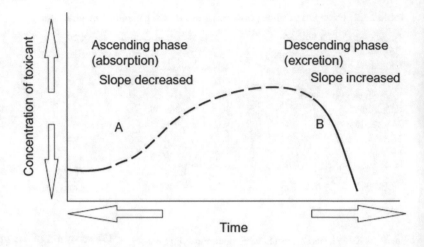

Ascending phase (absorption)
Slope decreased

Descending phase (excretion)
Slope increased

Concentration of toxicant

A

B

Time

Table 23.5 Methods of removal of poisons from the body

Poisoning	Suggested methods of removal
Ingested	Gut decontamination
Inhaled	Provide fresh air, artificial respiration
Injected	Give first aid, followed by specific antidote, diuretics, dialysis, etc.

to be absorbed (A). And increasing the slope of DP causes rapid elimination (B) in a short time (Fig. 23.1).

Q. What are the different methods of removal of poisons from the body?

The different methods of removal of poisons from the body are summarized in Table 23.5.

Q. What are the steps to be followed for general management of poisoning?

- The following concepts are central to approaching a toxicosis patient:
  (a) Ensure airway so that breathing and circulation are adequate.
  (b) Remove unabsorbed material.
  (c) Limit the further absorption of toxicant.
  (d) Hasten toxicant elimination.

The initial survey should always be directed at the assessment of and correction of the life-threatening problems; if present, attention must be paid to the airways, breathing, circulation (ABC), and CNS.

Q. Define the term envenomation.

- Envenomation is the infusion of venom into another creature by the means of biting or stinging.

Q. What is decontamination?

- Decontamination refers to:
  (a) Skin/eye decontamination
  (b) Gut evacuation
  (c) And administration of activated charcoal

Q. What are methods used to increase elimination of poisons from the body?

The following methods are used to increase elimination of poisons from the body:
  (a) Urinary alkalization
  (b) Multiple-dose activated charcoal
  (c) Extracorporeal techniques
  (d) Diaphoresis

Q. What are three aims of emergency care when someone is bitten or stung by a poisonous animal?

- The aims of the emergency care are:
  (a) To minimize systemic absorption of the venom
  (b) To maintain life support
  (c) To facilitate the neutralization of the toxins by the immune system

Q. What is a chelating agent?

- A substance that binds strongly to metal ions, facilitating its elimination.

Q. Which chelating agent is preferred for mild lead poisoning and what is the dose?

- Succimer is the agent of choice for asymptomatic, mild lead poisoning (45–70 mcg/dL in children, 70–100 mcg/dL in adults) because it is available PO and has a low side effect profile.

Table 23.6 Common antidotes and toxins based on the mode/mechanism of action

Toxin	Antidote
Acetaminophen	N-Acetylcystein
Benzodiazepines	Flumazenil
Ca channel blockers	Ca, IV insulin in high doses with IV glucose
Organophosphates and (cholinesterase inhibitors)	Pralidoxime, physostigmine
Carbamates	Atropine and protopam
Heparin	Protamine
Ethylene glycol	Ethanol fomepizole
Tricyclic antidepressants	NaHCO3
Isoniazid	Pyridoxine (vitamin B6
Digitalis glycosides(digoxin, digitoxin, oleander, fox glove)	Steroid binding resins; Potassium salts; beta adrenergic blocking agents; procaine amide
Formaldehyde	Ammonia (by mouth)
Cyanide	Methemoglobin (formed by nitrite administration), thiocyanide
Botulinum	Botulinum antitoxin; guanidine
Methyl alcohol	Ethanol
Selenocysthionine	Cystine
Fluoroacetate	Acetate; monoacetin
Bromide	Chloride
Strontium, radium	Calcium salts
Neuromuscular blocking agents, e.g., curare	Neostigmine; edrophonium
5-Fluorouracil and 6-mercaptopurine	Thymidine Purines
Morphine and other related narcotics (opioids)	Naloxone and other related
Coumarin anticoagulants	Vitamin K
Thallium	Potassium salts
Amino acid analogs	Amino acids
Carbon monoxide	Oxygen
Cyclopropane	Alpha adrenergic blocking agents, i.e., haloalkylamine; antihistamines
Histamine	Antihistamines
Agents that produce methemoglobinemia (e.g., aniline dyes, some local anesthetics, nitrites, nitrates, phenacetin, sulfonamides)	Methylene blue
Anti-tumor agents such as methotrexate and other folic acid antagonists	Glycine

Table 23.7 Metals that make complexes (inert complex formation) with poison. Guidelines for their therapy

Metal	Chelating drugs
Antimony, arsenic, bismuth, chromates, chromic acid, chromium trioxide, copper salts, gold, nickel, tungsten, zinc salts	Dimercaprol
Cadmium, lead, zinc, zinc salts	Edetate Ca disodium edathamil
Arsenic, copper salts, gold, lead, mercury, nickel, zinc salts	Penicillamine
Arsenic (occupational exposure), Bismuth, lead	Succimer
Lead (occupational exposure in adults)	
Mercury (occupational exposure in adults)	

Note: Iron and thallium salts are not chelated effectively
Note: Dosages depend on type and severity of poisoning

Q. What is an antidote?
- An antidote is a medicine taken or given to counteract a particular poison which may be chemical, pharmacological, or physiological in nature.

Q. Give some examples of some toxins and their antidotes.
  Important examples of some toxins and their antidotes are summarized in Tables 23.6 and 23.7.

Q. Which chelating agents are recommended for acute lead poisoning with signs of encephalopathy?
- Dimercaprol + Calcium EDTA.

Q. For what purpose ipecac syrup is used?
- To induce emesis.

Q. When gastric lavage should be performed?
- Can be performed 4–6 hours after intoxication when hepatic recirculation occurs.

Q. To increase the renal excretion of an alkaline substance, what should be done?
- Acidify the urine with and infusion of NH4Cl.

Q. The use of ethanol in methanol intoxication is an example of....
- A dispositional antidote.

Q. What is the antidote of copper poisoning?
- Stomach wash with potassium ferro cyanide 1% solution in water acts as an antidote by forming cupric ferro cyanide. Calcium EDTA or BAL is the recommended antidote. Maintain electrolyte and fluid balance.

Q. Name the agent(s) used in the treatment of poisoning by cyanide.
- Amyl nitrite, sodium nitrite, and sodium thiosulfate.

Q. Name the agent(s) used in the treatment of poisoning by mercury.
- Penicillamine.

Q. Name the agent(s) used in the treatment of poisoning by organophosphate pesticides.
- The organophosphate pesticides can be treated using atropine and pralidoxime iodide.

Q. Your neighbor visits you in an extremely distressed state. A young 3-year-old child has swallowed an unknown quantity of paracetamol tablets. What would you advise his/her parents to do and why?
- Contact the ambulance straight away. The child must be taken to hospital immediately. Paracetamol must be removed immediately to prevent liver damage.

If ipecac syrup is available, this may be administered to induce vomiting though it appears that this drug is not routinely used to remove drugs from the body because of problems such as aspiration.

Q. Farmer A, 60 years old, is brought into the emergency department with organophosphate poisoning. How would this form of poisoning be treated?
   (a) Respiratory support of the farmer by mechanical ventilation.
   (b) Blockade of the cholinergic receptors by the administration of atropine
   (c) The reactivation of the enzyme cholinesterase by the administration of pralidoxime iodide

Q. Which four principles underlying the management of acute clinical overdose should be used?

- There are four principles underlying the management of clinical over dosage:
   (a) Life support
   (b) Client assessment
   (c) Drug decontamination/detoxification and
   (d) Drug neutralization/elimination

Q. What are the main tools used in client assessment to identify the specific agent in a suspected drug overdose?
   (a) Taking a client history
   (b) Noting the set of clinical manifestations,
   (c) And laboratory testing of blood samples

Q. Name the specific antidote(s) for overdose of warfarin poisoning.
- Vitamin K.

Q. Name the specific antidote(s) for overdose of digoxin poisoning.
- Digoxin antibody fragments.

Q. Name the specific antidote(s) for overdose of pethidine poisoning.
- Narcotic antagonist, naloxone.

Q. Name the specific antidote(s) for overdose of heparin toxicity.
- Protamine sulfate.

Q. Describe in brief different mechanisms of specific antidotal therapy.
   (a) Agents which specifically interact with the toxicant, e.g., iron (desferrioxamine); silver nitrate (sodium chloride), etc.
   (b) Complex formation, e.g., methanol, fluoroacetate, heparin, etc.
   (c) Metabolic activation, e.g., enhance metabolic conversion
   (d) Pharmacological antidotes, e.g., morphine, warfarin, curare, etc.
   (e) Enhancement of excretion of the toxicants, e.g., bromide, copper, lead, arsenic, etc.

Q. Under what circumstances might you use gastric lavage or hemodialysis to facilitate the elimination of a drug in overdose?
- Where most of the drug dose is present in the bloodstream rather than in tissues or in interstitial fluid. The apparent volume of distribution (V_d), can be a useful indicator of this.

Q. Describe the management of a young woman admitted to the emergency department following ingestion of ecstasy at a street party. She is extremely agitated and anxious, but her fluid status and electrolyte levels are normal.
- In treating individuals suffering from the effects of stimulants, de-escalation techniques through verbal communication, group negotiation with affected individuals, and physical restraint. Sedation may also need to be administered to reduce the risk of the individuals harming themselves and others. In giving sedating medication, benzodiazepines are usually preferred compared with antipsychotic drugs because benzodiazepines are more sedating and have fewer side effects.

Q. What is the problem associated with the detection of some banned substances through urine testing of sports people?
- Some banned substances are naturally present in the body.

Q. Why ethylene toxicity causes renal toxicity?
- Ethylene glycol toxicity is caused by its conversion to oxalic acid, which causes renal toxicity.

Q. Why methanol toxicity causes renal and ocular toxicity?
- Methanol toxicity is caused by its conversion to formic acid, which causes both renal and ocular toxicity.

Q. Why fomepizole is good option for alcohol poisoning?
- Fomepizole is an alcohol dehydrogenase inhibitor, which blocks the initial conversion of ethylene glycol to glycoaldehyde and methanol to formaldehyde, thus decreasing the precursors to oxalic and formic acid which are responsible for toxicity.

Q. Which chelating agent is preferred for copper poisoning?
- Penicillamine.

Q. How do methemoglobinemia causes cyanosis?
- Methemoglobinemia causes cyanosis due to the oxidation of the iron molecule in hemoglobin, thereby reducing its oxygen carrying capacity.

Q. When removing an unabsorbed portion of a poison substance, which technique can be utilized?
(a) Gastric lavage
(b) Adsorption of the poison
(c) Cathartics
(d) Whole-bowel irrigation

Q. What is the factor on which the risk of intoxication from a toxicant depends upon in divided dose?
- Depends on the elimination rate.

Q. A drug combination whose toxic effect can be described as $3 + 0 = 8$ refers to?
- Potentiation.

Q. In 2003, the American Academy of Pediatrics issued a policy to stop the usage of a substance because research failed to show any benefit in children; name the substance?
- Ipecac.

Q. How do you detect corneal poisoning? How do you treat it?
(a) Look for green stain in the cornea.
(b) Use 2% fluorescein (orange dye under blue light).

Q. Name the substances that prevent absorption of poison by their presence (act locally and not systemically)
(a) Physical antidotes
(b) Demulcents
(c) Activated charcoal

Q. Which salt is preferred to prevent an arrhythmia?
- NHCO3 is preferred.

Q. The administration of phenobarbital in warfarin poisoning...?
- Increases the induction of microsomal enzymes that inactivate warfarin.

Q. British anti-Lewisite (BAL) is----?
- A chemical agonist/chelating agent that is used for heavy metal intoxication.

Q. Why does the lethal dose for chloroform have to be greater than toxic dose?
- The lethal dose is always greater than the toxic dose. A toxic dose causes physiological damage but does not cause death immediately.

Q. What is the purpose of advanced CNS support?
   (a) Aimed at avoiding coma
   (b) Aimed at avoiding convulsions

Q. Advanced respiratory life support includes-----?
   (a) Prolonged resuscitation over 20–30 minutes
   (b) Use of doxapram

Q. In the intoxicated patient, does hypothermia provide any information?
   • It is not informative.

4   Sample MCQ's

(Choose the correct statement; it may be one, two, or more or none)

Q.1. Toxicity associated with any chemical substance is referred to as -----.

   A. Poisoning
   B. Intoxication
   C. Over dosage
   D. Toxicology

Q.2. Clinical toxicity, which is secondary to accidental exposure-------.

   A. Toxicology
   B. Intoxication
   C. Poisoning
   D. Overdose

Q.3. Chest pain is related to -----.

   A. Neurological examination
   B. Cardiopulmonary examination
   C. Gastrointestinal examination
   D. Both cardiopulmonary examination and gastrointestinal examination

Q.4. Technique in which anticoagulated blood is passed through a column containing activated charcoal or resin particles is referred to as ------.

   A. Whole-bowel irrigation
   B. Forced dieresis
   C. Hemodialysis
   D. Hemoperfusion

Q.5. Which of the following substances is not easily adsorbed by activated charcoal?

   A. Iron
   B. Ethanol
   C. Methanol
   D. All of the above

Q.6. The effect of ipecac syrup starts within 30 minutes of administration and lasts for approximately.

   A. 30 minutes
   B. 1 hour
   C. 1 hour and 30 minutes
   D. 2 hours

Q.7. Which of the following procedure is contraindicated for patients who have ingested strong acids -----?

   A. Emesis
   B. Gastric lavage
   C. Whole-bowel irrigation
   D. Both emesis and gastric lavage

Q.8. Which of the following technique is helpful in removing ethanol from body?

   A. Dialysis
   B. Activated charcoal
   C. Diuresis
   D. Hemoperfusion

Q.9. The most effective treatment in GI decontamination with acetaminophen is -----.

   A. Emesis
   B. Gastric lavage
   C. Activated charcoal
   D. Dialysis

Q.10. Drug X is available as a 2.5% solution for intravenous administration. The desired dosage of this drug is 5 mg/kg. What volume of drug should be injected if the patient weighs 50 kg?

A. 0.2 ml
B. 1.0 ml
C. 2.0 ml
D. 10 ml
E. 20 ml.

Q.11. Thalidomide was accidentally discovered as ------.

A. Cardiotoxic agent
B. Liver tonic
C. A sedative/tranquilizer
D. Cough mixture

Q.12. With barbiturate and benzodiazepine abuse, dependency and sedative intoxication are generally associated with -------.

A. Slurred speech
B. Uncoordinated motor movements
C. Impairment attention
D. All of the above

Q.13. A target organ of toxicity is -------

A. Lung
B. Heart
C. Reproductive system
D. Kidney
E. Liver

Q.14. A single large dose of N-nitrosodimethylamine fails to induce cancer in rats, but repeated dosing induces cancer because ------

A. The single large dose is lethal, while the threshold for cancer induction can be exceeded by repeated smaller doses.

B. The main DNA lesion from a single large dose can be repaired readily by methyl transferase, while repeated smaller doses can deplete the available repair enzyme, induce mutations in DNA, and effectively induce cancer.

C. The enzyme system involved in detoxification of N-nitrosodimethylamine is depleted after repeated doses, allowing N-nitrosodimethylamine to build up and exceed the threshold for cancer induction.

D. The enzyme system involved in conversion of N-nitrosodimethylamine to the active carcinogen is induced and on subsequent repeated doses more active carcinogen is produced.

E. The initial dose of N-nitrosodimethylamine causes cell damage and, thus, high mitotic rates; subsequent small doses induce mutations in DNA and effectively induce cancer.

Q.15. Allergic contact dermatitis is -------

A. A nonimmune response caused by a direct action of an agent on the skin
B. An immediate type I hypersensitivity reaction
C. A delayed type IV hypersensitivity reaction
D. Characterized by the intensity of reaction being proportional to the elicitation dose
E. Not involved in photo-allergic reactions

Q.16. Duration of ultra-short acting barbiturate is -------.

A. 12 hours
B. 3 hours
C. 15–20 minutes
D. 0 minute

Q.17. Which of the following is most commonly used as a drug of sexual assault?

A. Narcotics
B. Amphetamines
C. Benzodiazepines
D. Ethanol
E. Antidepressants

Q.18. Which of the following criteria is *not* routinely used to check or adulteration of drug urine analysis?

A. Urea
B. pH
C. Color
D. Specific gravity
E. Creatinine

Q.19. Which blood alcohol concentration (BAC) is most commonly used as the statutory definition of driving under the influence (**DUI**) of alcohol?

A. 0.04
B. 0.06
C. 0.08
D. 0.12
E. 0.16

Q.20. Which of the following drugs is *not* properly matched with its most common analytic method?

A. Benzodiazepines—GC/MS
B. Ibuprofen—LC/HPLC

C. Amphetamines—immunoassays
D. Barbiturates—GC/immunoassays
E. Ethanol—immunoassays

Answers
1. B.   2. C.   3. B.   4. D.   5. D.   6. D.
7. A and B.   8. A.   9. C.   10. D.   11. C.
12. D.   13. D.   14. B.   15. C.   16. C.
17. D.   18. A.   19. C.   20. E.

Further Reading

Cantilena LR Jr (2015) Clinical toxicology. In: Klaassen CD, Watkins JB III (eds) Casarett & Doull's essentials of toxicology, 3rd edn. McGraw-Hill, USA, pp 471–480

Goldberger BA, Wilkins DG (2015) Analytical and forensic toxicology. In: Klaassen CD, Watkins JB III (eds) Casarett & Doull's essentials of toxicology, 3rd edn. McGraw-Hill, USA, pp 463–470

Gupta PK (2010a) Principles of non-specific therapy. In: Gupta PK (ed) Modern toxicology: the adverse effects of xenobiotics, vol 3., 2nd reprint. PharmaMed Press, Hyderabad, India, pp 210–243

Gupta PK (2010b) Mechanism of antidotal therapy. In: Gupta PK (ed) Modern toxicology: the adverse effects of xenobiotics, vol Vol. 3., 2nd reprint. PharmaMed Press, Hyderabad, India, pp 244–264

Gupta PK (2014) Essential concepts in toxicology. BSP Pvt Ltd, Hyderabad, India

Gupta PK (2016) Fundamental in toxicology: essential concepts and applications in toxicology. Elsevier / BSP, USA

Gupta PK (2018) Illustrative toxicology: 1st ed. Elsevier, San Diego.

Gupta PK (2019) Concepts and applications in veterinary toxicology: an interactive guide. Springer Nature, Switzerland

Gupta PK (2020) Brain storming questions in toxicology. Francis and Taylor CRC Press, USA

Occupational Toxicology

24

Abstract

Occupational toxicology is the application of the principles and methodology of toxicology toward understanding and managing chemical and biological hazards encountered at work. Diseases arising in occupational environments involve exposure primarily through inhalation, ingestion, or dermal absorption. This chapter briefly describes the overview, key points, and relevant text that are in the format of problem-solving study questions followed by multiple-choice questions (MCQs) along with their answers.

Keywords

Occupational toxicology · Occupational diseases · Exposure · Toxicology · Questions and answers · MCQs · Problem-solving questions

1 Introduction

Occupational (or industrial) toxicology is the application of the principles and methodology of toxicology to understanding and managing chemical and biological hazards encountered at work. The objective of the occupational toxicologist is to prevent adverse health effects in workers that arise from exposures in their work environment. This chapter briefly describes an overview, key points, and relevant text that is in the format of problem-solving study questions followed by multiple-choice questions (MCQ's) along with their answers.

2 Overview

The large number of chemicals, and modifying conditions, found at the workplace without adequate toxicological information argues for the continued presence of occupational toxicology programs. Many of the chemicals that occupational toxicologists must deal don't cause an appreciable risk to health when they are present at low levels in food, consumer products, and the environment. However, workers may be exposed to these chemicals at considerably higher levels than the general public, so the consequences of human exposure are potentially the most serious in the work place. Occupational toxicology is not only important in chemical factories but is just as relevant in high-street bakeries handling flour dust or hairdressers using hair dyes. They also advise government on legal controls necessary to ensure that chemicals are handled and used safely. A number of guiding policies and philosophies form the framework for the NIOSH's efforts in occupational toxicology.

P K Gupta, *Problem Solving Questions in Toxicology*, https://doi.org/10.1007/978-3-030-50409-0_24

Such programs should be the responsibility of industry, labor, and the government. Some of the details of what we perceive to be a program in occupational toxicology follow. The typical worker is not usually confronted with exposure to a single chemical. More often, exposure is to multiple chemicals or other conditions that may interact to modify a given chemical's toxicity. The NIOSH believes that the matter of toxic interactions needs to be emphasized.

Key Points

- Occupational toxicology is the application of the principles and methodology of toxicology toward understanding and managing chemical and biological hazards encountered at work.
- The work environment with its chemical and biological hazards plays a role in the occurrence of adverse human health effects.
- Diseases arising in occupational environments involve exposure primarily through inhalation, ingestion, or dermal absorption.
- There may be a long interval between exposure and the expression of disease.
- The objective of the occupational toxicologist is primary prevention, that is, to prevent adverse health effects in workers that could arise from exposures in their work environment.

---

3   Problem-Solving Study Questions

3.1   Workplaces, Exposures, and Standards

Q. What are important modifying factors for occupational diseases?

Some of the important modifying factors for occupational diseases include contemporaneous exposures, genetic susceptibility, age, gender, nutritional status, and behavioral factors.

Q. What are the important determinants of toxicant dose responsible for inhalation exposure in occupational environment?
- Airborne concentration
- Particle size distribution
- Respiratory rate
- Tidal volume
- Other host factors such as:
  - Duration of exposure
  - Chemical, physical, or biological properties of the hazardous agent
  - Effectiveness of personal protective devices

Q. What are the important determinants of toxicant dose responsible for dermal exposure in occupational environment?

Important determinants of toxicant dose responsible for dermal exposure include:
- Concentration in air, droplets, or solutions
- Degree and duration of wetness
- Integrity of skin
- Percutaneous absorption rate
- Region of skin exposed
- Surface area exposed
- Preexisting skin disease
- Temperature in the workplace
- Vehicle for the toxicant
- Presence of other chemicals on skin

Q. What are occupational exposure limits [OELS])?

An occupational exposure limit is an upper limit on the acceptable concentration of a hazardous substance in workplace air for a particular material or class of materials or as concentrations of a toxicant, its metabolites. It is typically set by competent national authorities and enforced by legislation to protect occupational safety and health.

Q. What are permissible exposure limits (PELS)?

In the United States, the occupational safety and health administration under the department of labor promulgates legally enforceable standards known as permissible exposure limits (PELS).

Q. What are the threshold limit values (*TLV*) of a chemical substance?

The threshold limit value (*TLV*) of a chemical substance is believed to be a level to which a worker can be exposed day after day for a working lifetime without adverse effects.

Q. What is the difference between TLV and TWA?

A time weighted average (TWA) is a TLV$^{(r)}$ based on an 8-hour workday and a 40-hour workweek. A short-term exposure limit (STEL) is a TLV$^{(r)}$ based on a 15-minute average. A ceiling is a TLV that should not be exceeded during any part of the work experience.

Q. What does immediately dangerous to life or health (IDLH) stand for?

IDLH is defined by the US National Institute for Occupational Safety and Health (NIOSH) as exposure to airborne contaminants that is "likely to cause death or immediate or delayed permanent adverse health effects or prevent escape from such an environment."

Q. Why do we calculate weighted average?

Weighted average is a kind of arithmetic mean in which some elements of the data set carry more importance than others. In mathematics and statistics, one calculates weighted average by multiplying each value in the set by its weight, and then one adds up the products and divides the products' sum by the sum of all weights.

Q. What are binding occupational exposure limit values (BOELV) and biological limit values (BlV)?

The European commission has established legally enforceable binding occupational exposure limit values (BOELV) and biological limit values (BLV) for the protection of health and safety in the workplace. Socioeconomic and technical feasibility factors are also considered in setting these values.

3.2   Occupational Problems

Q. What are routes of exposure in occupational environments?

- Diseases or problems arising in occupational environments involve exposure primarily through inhalation, ingestion, or dermal absorption.

- Exposures leading to occupational infections may arise through inhalation or ingestion of microorganisms, from needle sticks.

- In healthcare workers or from insect bites among those who work outdoors.

- Additionally, poisonings from toxic plants or venomous animals can occur through skin inoculation (e.g., zookeepers, horticulturists, or commercial skin divers).

Q. What kind of lung and airway problems can be encountered during occupational exposure?

Common lung and airway problems include acute pulmonary edema, bronchiolitis, obliterans, allergic rhinitis asphyxiation, asthma, asthma-like syndrome, bronchitis, pneumonitis, chronic bronchitis, emphysema, fibrotic lung disease, hypersensitivity pneumonitis, metal fume fever, mucous membrane irritation, organic dust toxic syndrome, upper respiratory tract inflammation, etc.

Q. What type of cancers can be encountered during occupational exposure?

Types of cancers that are common during occupational exposure include acute myelogenous leukemia, bladder cancer, gastrointestinal cancers, hepatic hemangiosarcoma, hepatocellular carcinoma, mesothelioma, lung carcinoma, and skin cancer.

Q. What are the common agents responsible for cancer in occupational health workers?

Common agents include benzene, ethylene oxide, benzidine, 2-naphthylamine, 4-biphenylamine, asbestos, vinyl chloride, aflatoxin, hepatitis B virus, asbestos, arsenic, radon, bis-chloro methyl ether, polycyclic aromatic hydrocarbons, and ultraviolet irradiation.

Q. What are the common agents responsible for immune suppression in occupational health workers?

Common agents include vinyl chloride, silica, TCDD, lead, mercury, pesticides, etc.

Q. What are the common agents responsible to affect nervous system in occupational health workers?
Common agents includeorganophosphate insecticides, methylmercury, carbon monoxide, carbon disulfide, n-hexane, trichloroethylene, and acrylamide.

Q. Which types of metal are known to cause cancer in occupationally exposed workers?
Arsenic, beryllium, cadmium and cadmium compounds, gallium arsenide, hexavalent chromium compounds, and nickel compounds

Q. What type of causative agents are involved to cause infections in occupational diseases?
Common causative organisms include alphavirus, bunyavirus, flavivirus, *Aspergillus niger*, *A. fumigatus*, *A. flavus*, *Cryptosporidium parvum*, hepatitis B virus, *Histoplasma capsulatum*, *Legionella pneumophila*, *Borrelia burgdorferi*, *Chlamydia psittaci*, and mycobacterium tuberculosis hominis.

Q. What types of chemical agents are involved to cause liver disease in occupational workers?
Carbon tetrachloride, toluene, arsenic, trichloroethylene, dimethylformamide, and TCDD

3.3   Evaluation of Occupational Risks

Q. What types of studies are under taken for the evaluation of occupational risks?
Five sources of data may be available to inform the occupational risk assessment process. These sources include in vitro assays, animal toxicology studies, human challenge studies, case reports, and epidemiology studies.

4   Sample MCQ's

(Choose the correct statement; it may be one, two, or more or none.)

Q.1. Which of the following lung diseases has the highest occupational death rate?

A. Asbestosis
B. Coal workers' pneumoconiosis
C. Byssinosis
D. Hypersensitivity pneumonitis
E. Silicosis

Q.2. Prolonged arsenic exposure could cause ----

A. Infertility
B. Cirrhosis
C. Cor pulmonale
D. Skin cancer
E. Nephropathy

Q.3. Which would increase the likelihood of toxic dosage through dermal exposure?

A. No preexisting skin disease
B. Toxic exposure to thick skin
C. Increased percutaneous absorption rate
D. Low surface area of exposure
E. High epidermal intercellular junction integrity

Q.4. Which of the following is least likely to increase occupational inhalation of a chemical?

A. Increased airborne concentration
B. Increased respiratory rate
C. Increased tidal volume
D. Increased particle size
E. Increased length of exposure

Q.5. Which of the following is not a modifying factor that can influence the likelihood of disease?

A. Age
B. Dose
C. Nutritional status
D. Gender
E. Genetic susceptibility

Q.6. Lyme disease is caused by which of the following?

A. *B. burgdorferi*
B. *H. capsulatum*
C. *M. tuberculosis*
D. *L. pneumophila*
E. *C. psittaci*

Q.7. Which of the following infectious agents can cause hepatocellular carcinoma?

A. Flavivirus
B. Bunyavirus
C. Alphavirus
D. Hepatitis C virus
E. Hepatitis B virus

Q.8. Which of the following might be linked to parkinsonism?

A. Nitrogen dioxide
B. Zinc
C. Copper
D. Magnesium
E. Carbon monoxide

Q.9. Exposure to which of the following can cause autoimmune disease?

A. Mercury
B. Nitrogen dioxide
C. Vinyl chloride
D. Lead
E. Flavivirus

Q.10. Asbestos exposure is unlikely to cause ------

A. Lung cancer
B. GI cancer
C. Emphysema
D. Pulmonary fibrosis
E. Mesothelioma

Answers
1. D.   2. B.   3. C.   4. C.   5. D.   6. B.
7. D.   8. A.   9. B.   10. D.

Further Reading

Joseph LaDou ed. (2007) Current occupational & environmental medicine (Lange Medical Books), McGraw-Hill, USA

Bourgeois MM, Harbison RD, Johnson GT (eds) (2015) Industrial toxicology. John Wiley, USA

Thorne PS (2015) Occupational toxicology. In: Klaassen CD, Watkins JB III (eds) Casarett & Doull's essentials of toxicology, 3rd edn. McGraw-Hill, USA, pp 480–490

Thorne PS (2019) Occupational toxicology. In: Klaassen CD (ed) Casarett & Doull's basic science of poisons, 9th edn. McGraw-Hill, USA, pp 1551–1572

Index

Printed in the United States
by Baker & Taylor Publisher Services